SAUNDERS SOLUTIONS IN
VETERINARY PRACTICE

SMALL ANIMAL

EMERGENCY MEDICINE

Commissioning Editor: Robert Edwards
Development Editor: Ewan Halley
Project Manager: Kiruthiga Kasthuriswamy
Designer: Charles Gray

SAUNDERS SOLUTIONS IN
VETERINARY PRACTICE

SMALL ANIMAL

EMERGENCY MEDICINE

Series Editor: **Fred Nind** BVM&S, MRCVS

Shailen Jasani

VetMB MA MRCVS (ACVECC Diploma eligible)

CHURCHILL LIVINGSTONE

ELSEVIER

Edinburgh London New York Oxford Philadelphia St Louis Sydney Toronto 2010

SAUNDERS
ELSEVIER

First published 2011

ISBN: 978-0-7020-2984-4

British Library Cataloguing in Publication Data
A catalogue record for this book is available from the British Library

Library of Congress Cataloging in Publication Data
A catalog record for this book is available from the Library of Congress

Notice

Knowledge and best practice in this field are constantly changing. As new research and experience broaden our understanding, changes in research methods, professional practices, or medical treatment may become necessary.

Practitioners and researchers must always rely on their own experience and knowledge in evaluating and using any information, methods, compounds, or experiments described herein. In using such information or methods they should be mindful of their own safety and the safety of others, including parties for whom they have a professional responsibility.

With respect to any drug or pharmaceutical products identified, readers are advised to check the most current information provided (i) on procedures featured or (ii) by the manufacturer of each product to be administered, to verify the recommended dose or formula, the method and duration of administration, and contraindications. It is the responsibility of practitioners, relying on their own experience and knowledge of their patients, to make diagnoses, to determine dosages and the best treatment for each individual patient, and to take all appropriate safety precautions.

To the fullest extent of the law, neither the Publisher nor the authors, contributors, or editors assume any liability for any injury and/or damage to persons or property as a matter of products liability, negligence or otherwise, or from any use or operation of any methods, products, instructions, or ideas contained in the material herein.

The Publisher

The publisher's policy is to use **paper manufactured from sustainable forests**

Printed in China

Contents

Introduction

Saunders Solutions in Veterinary Practice series is a new range of veterinary textbooks that will grow into a mini library over the next few years, covering all the main disciplines of companion animal practice.

Readers should realise that it is not the authors' intention to cover all that is known about each topic. As such the books in the *Saunders Solutions* series are not standard reference works. Instead they are intended to provide practical information on the more frequently encountered conditions in an easily accessible form based on real-life case studies. They cover that range of cases that falls between the boringly routine and the referral. The books will help practitioners with a particular interest in a topic or those preparing for a specialist qualification. The cases are arranged by presenting sign rather than by the underlying pathology as this is how veterinary surgeons will see them in practice.

Each case also includes descriptions of underlying pathology and details of the nursing required both in the veterinary clinic and at home. It is hoped that the books will also, therefore, be of interest to veterinary students in the later parts of their course and to veterinary nurses.

Continuing professional development (CPD) is mandatory for many veterinarians and a recommended practice for others. The *Saunders Solutions* series will provide a CPD resource that can be accessed economically, shared with colleagues and used anywhere. They will also provide busy veterinary practitioners with quick access to authoritative information on the diagnosis and treatment of interesting and challenging cases. The robust cover has been made resistant to some of the more gruesome contaminants found in a veterinary clinic because this is where we hope these books will be used.

Joyce Rodenhuis, Mary Seager and subsequently Robert Edwards were the inspiration for the series and both the series editor and the individual authors are grateful for their foresight in commissioning the series and their unfailing support and guidance during their production.

EMERGENCY VETERINARY MEDICINE

In recent years a cadre of the veterinary profession has appeared that works only outside normal practice hours and this has helped develop the provision of emergency veterinary care as a distinct professional discipline. However, we should not forget that emergency cases can present during the normal working day as well as out of hours.

A proportion of these cases will be truly life-threatening illnesses or animals with severe pain. Diagnosis needs to be quick and accurate and treatment urgent. In some cases treatment may be technically difficult and sophisticated. It may involve procedures with which the practitioner is relatively unfamiliar, or the use of equipment that is rarely needed in routine veterinary care.

This book has been written in a clear and concise way, by an author with extensive experience, as a practical guide to the care of these cases and should become the handbook of the emergency team. Information is easy to find with a plethora of practical clinical tips being highlighted.

A successful outcome for a severely ill emergency case can give the practitioner a warmer inner glow than almost any other case. We hope this book will help you achieve that glow more confidently and more often.

Fred Nind, Series Editor
2010

Preface

In essence, whether or not an animal presents as an emergency is ultimately at the discretion of its owner. A significant proportion of dogs and cats seen as emergencies are afflicted by some of the same non urgent disorders that are seen during routine practice; the urgency stems more from the owner's concern than the patient's clinical status. However, there are also a significant number of dogs and cats presented for veterinary attention that are legitimately considered to be emergencies. These animals present with a diverse variety of abnormalities, some of which are imminently life-threatening, while others are associated with variable levels of pain or other morbidity. Some of the challenges, and appeals, of emergency medicine are the need to have a wide breath of knowledge and expertise covering all body systems, to know how to prioritize individual patients and specific problems within a single patient, and to be prepared to see and embrace the unknown and sometimes unexplainable!

Dogs and cats are seen as emergencies in a variety of environments – general practice, non-referral dedicated emergency clinics, and referral hospitals. The same cases may therefore be seen by individuals with varying degrees of experience and with access to different levels of facilities. This book has been written by a clinician who has worked in all of these environments over the last 10 years and it is very much intended to demonstrate how excellent emergency medicine can be provided in a non-referral environment by adhering to certain fundamental principles (Section 1). In particular, the author cannot stress enough how much invaluable information can be obtained from astute physical examination, which does not require any special equipment, and how important a logical and rational approach is in emergency medicine in particular.

In Section 2, the author presents common problems identified in emergency patients, including clinical signs and other findings, and in Section 3 the approach to common disorders is illustrated using case examples. By necessity there is a degree of overlap between these two sections. The author hopes that Section 3 in particular will demonstrate the application of the fundamental principles described in Section 1 and allow the reader to become more comfortable with early assessment of emergency patients. As such, the author would strongly encourage the reader to read the whole of Section 1 first and cannot stress enough how much emergency medicine is about applying these fundamental principles to a limitless array of different disorders.

The reader is reminded that this book is not intended to be a reference text. The author has purposely chosen only relatively common emergencies to cover in enough detail as to be useful in the management of these cases. In addition, in contrast to some other areas of veterinary medicine, it is very common for initial management to be required in emergency patients in which a definitive diagnosis has not been obtained. Again, this is one of the challenges, and appeals, of emergency medicine!

SJ
Hatfield, 2010

Acknowledgements

The author would like to thank all of the following who in some way have contributed to the writing of this book:

Dez Hughes for his expert teaching and 'keep it simple, stupid!' ethos that laid the foundations for the emergency clinician I am today.

Chiara Valtolina for her advice and support throughout my book-writing journey, and Dan Lewis and Dom Barfield for the many impromptu discussions about the book's contents.

My long-term friend, Simon Ripoll, for co-authoring the chapter on sedation and general anaesthesia.

All my colleagues who provided me with many of the photographs in this book, in particular Kate English.

My family for their support over the years and tolerating being neglected while I have endeavoured to take care of *mungu prani* (God's animals) as my mum likes to call them.

Last, but definitely not least, my dad for showing immense willpower in the face of prolonged adversity and being a huge source of inspiration; may God rest his soul.

SECTION 1

THE FUNDAMENTALS

1 Major body system examination

CLINICAL TIPS

- The initial physical examination should focus on the major body systems, namely the cardiovascular, respiratory and central nervous systems, as severe abnormalities in these systems have the potential to be rapidly fatal. This approach is somewhat different from the head-to-tail physical examination commonly performed that is only appropriate for non-emergency patients.
- Pain assessment is also a high priority in the initial evaluation.

A considerable amount of invaluable information can be obtained from the physical examination of the emergency patient. The initial priority is to identify any potentially life-threatening problems so that immediate intervention can be provided. As such the initial physical examination (primary survey) should focus on the major body systems, namely the cardiovascular, respiratory and central nervous systems, as severe abnormalities in these systems have the potential to be rapidly fatal. Abdominal palpation and measurement of body temperature are also important. Once measures have been taken to stabilize abnormalities in the major body systems a more comprehensive physical examination (secondary survey) can be performed. This approach is somewhat different from the head-to-tail physical examination commonly performed that is only appropriate for non-emergency patients.

CARDIOVASCULAR SYSTEM

The most important questions to be answered when examining the cardiovascular system are, does the patient have signs of compromised systemic perfusion, and is there any evidence of primary cardiac disease? The following should be examined during evaluation of the cardiovascular system:

- Heart rate, sounds and rhythm
- Pulse quality and rate (are there pulse deficits?)
- Mucous membrane colour and capillary refill time
- (Mentation)
- (Temperature of the extremities).

All of the information obtained from this evaluation should be used to guide subsequent therapy. For example, a patient with severe hypovolaemia will require aggressive fluid administration (see Ch. 4). However a more conservative approach may need to be taken if a non-physiological heart murmur is detected during initial evaluation. The most common cause of hypoperfusion in the emergency patient is hypovolaemia (see Ch. 2). Cardiovascular abnormalities may also be seen for example with heart failure (see Ch. 31), anaemia (see Ch. 19) and systemic inflammatory response syndrome (SIRS) or sepsis.

RESPIRATORY SYSTEM

Animals with respiratory embarrassment are amongst the most unstable emergency patients and in some cases even a brief major body system examination will not be tolerated. Oxygen supplementation and potentially other empirical intervention (e.g. sedation of a dog with severe upper respiratory tract dyspnoea, see Ch. 32) may have to be performed prior to examination of these patients. This is especially true for cats (see Ch. 23). The following should be examined during evaluation of the respiratory system:

- Respiratory rate
- Respiratory effort
- Respiratory pattern and noise.

Respiratory rate in a normal adult dog or cat is usually 15–30 breaths per minute although a certain degree of

BOX 1.1 Postural adaptation to dyspnoea

- Open-mouth breathing
- Neck extension
- Repeated changing of position
- Abduction of elbows (dogs)
- Sternal recumbency (cats)

normal variation occurs due to factors such as anxiety and excitement.

CLINICAL TIP

- Panting in dogs is often an innocuous finding. However, occasionally it is the earliest sign of compensation in a dog with respiratory compromise and must not therefore be automatically ignored.

Respiratory effort

Dyspnoeic animals may show postural adaptation as described in Box 1.1. Some dyspnoeic animals demonstrate increased abdominal effort (increased contraction of abdominal muscles) that assists with expiration only. Paradoxical abdominal breathing, whereby the thoracic and abdominal walls move in opposite directions, is generally associated with severe respiratory distress (during normal inspiration the thoracic wall moves out and the abdominal wall also moves out passively).

Respiratory pattern and noise

Respiratory distress can occur as a result of an abnormality affecting any one or more of the following areas:

- Upper respiratory tract (URT) (e.g. laryngeal neoplasia)
- Lower respiratory tract (e.g. feline bronchial disease)
- Lung parenchyma (e.g. pulmonary contusions, pulmonary oedema)
- Pleural space (e.g. pleural effusion, pneumothorax)
- Thoracic wall and diaphragm (e.g. traumatic diaphragmatic rupture).

Being able to identify the area affected is extremely important with respect to patient management. Depending on the case in question, a combination of observation and listening may allow reliable localization of the affected area. This is described further in Box 1.2. Lung sounds are typically louder cranioventrally and may not be audible in a normal cat at rest.

BOX 1.2 Interpretation of respiratory pattern and noise findings

- Inspiratory stridor/stertor; prolonged inspiration: dynamic extrathoracic upper respiratory tract (URT) obstruction (e.g. laryngeal paralysis)
- Inspiratory and expiratory stridor: fixed URT obstruction (e.g. mass lesion) (or diffuse tracheal disease)
- Expiratory stridor: intrathoracic tracheal abnormality
- Prolonged expiration with increased abdominal effort: lower airway disease
- Muffled lung sounds ventrally: pleural effusion (lung sounds may be louder than normal dorsally)
- Muffled lung sounds dorsally: pneumothorax (lung sounds may be louder than normal ventrally)
- Louder than normal lung sounds (harshness, wheezes, crackles): small airway or parenchymal disease

CENTRAL NERVOUS SYSTEM

Initial examination of the central nervous system (CNS) focuses on mentation and ability to stand and ambulate. If the animal is ambulatory, then gait is assessed. Mentation may be affected by cardiovascular and respiratory abnormalities and if such abnormalities are present, it is important to decide whether the animal's mentation is appropriate. Inappropriately altered mentation should raise the index of suspicion for a primary CNS disorder. In some cases mentation cannot be reliably evaluated until other abnormalities have been resolved or improved (e.g. fluid therapy to correct systemic hypoperfusion, warming to treat hypothermia).

Similarly, animals may be recumbent as a result of primary CNS disorders but also due to cardiovascular and respiratory compromise. Gait abnormalities in ambulatory animals are most likely to be related to the nervous systems (central or peripheral) and multiple limb involvement often suggests a more serious disease.

2 Shock and dehydration

Shock and dehydration are both commonly seen in emergency practice and both require fluid therapy as a crucial part of their management (see Ch. 4). However, they represent different pathophysiological processes and have different clinicopathological findings. Understanding these differences is essential to ensuring that the most appropriate management is implemented.

BODY FLUID COMPARTMENTS

Total body water typically constitutes approximately 60% of a healthy non-obese adult dog or cat's body weight. A basic understanding of the way in which the total body water is distributed is central to appreciating the concepts of perfusion, volume status, shock and hydration. The total body water is distributed as follows:

- Intracellular compartment (40% body weight)
- Extracellular compartment (20% body weight):
  - Interstitial space including lymph (15% body weight)
  - Intravascular space (4% body weight)
  - Transcellular compartment (e.g. cerebrospinal and synovial fluid; approximately 1%).

Active and/or passive movement of fluid occurs continuously between the intravascular and interstitial compartments at the capillary membrane. The most important factor that determines the size of each fluid compartment is the amount of solutes it contains.

HYPOPERFUSION AND SHOCK

Organs and peripheral tissues rely on an adequate intravascular fluid space (adequate perfusion) for the delivery of oxygen and nutrients and the removal of by-products of tissue metabolism. 'Hypoperfusion' describes a situation in which there is a decrease in the blood supply to an organ or tissue. Although this can occur solely on a local level, it is seen most commonly in the context of a global (systemic) reduction in blood supply.

The term 'shock' is used clinically to describe the condition of a patient in which this global hypoperfusion has reached a certain level of severity, sufficient for the patient to manifest a number of characteristic clinical findings. This usually occurs when the reduction in blood supply is severe enough to cause inadequate oxygen delivery to the cells and thereby inadequate energy production. If the degree of shock is sufficiently severe or prolonged, irreversible cell damage can occur and treatment is invariably unsuccessful.

CLINICAL TIP

- Systemic hypoperfusion is common in emergency patients and being able to recognize and treat this abnormality is crucial for successful stabilization.

Causes of hypoperfusion

The mechanisms of hypoperfusion and shock can be divided into four categories. However, it is important to remember that more than one type can exist in the same patient at the same time, and that they share some common changes and derangements at a cellular level.

Hypovolaemic shock

Hypovolaemia is a reduction in the effective circulating intravascular volume and is the most common cause of hypoperfusion in companion animals. It can be subdivided into absolute and relative hypovolaemia. Absolute hypovolaemia is the most common type and occurs as a result of loss of fluid from the intravascular space. This fluid loss may affect just the intravascular space (e.g. haemorrhage) or the extravascular space as well (e.g. salt and water loss, for example in vomiting and diarrhoea).

Maldistributive shock

With maldistributive shock, the fluid in the intravascular space (the absolute volume of which may or may not be reduced) is distributed across the body in an abnormal way. This occurs as a result of inappropriate generalized vasodilation and can potentially be viewed as a form of relative hypovolaemia. Maldistributive shock is seen in animals with systemic inflammatory response syndrome (SIRS) which may occur for example in sepsis, severe pancreatitis or major tissue injury. Maldistribution also occurs in anaphylactic/anaphylactoid shock.

Cardiogenic shock

Primary cardiac dysfunction (e.g. from organic heart disease or severe dysrhythmia) results in failure of the heart to pump adequately. This compromises cardiac output causing hypoperfusion (see Ch. 31).

Obstructive shock

Systemic hypoperfusion occurs due to obstruction of blood flow from the heart or venous return to the heart; the most common example of this in small animals is pericardial tamponade.

Causes of systemic hypoperfusion in companion animals are listed in Table 2.1.

Table 2.1 Causes of systemic hypoperfusion in dogs and cats

Type of hypoperfusion	Causes
Hypovolaemia	Blood loss (trauma, coagulopathy, ruptured neoplasm) Vomiting and diarrhoea Severe dehydration Third space fluid loss (peritoneal, pleural, interstitial, gastrointestinal) Neoplasia Burn injury Severe polyuria
Maldistributive	Systemic inflammatory response syndrome (SIRS): • Sepsis • Severe pancreatitis • Major tissue trauma • Neoplasia • Burn injury Anaphylaxis/anaphylactoid reaction
Cardiogenic	Cardiomyopathy (especially dilated and hypertrophic) Valvular disease Severe dysrhythmia
Obstructive	Pericardial tamponade Constrictive pericarditis Pulmonary thromboembolism (PTE)

HYPOVOLAEMIA

The two most common causes of hypovolaemia in companion animals are haemorrhage and salt and water loss. Haemorrhagic hypovolaemia may cause some extravascular fluid deficits, while animals presenting with hypovolaemia due to salt and water loss (e.g. from vomiting and diarrhoea) will certainly have extravascular fluid deficits.

Assessing perfusion and volume status

CLINICAL TIP

- Physical examination is undoubtedly the most valuable and readily available means of assessing systemic perfusion in companion animals. The amount of information that can be derived from this examination should not be underestimated. Following initial assessment, repeated physical examination allows response to therapy and ongoing progress to be readily evaluated.

A number of physical examination parameters are used to assess perfusion:

- Heart rate (HR)
- Arterial (usually femoral and dorsal pedal) pulse quality
- Mucous membrane (MM) colour
- Capillary refill time (CRT)
- (Mentation)
- (Temperature of extremities.)

The dorsal pedal artery is located just distal to the hock on the craniomedial aspect of the pelvic limb. Being confident in palpating the arterial pulse at this site is useful for a number of reasons in addition to assessing perfusion status.

In animals with uncomplicated hypovolaemia, the perfusion parameters listed above are reliable indicators of volume status and tend to follow predictable trends both as hypovolaemia progresses, from compensatory through to early and then late decompensatory phases, and as normal perfusion is restored.

Dogs

Compensatory phase of hypovolaemia In this phase, hypovolaemia is mild. A compensatory increase in sympathetic activity causes both an increase in heart rate and cardiac contractility, and peripheral vasconstriction. The corresponding clinical picture is hyperdynamic:

- HR 120–150 beats per minute
- MM normal or pinker than normal with a rapid CRT of 1 second or less
- Femoral pulses are bounding or snappy (hyperdynamic) with dorsal pedal pulses that are readily palpable
- (Mentation and extremity temperature are typically normal.)

Note that most healthy adult dogs have a heart rate in the practice setting of 70–120 beats per minute. There is some variation in heart rate amongst dogs of different size (with bigger dogs usually having slower heart rates) and resting heart rate is also dependent on factors such as the individual animal's level of fitness. It would be highly unusual to detect a resting heart rate in a calm healthy greyhound of 110 beats per minute; likewise a resting heart rate of 70 beats per minute in a Chihuahua. Thus the heart rate identified must be interpreted in the context of the patient in question as a heart rate within the normal range may in fact be an inappropriate finding.

Early decompensatory phase of hypovolaemia

In this phase, hypovolaemia is moderate and systemic perfusion has become compromised due to progressive failure of compensatory mechanisms:

- HR 150–170 beats per minute
- MM pale pink with an apparently normal CRT of 1–2 seconds
- Femoral pulses are weak with dorsal pedal pulses that are only just palpable
- (Mentation is depressed and extremity temperature is normal or cool.)

Late decompensatory phase of hypovolaemia

In this phase, hypovolaemia is severe and systemic perfusion is severely compromised. The corresponding clinical picture is markedly hypodynamic:

- HR 170–220 beats per minute
- MM extremely pale/white with a CRT that, if detectable, is more than 2 seconds
- Femoral pulse very weak or 'thready' with a dorsal pedal pulse that is no longer palpable
- (Mentation is severely depressed and extremities are cold.)

Some dogs in this final stage of hypovolaemic shock present with a heart rate that is inappropriately within normal limits or bradycardic. This is because the heart can no longer sustain its compensatory chronotropic response.

CLINICAL TIP

- A heart rate in a dog of more than 220–240 beats per minute (more than 300 beats per minute in a cat) is unlikely to represent a physiological sinus tachycardia and is most likely to be the result of a tachydysrhythmia (see Ch. 12).

Cats

There are a number of important differences with respect to perfusion assessment and hypovolaemia in cats that lend further support to the notion that 'cats are not small dogs'.

- The heart rate of healthy cats in the veterinary setting is usually 160–200 beats per minute. However, cats are more susceptible to the stress of this environment and much higher heart rates (even up to 240 beats per min) can be seen in cats that are completely healthy.
- Hypovolaemic cats are often found to have a hypodynamic clinical picture (inappropriate bradycardia, weak or absent pulses, pallor, prolonged or undetectable CRT, depression and hypothermia).
- The oral mucous membranes can appear pale in normal cats and another site (usually the conjunctival membranes) should be used to clarify this finding.
- Peripheral pulse assessment is not as reliable and repeatable in cats.

Assessing perfusion – the holistic approach

Animals with hypovolaemia may have concurrent abnormalities that preclude their perfusion parameters changing in the predictable way described above. When assessing a patient's perfusion status it is therefore important to adopt a holistic approach that takes changes in all the perfusion parameters into account and correlates them in the context of the patient in question. For example:

- A dog in an Addisonian crisis may have a heart rate in the normal range despite other findings suggestive of moderate or severe hypovolaemia. This heart rate is in fact an inappropriate bradycardia due to hyperkalaemia that would be overlooked were it not interpreted in the context of all the other perfusion parameters.
- Mucous membranes may remain pale despite appropriate fluid therapy in an animal with severe anaemia.
- Mentation may remain depressed in an animal with head trauma despite appropriate fluid therapy as a result of raised intracranial pressure.

In addition to physical examination, other measures of perfusion, if available, include blood pressure measurement, venous lactate concentration and urine output. Again these findings must be interpreted in the context of the patient's physical examination parameters.

CLINICAL TIP

- Bradycardia in dogs with signs of hypoperfusion is usually the result of primary heart disease (primary cardiac bradydysrhythmia – see Ch. 12), brain disease, severe hyperkalaemia (or hypocalcaemia) or drug toxicity (e.g. digoxin).

Pain management

The majority of causes of hypovolaemia will also result in pain that can interfere with cardiovascular and respiratory function, and confuse clinical assessment. Adequate analgesia is therefore extremely important. The use of opioids initially is the mainstay of pain management and nonsteroidal antiinflammatory agents should be avoided until hypovolaemia and dehydration have been corrected (see Ch. 5).

Maldistributive shock

Early on when intravascular volume remains adequate, dogs in maldistributive shock typically have a hyperdynamic vasodilatory cardiovascular picture, i.e. tachycardia, hyperdynamic pulses, markedly hyperaemic mucous membranes and a fast capillary refill time. With the onset of concurrent severe hypovolaemia, tachycardia progresses but pulses become weaker and CRT more prolonged. However, unlike dogs with uncomplicated severe hypovolaemia, dogs in severe hypodynamic maldistributive shock are likely to retain colour in their mucous membranes that may be normal in appearance or hyperaemic. By cross-referencing perfusion findings it is often possible to identify this retained mucous membrane colour as a discrepant finding that suggests the presence of a distributive component to the hypoperfusion.

Cats in maldistributive shock are more likely to present with a hypodynamic cardiovascular picture.

DEHYDRATION

For clinical purposes, dehydration can be defined as the process whereby an animal loses more salt and water from its body than it takes in. This loss of body fluid is predominantly extravascular and the effect on intravascular volume depends on both the degree of fluid loss and the tonicity (isotonic or hypotonic) of the fluid. The tonicity is related to the sodium concentration.

Assessing hydration status

The physical examination parameters that are used to assess hydration are related to interstitial volume. They are the moistness of the mucous membranes, skin turgor (elasticity), and the presence and degree of globe retraction. The perfusion parameters described above also become relevant if dehydration is severe enough to cause hypovolaemia.

CLINICAL TIP

- Guidelines for estimating dehydration on the basis of physical examination findings must only be used as an approximation of fluid loss in the dehydrated patient to facilitate the initial fluid plan as there are a number of potential inherent inaccuracies.

Guidelines similar to those in Table 2.2 are generally used to estimate dehydration on the basis of physical examination findings. However, these guidelines must only be used as an approximation of fluid loss in the dehydrated patient to facilitate the initial fluid plan (see Ch. 4) as there are a number of potential inherent inaccuracies. For example, skin turgor can be affected by the degree of subcutaneous fat present (with obese animals having increased turgor), and mucous membrane moistness can be affected by salivation (e.g. due to nausea).

Table 2.2 Guidelines for estimating dehydration on the basis of physical examination

Severity of dehydration (estimated % of body weight)	Progression of physical examination findings
<5%	Normal
Mild (5–6%)	Skin turgor mildly reduced
Moderate (6–10%)	Skin turgor progressively reduced Mucous membranes dry Eyes sunken
Severe (10–15%)	Complete loss of skin turgor Mucous membranes very dry Eyes severely sunken and dull Progressive signs of hypovolaemia, ultimately leading to shock and death

Additional measures of dehydration

In addition to physical examination, a number of other parameters can readily be evaluated to determine the presence and severity of dehydration. Given the inaccuracies of assessing hydration status based on physical examination, it is recommended that these additional measures are utilized as much as possible especially for monitoring rehydration (see Ch. 3). They include:

- Packed cell volume and serum total solids
- Blood urea and creatinine concentrations in conjunction with urine specific gravity.

Short-term changes in body weight may also provide useful information with respect to fluid balance in hospitalized patients.

3 Emergency database interpretation

Together with an astute major body system examination, an immense amount of useful information can be derived from an emergency database. Traditionally the minimum emergency database consists of manual packed cell volume (PCV), plasma total solids (TS), blood glucose concentration and blood urea nitrogen (BUN) concentration. Where possible the author prefers to measure plasma creatinine concentration alongside BUN as creatinine is less prone to acute fluctuations. Gross plasma appearance may also provide valuable information.

In addition to the minimum emergency database, it is often appropriate to perform additional measurements or tests as part of the emergency database for specific patient populations. These include:

- Peripheral blood smear examination
- Plasma electrolytes (potassium, sodium, calcium)
- Urinalysis: gross appearance; specific gravity, dipstick analysis, sediment examination.

Depending on the facilities available, it may be possible to obtain all the blood required for the emergency database from an intravenous catheter at the time of placement.

PACKED CELL VOLUME AND PLASMA TOTAL SOLIDS

Manual PCV and TS should always be interpreted together and the changes identified will raise the index of suspicion for particular causes (see Table 3.1).

> **CLINICAL TIP**
>
> - In the majority of cases, reference ranges for normal plasma total protein concentration may be applied to plasma total solids. Synthetic colloid administration and hyperglycaemia may artefactually increase plasma total solids measured by refractometry.

Reduction in PCV and TS following haemorrhage is the result of dilution by fluid moving into the bloodstream from the interstitium. However, this decrease does not occur immediately as there is a lag for fluid movement to occur. Furthermore, in dogs, but not cats, splenic contraction occurs following acute haemorrhage to increase circulating red blood cell mass. Therefore PCV may be normal in the face of low TS following acute haemorrhage and these findings must be interpreted in light of the patient's history and physical examination findings.

With the exception of haemorrhage and protein-losing enteropathy (PLE), most causes of hypoproteinaemia relate to hypoalbuminaemia. Causes of hypoalbuminaemia include protein-losing nephropathy (PLN), liver failure, malnutrition/malabsorption, chronic effusions and exudative skin lesions. Hyperglobulinaemia may occur secondary to dehydration but also inflammation, monoclonal gammopathy (e.g. due to plasma cell myeloma) and polyclonal gammopathy (e.g. due to chronic inflammatory disease, inflammatory bowel disease, feline infectious peritonitis).

When interpreting changes in all laboratory parameters, including PCV and TS, it is important to remember that normal ranges cited for adult dogs and cats may not be applicable to puppies and kittens (see Ch. 41).

GROSS PLASMA APPEARANCE

Common abnormalities of plasma appearance and possible causes are listed in Table 3.2. In addition to plasma appearance, samples can be evaluated for the size of the buffy coat following centrifugation, with a large buffy coat suggestive of leukocytosis.

BLOOD GLUCOSE CONCENTRATION

Clinically significant hyperglycaemia requiring specific therapy is typically only associated with patients suffering from diabetes mellitus. Hyperglycaemia not requiring

Table 3.1 Interpretation of manual packed cell volume and plasma total solids

Packed cell volume (%)	Plasma total solids (g/L)	Causes to consider
Decreased	Normal	Chronic anaemia Acute haemolytic anaemia
Decreased	Decreased	Haemorrhage Chronic anaemia + additional cause of hypoproteinaemia Aggressive fluid therapy
Normal	Increased	Hyperglobulinaemia Artefactual increase
Normal	Decreased	Acute haemorrhage Hypoproteinaemia Severe vasculitis
Increased	Normal	Breed-related normal variation Absolute polycythaemia Dehydration with concurrent protein loss
Increased	Increased	Dehydration

Table 3.2 Possible causes of abnormalities in gross plasma appearance

Plasma appearance	Possible causes
Haemolysed	Poor sampling technique Intravascular haemolysis
Icteric	Prehepatic causes, especially haemolytic anaemia Hepatic disorders causing intrahepatic cholestasis Posthepatic disorders (e.g. obstructive biliary tract disease)
Lipaemic	Postprandial lipaemia Pancreatitis Hyperadrenocorticism

treatment may also be seen in other endocrine disorders (hyperadrenocorticism and acromegaly), secondary to stress (especially cats) and following seizures and head trauma.

Clinically significant hypoglycaemia requiring treatment is seen most commonly as a result of hyperinsulinism, iatrogenic causes or neoplasia, and in very young animals or toy breed dogs. Hypoglycaemia may also be identified in hypoadrenocorticism, liver failure, sepsis and heatstroke.

AZOTAEMIA

The causes of azotaemia may be divided into prerenal, renal or postrenal.

Prerenal azotaemia

Prerenal azotaemia occurs as a result of reduced renal perfusion and a consequent functional decrease in glomerular filtration rate (GFR). Causes include dehydration, hypovolaemia and heart failure. Prerenal azotaemia is characterized by increased PCV, TS and urine specific gravity (USG), and is usually only mild. It is typically reversible but structural renal injury and renal azotaemia may develop if renal hypoperfusion is protracted.

Renal azotaemia

Renal azotaemia occurs as a result of reduced GFR secondary to structural renal changes. Urine specific gravity is isosthenuric (1.007–1.015) as the kidneys are no longer able to concentrate or dilute the urine and azotaemia may be mild, moderate or severe. Anaemia may be present with chronic renal insufficiency.

CLINICAL TIP

- Blood urea nitrogen (BUN) concentration may be affected by a number of extrarenal factors, being increased for example by increased dietary protein intake, gastrointestinal haemorrhage and increased protein catabolism. Thus BUN concentration should ideally be interpreted together with serum creatinine concentration as the latter is considered a more reliable indicator of renal function.

Postrenal azotaemia

Postrenal azotaemia occurs due to urinary tract obstruction or rupture which prevents excretion of urea and creatinine from the body. Azotaemia in these cases may be very severe but frequently will fully resolve with appropriate correction of the underlying disorder. Protracted urinary outflow obstruction can result in damage to the renal parenchyma and consequent intrinsic acute renal failure.

PERIPHERAL BLOOD SMEAR EXAMINATION

Peripheral blood smear examination is recommended for the majority of emergency patients. Cytology allows cell morphology to be evaluated and abnormal cell populations to be identified; a degree of quantitative information can also be obtained. Red blood cells, white blood cells and platelets are evaluated (Figures 3.1 and 3.2).

Red blood cells

Red blood cells are examined for variability in size (anisocytosis) and colour (polychromasia) (Figure 3.3), both of which are suggestive of regenerative anaemia. When stained using a Romanowsky stain such as Diff-Quik, immature red blood cells (polychromatophils), which are larger than mature cells, have a purplish- or bluish-tinged appearance.

Red blood cells should also be examined for additional features such as spherocytosis (Figure 3.4) and the presence of increased numbers of nucleated red cells (Figure 3.5). Spherocytes are smaller, more rounded and denser staining than normal red blood cells and they lack central pallor. They are formed when red blood cells undergo partial phagocytosis and are characteristic of immune-mediated haemolytic anaemia (see Ch. 33). Nucleated red cells may be seen for example with strongly regenerative anaemia or heatstroke (see Ch. 38).

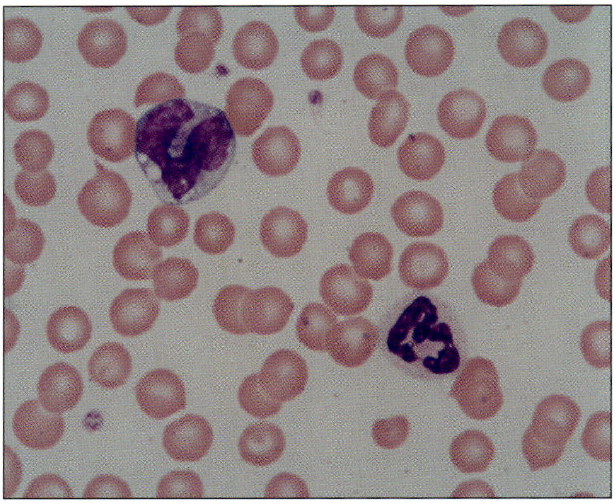

Figure 3.1 Normal canine red blood cells, neutrophil, monocyte and platelets (×1000) (Photograph courtesy of Kate English).

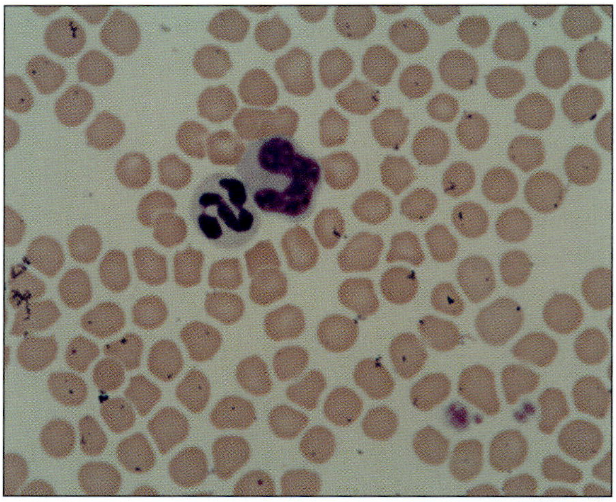

Figure 3.2 Normal feline red blood cells, neutrophil, monocyte and platelets (×1000) (Photograph courtesy of Kate English).

White blood cells

Neutrophils are the white blood cells of main concern in most cases and it is generally acceptable in the emergency setting to make a subjective assessment of neutrophilia or neutropenia in the context of the patient in question. The proportion of band neutrophils (Figure 3.6) should be estimated. These are immature neutrophils with unsegmented nuclei released early from the

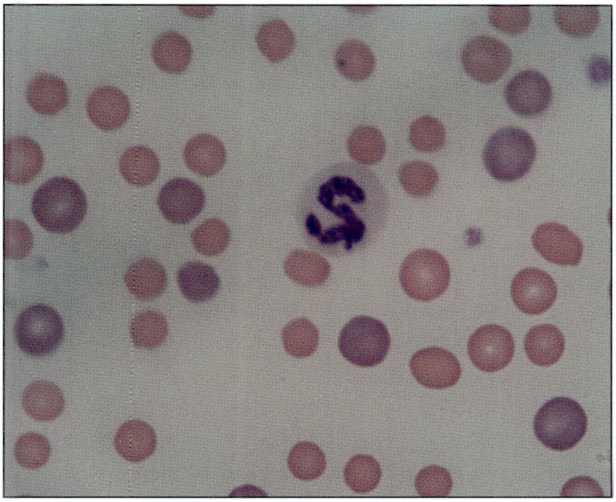

Figure 3.3 Peripheral blood smear from a dog showing regenerative anaemia (×1000). Marked polychromasia (large purplish-tinged red blood cells) and anisocytosis (variation in red blood cell size) is present; a neutrophil and two platelets can also be seen. (Photograph courtesy of Kate English)

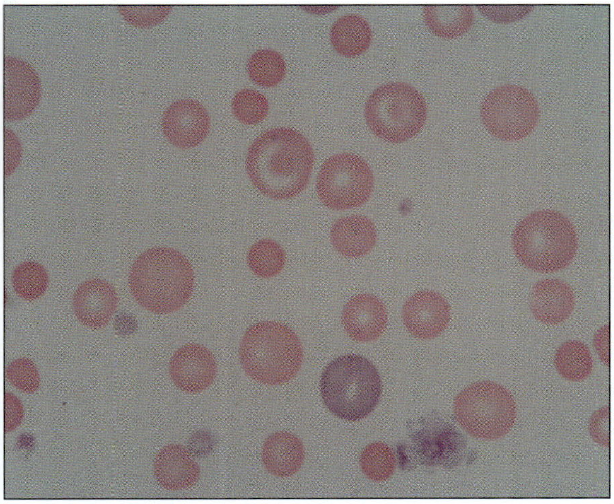

Figure 3.4 Spherocytes in peripheral blood smear from a dog (×1000). Spherocytes are smaller, more rounded and denser staining than normal red blood cells and they lack central pallor. (Photograph courtesy of Kate English)

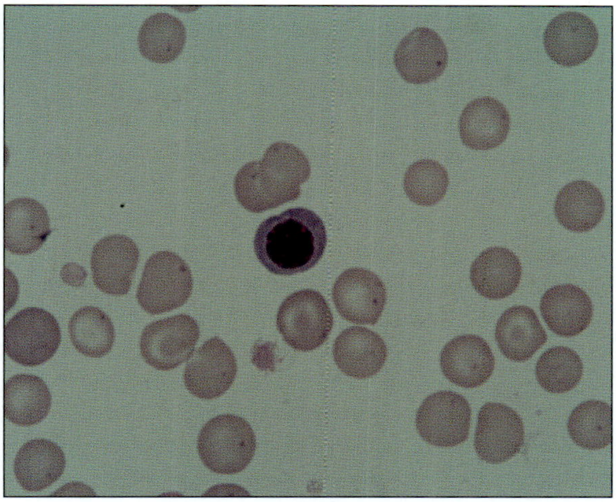

Figure 3.5 Nucleated red blood cell in peripheral blood smear from a dog (×1000); other red blood cells and two platelets can also be seen. (Photograph courtesy of Kate English)

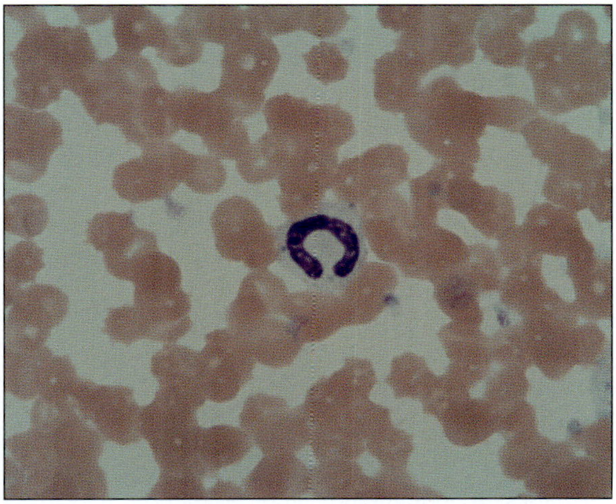

Figure 3.6 Canine band neutrophil (×1000). (Photograph courtesy of Kate English)

bone marrow in response to acute demand. A normal or low neutrophil count with a high proportion of band cells is referred to as a degenerate left shift and indicates severe pathology. Neutrophils should also be examined for toxic changes (Figure 3.7) which are morphological abnormalities that occur during intensified neutrophil maturation in severe inflammation.

Leukopenia may be the result of reduced production (e.g. parvovirus, immunosuppressive therapy) or sequestration (e.g. severe infection or inflammation).

Platelets

A manual platelet count should be performed under high power (×1000, under oil immersion) in the monolayer of the smear. Guidelines vary but 1 platelet per high power field may be considered equivalent to 15–20 × 10^9 platelets/litre. Prior to performing the count, the

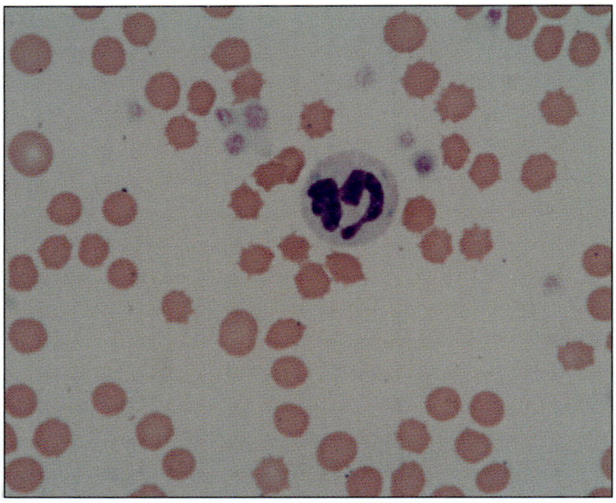

Figure 3.7 Canine toxic neutrophil showing cytoplasmic basophilia, toxic granulation and three Döhle bodies (×1000). (Photograph courtesy of Kate English)

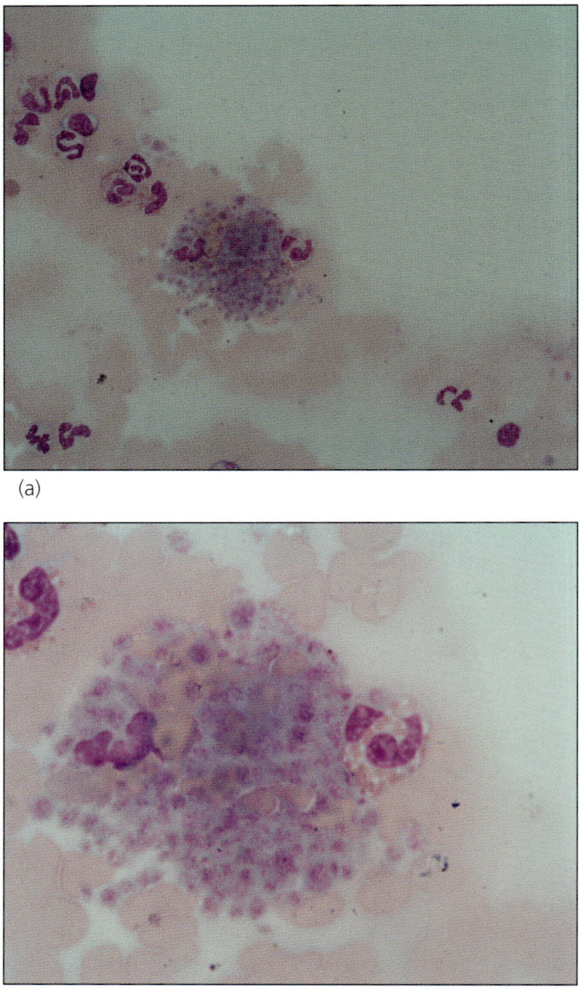

(a)

(b)

Figure 3.8 Canine platelet clump: (a) ×400 magnification; (b) ×1000 magnification. (Photographs courtesy of Kate English)

feathered edge should be examined for the presence of platelet clumps (Figure 3.8) which will reduce the number of platelets in the monolayer and if missed, may lead to a misdiagnosis of thrombocytopenia. Platelet clumping implies an adequate platelet count. Large platelets may be seen as part of a regenerative platelet response for example following haemorrhage. In addition, macrothrombocytopenia is recognized in Cavalier King Charles spaniels.

Spontaneous haemorrhage secondary to thrombocytopenia is unlikely to be seen in patients with two or more platelets per high power field although it must be remembered that this is only a guideline. It can be difficult to identify even a single platelet in smears from animals with immune-mediated thrombocytopenia (see Ch. 33).

PLASMA ELECTROLYTES

Potassium

Hyperkalaemia

Some of the more common causes of hyperkalaemia are listed in Box 3.1.

Hypokalaemia

Hypokalaemia in emergency patients is most commonly the result of reduced intake due to inappetence, and concurrent increased loss via the gastrointestinal tract due to vomiting and/or diarrhoea. Excessive loss may also occur via the urinary system, for example in some animals (especially cats) with chronic renal failure or secondary to loop or thiazide diuretic administration.

Sodium

Sodium metabolism and water balance are closely interconnected via complex mechanisms involving a number of different receptors and hormones, and it is therefore essential to consider the patient's intravascular volume status when interpreting measured serum sodium concentration. Some causes of hyper- and hyponatraemia are listed in Tables 3.3 and 3.4.

BOX 3.1 Causes of hyperkalaemia

Decreased urinary excretion

- Urethral obstruction
- Uroperitoneum
- Hypoadrenocorticism (Addison's disease)
- Anuric or oliguric renal failure
- Certain gastrointestinal disorders (e.g. trichuriasis (whipworm), salmonellosis)
- Effusions
- Drug-related (e.g. angiotensin converting enzyme inhibitors, potassium-sparing diuretics)

Release of intracellular potassium

- Insulin deficiency (e.g. diabetic ketoacidosis)
- Acute mineral acidosis
- Significant cell death (e.g. heatstroke, severe trauma, reperfusion following thromboembolism, acute tumour lysis syndrome)
- Pseudohyperkalaemia (e.g. haemolysis, especially in certain breeds like the Japanese Akita; thrombocytosis)

Contamination of plasma sample with potassium EDTA during transfer into blood tubes

Table 3.3 Causes of hypernatraemia

Hypovolaemia (water loss is greater than sodium loss, i.e. hypotonic fluid loss)	Extrarenal: • Vomiting • Diarrhoea • Third space loss • Cutaneous burn injury Renal: • Osmotic diuresis (diabetes mellitus, mannitol administration) • Diuretic therapy • Chronic renal failure • Polyuric acute renal failure • Postobstructive diuresis
Normovolaemia (pure water deficit)	Hyperthermia Diabetes insipidus (central, nephrogenic) Water restriction Primary hypodipsia
Hypervolaemia (impermeant solute gain)	Hypertonic saline administration Salt poisoning

Table 3.4 Causes of hyponatraemia

Hypovolaemia (sodium loss is greater than water loss)	Vomiting Diarrhoea Hypoadrenocorticism (Addison's disease) Diuretic therapy Third space loss Cutaneous burn injury
Normovolaemia (pure water deficit)	Hypotonic fluid administration Psychogenic polydipsia Syndrome of inappropriate ADH secretion (SIADH)
Hypervolaemia (water excretion reduced)	Congestive heart failure Severe hepatic failure Nephrotic syndrome Oliguric/anuric renal failure

CLINICAL TIP

- Glucose is an osmotically active substance drawing water from the interstitium into the intravascular space. A 1 mmol/l increase in blood glucose concentration is expected to cause a reduction in serum sodium concentration of 0.3–0.4 mmol/l secondary to dilution. This must be borne in mind when interpreting sodium levels in diabetic animals.

Calcium

In the blood, calcium is found in three forms: ionized, protein-bound and complexed (e.g. with phosphate, bicarbonate). Ionized calcium is the most important biologically active form and accounts for 50–60% of total serum calcium in normal dogs. Measurement of total calcium is more widely available but may not reliably correlate with ionized calcium concentration.

CLINICAL TIP

- The use of albumin-based adjustment formulas to convert total serum calcium to ionized calcium is no longer considered reliable. Measurement of serum ionized calcium is recommended in all cases in which a clinically significant serum calcium abnormality is suspected.

Table 3.5 Common conditions associated with hypercalcaemia

Cause	Notes
H: primary Hyperparathyroidism	
A: hypoadrenocorticism (Addison's disease)	Transient, clinically insignificant
R: Renal failure	Chronic or polyuric acute renal failure
D: hypervitaminosis D	Vitamin D promotes intestinal absorption and renal reabsorption of calcium Usually due to intoxication (e.g. rodenticides containing cholecalciferol, antipsoriasis cream containing calcipotriol or calcipotriene)
I: Idiopathic	Most common form in cats
O: Osteolysis	
N: Neoplasia	Humoral hypercalcaemia of malignancy most common cause in dogs; commonly due to lymphoma or anal sac apocrine gland adenocarcinoma
S: granulomatouS disease	e.g. panniculitis and angiostrongylosis

Young dogs (typically less than 1 year old) may have serum calcium concentrations that are greater than quoted reference ranges for adult dogs. This is presumed to be due to normal bone growth and should not be overlooked when interpreting results from this patient population.

Hypercalcaemia

Hypercalcaemia may occur secondary to a number of disorders and may in turn have adverse pathophysiological effects, most notably on the kidneys, heart, central nervous system and gastrointestinal tract. A useful acronym for remembering the most common conditions associated with hypercalcaemia is HARDIONS and is explained further in Table 3.5. Transient mild hypercalcaemia has also been associated with haemoconcentration, hyperproteinaemia and severe hypothermia.

Hypocalcaemia

A large number of conditions are associated with hypocalcaemia and the more common ones are listed in Box 3.2.

BOX 3.2 Conditions associated with hypocalcaemia

- Hypoalbuminaemia
- Renal failure (chronic, acute)
- Acute pancreatitis
- Puerperal tetany (eclampsia)
- Hypoparathyroidism
- Soft tissue trauma
- Rhabdomyolysis
- Ethylene glycol intoxication
- Transfusion of blood in citrated anticoagulant

URINALYSIS

Urinalysis is recommended in all emergency patients found to be azotaemic or where there are concerns for example regarding urinary tract infection. It is preferable to obtain urine for analysis prior to administration of intravenous fluid therapy or other drugs (e.g. diuretics, glucocorticoids) that may alter urine production. However, treatment that is urgently required should not be withheld purely for the purposes of obtaining a urine sample. Urine may be collected by voiding (midstream sample), catheterization or cystocentesis as appropriate. Voided samples are preferred for detection of haematuria due to risk of traumatic haemorrhage with the other techniques, and cystocentesis is arguably preferred for collection of samples for microbiology as it avoids possible urethral and/or genital contamination of the sample.

Gross discoloration

Gross appearance may be suggestive of certain disorders. Haematuria, haemoglobinuria and myoglobinuria are variably associated with urine that is pink, red, red-brown or brown in appearance. Methaemoglobinuria is also associated with brown urine. Significant bilirubinuria is associated with orangey urine while cloudy urine is typically the result of pyuria, crystalluria or mucus.

Specific gravity

USG is a measure of total solute concentration and reflects the ability of the kidneys to concentrate or dilute glomerular filtrate derived from plasma. Normal USG varies widely amongst dogs and cats. Isosthenuria is defined as USG of 1.007–1.015. This reflects the same total solute concentration as plasma and suggests inability of the kidneys to modify the initial filtrate. Isosthenuria is usually associated with renal azotaemia.

CLINICAL TIP

- Isosthenuria does not necessarily indicate structural renal injury in all cases. In disorders such as diabetes mellitus or hypercalcaemia, or following the administration of drugs such as furosemide or glucocorticoids, the ability of the kidneys to concentrate urine may be lost. Isosthenuria may therefore be identified in a clinically dehydrated animal for example.

Concentrated urine (USG more than 1.015) and hyposthenuria (USG less than 1.007) suggest some renal tubular function. Increased USG is expected in animals with prerenal azotaemia.

Dipstick analysis

With respect to emergency patients, dipstick analysis is most likely to be useful for detection of glucosuria and ketonuria. Glucosuria is diagnostic for diabetes mellitus when accompanied by significant hyperglycaemia. However, glucosuria is occasionally detected without hyperglycaemia in conditions involving renal tubular dysfunction (e.g. seen with some nephrotoxins). Glucosuria and hyperglycaemia may also be seen in stressed or excited cats.

Ketones are produced as a result of incomplete fatty acid oxidation and ketonuria is most commonly due to diabetic ketoacidosis. Other less common causes of increased ketone production and ketonuria include starvation, prolonged fasting or persistent hypoglycaemia. Acetone, acetoacetate and β-hydroxybutyrate are the three ketones produced and it is of note that the reagents in commercial urine dipsticks will not detect β-hydroxybutyrate.

CLINICAL TIP

- Although ketones are ideally detected in urine, ketonuria implies ketonaemia and it is possible to use the same urine reagent strips to detect ketones in plasma. This technique may be less sensitive but it is extremely useful in dehydrated patients in which obtaining urine may require some delay. This is very much the case for dogs and cats presenting in a diabetic ketoacidotic crisis. At least two haematocrit tubes are typically filled and centrifuged when measuring PCV and TS as part of the emergency database; the plasma from one of these tubes is then used for ketone detection.

Dipsticks are unable to differentiate haematuria, haemoglobinuria and myoglobinuria. Haematuria and haemoglobinuria can be differentiated by sediment examination. In contrast to animals with haemoglobinuria in which plasma is also likely to be discoloured secondary to haemoglobinaemia, plasma in animals with myoglobinuria is likely to be clear. Some causes of haematuria, haemoglobinuria and myoglobinuria are listed in Box 3.3.

Dipsticks should not be used to diagnose the presence of leukocytes in canine or feline urine as the methodology employed is unreliable in these species. Sediment examination is the diagnostic technique of choice. Mild to moderate bilirubinuria may be normal in dogs, especially males, but is always considered an abnormal finding in cats. Causes of bilirubinuria include haemolysis, hepatobiliary disorders, pyrexia and starvation.

Sediment examination

Urine sediment should be examined as quickly as possible after collection to minimize degeneration of casts and cells. Sediment may be examined unstained or can be stained with a commercial stain specifically intended for use with urine (e.g. Sedi-Stain™). The author, however, prefers to stain urine sediment with Diff-Quik. Sediment is examined for the number of red and white blood cells per high power field, infectious organisms

BOX 3.3 Causes of haematuria, haemoglobinuria and myoglobinuria

Haematuria

- Urinary tract trauma (e.g. blunt trauma; iatrogenic – urine sampling, renal biopsy)
- Urolithiasis
- Urinary tract inflammation (e.g. infection, feline lower urinary tract disease)
- Urinary tract neoplasia
- Systemic coagulopathy
- Renal infarction
- Renal pelvic haematoma
- Idiopathic renal haematuria
- Genital tract causes (e.g. inflammation, neoplasia, trauma, oestrus)

Haemoglobinuria

- Immune-mediated haemolytic anaemia
- Transfusion-associated haemolysis
- Splenic torsion
- Heatstroke

Myoglobinuria

- Significant rhabdomyolysis (e.g. status epilepticus, heatstroke, severe crush injury)

(typically bacteria), crystals, and number of casts per low power field.

Especially in the presence of haematuria and proteinuria, more than five white blood cells per high power field are suggestive of inflammation (infectious or non-infectious in origin) in a sample obtained via catheterization. A lower cut-off may be more appropriate in a sample obtained via cystocentesis and a higher cut-off in a voided sample. Urine should be submitted for culture and sensitivity if bacteriuria or pyuria is identified.

4 Parenteral fluid therapy

Parenteral fluid therapy is the most common therapeutic intervention performed in veterinary emergency practice. A thorough understanding of the indications for the use of parenteral fluids, the types of therapeutic fluid available, and the most appropriate protocol for their administration is mandatory both to maximize the benefit and minimize the potential harm associated with this therapy.

Hypovolaemia and dehydration are the most common indications for the use of fluid therapy and it is essential to understand their differences with respect to pathophysiology and clinical assessment in order to administer appropriate fluid therapy (see Ch. 2). This chapter focuses on the different types of parenteral fluid commonly available in nonreferral emergency practice and their appropriate use in hypovolaemia and dehydration.

TYPES OF PARENTERAL FLUID

Crystalloids

Crystalloids are electrolyte solutions that can pass freely out of the bloodstream through the capillary membrane. Crystalloid solutions are described as isotonic, hypertonic or hypotonic based on how their tonicity compares to that of plasma. The tonicity is related to the sodium concentration and it is the tonicity that determines how the crystalloid solution is distributed between fluid compartments following administration into the bloodstream.

The two most commonly used crystalloid solutions are buffered lactated Ringer's solution (Hartmann's solution, compound sodium lactate) and 0.9% sodium chloride (normal strength or physiological saline). Both these solutions are examples of replacement isotonic crystalloids as their tonicity and electrolyte composition are similar to that of extracellular fluid. Following intravascular administration, these fluids equilibrate relatively quickly with the interstitial space and 75–85% of the administered volume is likely to have left the bloodstream 30–60 min after infusion. This is why large volumes are required to expand the intravascular compartment effectively in hypovolaemia and is also the reason why these solutions are used to replenish extravascular fluid losses in dehydration (see below).

Hypertonic (e.g. 7.2–7.5% sodium chloride (hypertonic saline)) and hypotonic (e.g. 0.45% sodium chloride (half strength saline)) crystalloid solutions are also available but their use is much less commonly indicated. Hypertonic saline administration causes plasma volume expansion mainly by drawing water out of cells into the extracellular space down an osmotic gradient. Most of this fluid remains in the interstitial space but a proportion diffuses into the vasculature. The recommended dose is 4 ml/kg i.v. (dogs 4–7 ml/kg, cats 2–4 ml/kg) over a minimum of 5 minutes and a rapid though short-lived effect is typically seen (within 5 minutes). Hypertonic saline is indicated in volume resuscitation, especially in large or giant breed dogs where rapid administration of large volumes of isotonic crystalloids may be impossible. Administration of hypertonic saline must be followed by the use of a replacement isotonic crystalloid due to the osmotic diuresis and rapid sodium redistribution that occur with this treatment. Hypertonic saline is often administered in combination with a colloid solution to prolong intravascular volume expansion. Hypertonic saline is also indicated in the treatment of raised intracranial pressure, especially with concurrent hypovolaemia, where it causes fluid to move out of the brain parenchyma and into the vasculature (see Ch. 28).

Hypotonic saline is most often used in combination with 0.9% sodium chloride to correct hyponatraemia gradually. It is also occasionally used in dehydrated animals with cardiac disease to provide rehydration while limiting the amount of sodium administered.

CLINICAL TIP

- A 0.18% sodium chloride (with 4% glucose) solution is commercially available. This solution is markedly hypotonic compared to plasma and in the author's opinion there is no indication for its routine use. It may occasionally be required to treat animals with severe acute hypernatraemia but this is rare in companion animals. If this solution is used, animals must be monitored very closely for electrolyte abnormalities (hyponatraemia in particular) that may be severe with potentially very serious clinical consequences.
- The author is aware of cases in which this solution has been used as a convenient way of administering intravenous glucose supplementation. However, other proprietary glucose solutions (e.g. 5% glucose in 0.9% sodium chloride solution) are available and glucose solutions can also readily be formulated (see Appendix 1, Drug Formulary). The author would therefore strongly discourage the use of the 0.18% sodium chloride solution as a means of administering glucose supplementation.

Uses of isotonic crystalloid solutions

Isotonic crystalloid solutions are used in two main ways:

- High rate isotonic crystalloid therapy is used to treat hypovolaemia either alone or in combination with other fluid types (colloid, hypertonic saline)
- Low rate isotonic crystalloid therapy is used to treat dehydration.

Synthetic colloids

Colloid solutions consist of large (macro) molecules that do not readily leave the intravascular space (through capillary pores) and are hyperoncotic relative to normal animals. Synthetic colloids therefore draw fluid into and hold fluid in the vasculature, causing plasma volume expansion. Commercially available synthetic colloid preparations are often made up in a 0.9% sodium chloride solution. Nonsynthetic (natural) colloid solutions that are currently used therapeutically include plasma and human serum albumin solutions.

The three types of synthetic colloid solution currently in veterinary use are:

- Hydroxyethyl starches: tetrastarch (e.g. Voluven 130/0.4®, Fresenius Kabi); hetastarch (e.g. Hetastarch 600/0.7®, Baxter); pentastarch (e.g. HAES-Steril 200/0.5®, Fresenius Kabi)
- Gelatins (e.g. Gelofusine®, Braun; Haemaccel®, Intervet)
- Dextrans (e.g. Dextran-70®, Pharmacosmos).

The volume and duration of plasma expansion that follows colloid administration depend in part on the specific colloid used (its colloid osmotic pressure (COP)), as well as the dose given and the species in question.

Indications for synthetic colloid use

Synthetic colloids are usually used in hypovolaemic patients in one of two scenarios:

1. When fluid resuscitation with an isotonic crystalloid solution has proved to be ineffective; this is because colloids are more efficient at intravascular volume expansion.
2. When there are specific reasons that warrant the inclusion of a colloid; this might be the case for example in animals that are hypoproteinaemic (e.g. from gastrointestinal or renal loss). Isotonic crystalloids will remain in the circulation for even less time in these animals as plasma proteins (albumin in particular) are partly responsible for retaining these fluids in the intravascular space.

Synthetic colloids are not generally used alone when employed in the treatment of hypovolaemia and are typically discontinued earlier on than the replacement crystalloid solution. It is much less common for patients to remain on long-term colloid therapy (although ongoing hypoproteinaemia or the presence of systemic vasculitis or capillary-leak syndrome for example may warrant this treatment).

Adverse effects of synthetic colloids

The most important adverse effect to consider when using synthetic colloids is their effect on coagulation that is likely to be multifactorial in origin. Allergic reactions are also rarely identified.

Haemoglobin-based oxygen-carrying solutions

Haemoglobin-based oxygen-carrying solutions (HBOC) are not blood replacement solutions. They increase plasma haemoglobin concentration and therefore oxygen-carrying capacity but do not contain other blood constituents. The only HBOC currently available for veterinary clinical use is Oxyglobin® (Biopure Corporation; www.biopure.com). This solution is based on polymerized modified bovine haemoglobin and is administered using standard intravenous fluid administration sets. It is currently only licensed for use in dogs but has been used extensively off-licence in cats with great success.

The main indication for Oxyglobin® is in euvolaemic anaemia where it can act as a substitute for the deficient red blood cells and allow improved tissue oxygenation. Unlike with blood transfusions, there are no cellular antigens in Oxyglobin® so typing and crossmatching do not need to be performed. The product as supplied in foil by the manufacturer also has a long shelf-life of 3 years. Oxyglobin® is used in these cases to support the patient while diagnosis is achieved and treatment is instituted and given time to take effect.

CLINICAL TIP

Administration of Oxyglobin® typically causes a fall in packed cell volume (PCV) due to intravascular volume expansion. Ideally, therefore, plasma haemoglobin concentration should be used to monitor increase in oxygen-carrying capacity in lieu of packed cell volume. An approximately equivalent PCV can be calculated as follows:

$$\text{PCV (\%)} = \text{haemoglobin concentration (g/dl)} \times 3$$

However, a haemoglobinometer is required to measure free plasma haemoglobin concentration as in-house machines typically calculate haemoglobin concentration from haematocrit. Regardless of whether a haemoglobinometer is available or not, positive clinical response to treatment is the best guide of effective therapy.

As Oxyglobin® contains large molecules it is also a potent colloid solution and can therefore be used very effectively to provide intravascular volume expansion in animals with hypovolaemia. Despite the unique oxygen-carrying benefits of this modified biological colloid, the much greater cost of Oxyglobin® over other available colloids means that its use in hypovolaemia is typically restricted to animals that have suffered significant blood loss.

CLINICAL TIP

- The volume expanding properties of Oxyglobin® must be borne in mind when it is used to treat anaemia in patients without hypovolaemia as there is a very real risk of fluid overload if inappropriately high rates are used, especially in cats.
- Typical rates for Oxyglobin® use in euvolaemic anaemic patients are 0.5–1 ml/kg/hr in cats and 1–2 ml/kg/hr in dogs.
- Caution is also warranted in disease states associated with an increased risk of fluid overload such as cardiac disease, pulmonary parenchymal disease and cerebral oedema

As with all colloids, Oxyglobin® will interfere with serum total solids measurement via refractometry and results must be interpreted cautiously. Oxyglobin® will also interfere with colorimetric serum biochemistry analysis although the parameters affected will depend on both the analyser and the methodology. Peripheral blood smear evaluation is not affected.

THE FLUID PLAN

On the basis of the physical examination, and subsequently other findings, it should be possible to answer the following questions (see Ch. 2):

- Is the animal hypovolaemic and if so, is this mild, moderate or severe?
- Is the animal dehydrated and if so, what is the estimated percentage dehydration?

Hypovolaemia

The basic objective is to restore the effective circulating intravascular volume and thereby restore adequate tissue perfusion. Appropriate fluid therapy is therefore provided until end-points suggestive of acceptable systemic perfusion are achieved. This volume expansion is performed over a short period of time – usually a few minutes to an hour but sometimes longer – and may involve the use of both isotonic crystalloids and colloids including Oxyglobin® (plus whole blood and hypertonic saline if available). Isotonic crystalloids are the first choice in the majority of cases.

How?

Hypovolaemia is treated via the intravenous route using one or more of the shortest but largest bore catheters possible. If a peripheral vein cannot be catheterized and a central venous catheter is not available or inappropriate, the intraosseous route may be used initially.

How much and for how long?

Isotonic crystalloids

See Table 4.1 for guidelines for initial rates of isotonic crystalloid fluid therapy in dogs and cats with uncomplicated hypovolaemia. Initial boluses are usually given over 15–20 minutes. For some bigger dogs the use of a pressure infusor (Figure 4.1) around the crystalloid bag can be invaluable in delivering the fluid within a suitable period of time.

Table 4.1 Guidelines for isotonic crystalloid therapy for hypovolaemia in dogs and cats. Initial boluses are usually given over 15–20 minutes

	SIZE OF INITIAL FLUID BOLUS	ANTICIPATED SIZE OF TOTAL FLUID BOLUS (ml/kg)		
Severity of hypovolaemia		**Mild**	**Moderate**	**Severe**
Dogs	10–40	20–40	40–60	60–90
Cats	5–20	10–20	20–40	40–60

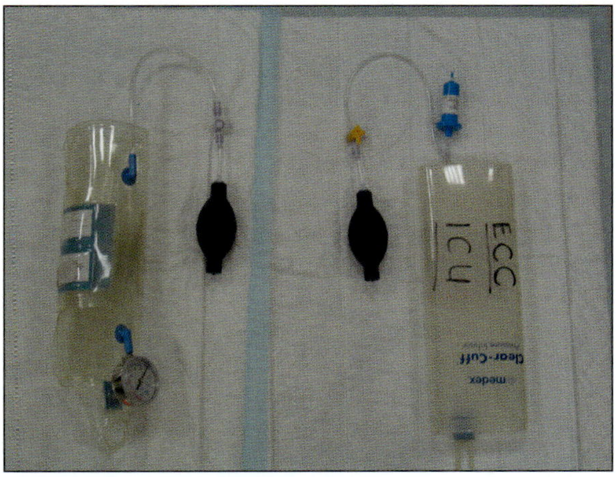

Figure 4.1 Two different types of pressure infusor for large volume rapid fluid administration.

Colloids

In moderate to severe hypovolaemia, the following rates of colloid administration are applicable:

- Dogs: 5 ml/kg boluses up to a total of 20 ml/kg
- Cats: 5 ml/kg boluses up to a total of 10 ml/kg
- Oxyglobin®: 10–30 ml/kg total dose.

Whenever a synthetic colloid is added to an animal's fluid regime, due attention must be paid to whether this affects the rate of crystalloid therapy, with the latter being reduced if appropriate (often by about 50%).

Approach to fluid resuscitation

Initial rates of fluid therapy for volume expansion were traditionally quoted per hour. However, it is more appropriate to think in terms of bolus administration and constant reassessment.

CLINICAL TIP

- Although it is possible to perform safe and successful volume resuscitation without the use of infusion pumps, these devices greatly facilitate acute fluid therapy in smaller dogs and cats. Their use is often inappropriate initially in medium- to larger-size hypovolaemic dogs (i.e. where the maximum infusion rate of the pump may be too slow). Most infusion pumps are designed to facilitate a bolus approach by allowing a set volume of fluid to be infused before an alarm sounds.
- In addition, the use of infusion pumps greatly enhances the reliability, accuracy and safety of more chronic rehydration and maintenance fluid therapy. In the author's opinion, access to adequate numbers of infusion pumps is extremely important in emergency practice.

A dog with hypoperfusion secondary to severe hypovolaemia for example may be given an initial intravenous isotonic crystalloid bolus of 40 ml/kg over 20 minutes:

- At the end of the initial bolus, the dog's perfusion parameters should be reassessed. If the dog is now normovolaemic, no further boluses are administered but the dog continues to be monitored closely for deterioration; if there has been some improvement but the dog remains hypovolaemic, a second smaller bolus (e.g. 20 ml/kg) is administered, perhaps over a longer period of time; if there has been no improvement, another 40 ml/kg bolus is administered.

- At the end of the second bolus, the dog's perfusion parameters should be reassessed. If the dog is now normovolaemic, no further boluses are administered but the dog continues to be monitored closely for deterioration; if there has been some improvement but the dog remains hypovolaemic, a third smaller bolus (e.g. 10 ml/kg) is administered, perhaps over a longer period of time; if there has been no improvement, a colloid may be introduced and the crystalloid rate modified if appropriate.
- This process is repeated continually until the dog's perfusion parameters reach end-points suggestive of adequate perfusion and it is on an appropriate rate and combination of fluid therapy to maintain this perfusion.
- The regular monitoring must then continue to detect any sudden deterioration.
- If the patient's presenting history and subsequent assessment suggest concurrent dehydration, this must be taken into account with respect to on-going fluid therapy (see below).

CLINICAL TIP

- There is no standard fluid combination, rate or period of administration in the treatment of hypovolaemia. Depending on the individual patient in question and the nature of the problems, acute volume expansion can be achieved in a matter of minutes using isotonic crystalloids alone or can take several hours and require the use of two or more types of parenteral fluid. Fluid therapy must therefore always be tailored to the needs of the individual patient.

Dehydration

The basic objective in the treatment of dehydration is to replenish the deficit from all fluid compartments that are affected. A significant proportion of dehydrated animals have minimal intravascular deficits (i.e. they are not hypovolaemic) and the aim of fluid therapy in these cases is therefore to replace fluid losses from the extravascular (interstitial and intracellular) compartments.

Dehydration is corrected over a longer period of time than hypovolaemia – typically 12–48 hours depending on the severity and rate of onset – and is usually achieved through the use of replacement isotonic crystalloids alone. In animals that have a normal intravascular volume, excessively aggressive rehydration will overexpand the interstitial compartment. This is manifested clinically as increased skin turgor, chemosis, subcutaneous pitting oedema and pulmonary oedema. Once pulmonary oedema (i.e. fluid overload of the pulmonary interstitial space) has developed, and despite the extensive protective lymphatic drainage available, alveolar flooding may occur and can be very severe if not addressed early enough. Cerebral oedema is another possible and extremely serious consequence of overexpansion of the interstitial compartment.

How?

Fluid therapy for rehydration is also usually given by the intravenous route. In some cases, the use of the subcutaneous route may be a reasonable option. Examples include:

- Animals with mild dehydration
- Animals whose owners are unable (or unwilling) to pay for intravenous fluid therapy
- Cases where owners are reluctant to leave their pets at the clinic.

Subcutaneous fluid therapy is also used intermittently to provide fluid support in chronic illnesses such as chronic renal failure. Its sole use is inappropriate in patients with hypovolaemia as absorption is too slow due to poor peripheral perfusion. An empirical total volume of 10 ml/kg of an isotonic crystalloid is usually given distributed over multiple sites; this clearly is highly dependent on patient compliance.

How much?

The equation that is traditionally used to calculate the fluid requirement of a dehydrated patient over a chosen period of time is:

Fluid requirement = Replacement volume +
Maintenance requirement +
On-going losses

Replacement volume

The volume of fluid required to replace the deficit in a dehydrated animal is calculated as follows:

$$\text{Fluid deficit (ml)} = \%\ \text{dehydration} \times \text{body weight (kg)} \times 10$$

Despite the inherent inaccuracies (see Ch. 2), estimating the patient's percentage dehydration on the basis of physical examination is useful as it allows the above calculation to be made.

Maintenance requirement

CLINICAL TIP

- Maintenance fluid requirements are related to metabolic rate which is a function of body surface area and varies with species and breed, and especially with age and size. In particular it is important to remember that maintenance requirements for puppies, kittens and toy canine breeds are higher than for adult animals and larger breeds.
- Although formulas are available for calculating maintenance intravenous fluid requirements based on body weight, there is some disagreement between them and the author prefers a more empirical approach with regular reassessment.

The commonly cited figures for maintenance crystalloid requirements are 2 ml/kg/hr or 50 ml/kg/day. While these rates may be appropriate for the majority of fully grown dogs and cats, the notion that all dogs and cats have the same maintenance fluid requirements is counterintuitive when one considers, for example, a 3-year-old Great Dane versus a 6-week-old Yorkshire terrier. It is more appropriate therefore to use a range for fully grown dogs of 1.5 ml/kg/hr (larger dogs) up to 4 ml/kg/hr (very small dogs), and a range for fully grown cats of 2–3 ml/kg/hr. Maintenance requirements for puppies and kittens are higher than for adult dogs and cats. Maintenance rates as high as 8 ml/kg/hr have been described by some authors, for example for paediatric animals of toy breeds. In addition, maintenance requirements for overweight animals should be calculated using a reduced body weight.

On-going losses

The practicalities of accurately quantifying on-going losses (e.g. vomitus, diarrhoea) in addition to those assumed in maintenance requirements preclude this as a realistic option in most settings. In order to allow initial fluid requirements to be calculated, a useful technique is to estimate the contribution from these on-going losses in terms of multiples of the patient's maintenance requirements. Thus some animals may have no additional contribution here; a vomiting animal may have an extra maintenance requirement added; and an animal with profuse vomiting and diarrhoea may have or more extra maintence requirement added to the initial calculation.

For how long?

The initial fluid plan calculated for a dehydrated patient is an approximation and must be approached dynamically; both the rate and the type of fluid used need to be reassessed. A range of different factors are taken into account, including:

- Changes in both the physical examination and emergency database parameters of hydration including body weight
- Whether the animal is eating/drinking (if allowed)
- A subjective assessment of the degree of on-going losses.

Due attention must also be paid to the provision of supplementary potassium in particular in appropriate cases.

FLUID THERAPY CASE EXAMPLES

The rest of this chapter will use some common canine and feline emergencies to highlight situations in which a more conservative approach is recommended in the aggressive fluid resuscitation of hypovolaemic patients. There is no set protocol for fluid therapy in any given situation and what follows are merely suggestions intended as a guide and to prompt discussion of other available options in each case. In addition to the case examples presented here, it is noteworthy that recent or active haemorrhage may be a reason to be more conservative with fluid therapy as overzealous volume expansion has the potential to exacerbate bleeding by disrupting blood clots at sites of haemostasis. Providing only sufficient fluid therapy to restore perfusion to minimum end-points may be most sensible in these cases but it must be remembered that restoration of effective circulating volume is essential.

Use of parenteral fluid therapy is further demonstrated by the case examples referred to throughout the book.

Case example 1 – pulmonary pathology

CLINICAL TIP

- Pulmonary parenchymal pathology, including pulmonary contusions (see Ch. 28), is a reason to be more conservative with fluid therapy. Despite the extensive lymphatic drainage available, pathological lungs may be more prone to oedema than healthy lungs. Animals suffering from severe trauma (thoracic or nonthoracic) or from other causes of shock may also develop acute lung injury (ALI) or acute respiratory distress syndrome (ARDS); this is especially true for cats.

PRESENTING SIGNS AND CASE HISTORY

A 3-year-old male neutered domestic short hair cat presented shortly after a suspected motor vehicle accident. The incident was estimated to have occurred within the 2 hours prior to presentation. The cat was initially found collapsed under a hedge. He had subsequently been seen to take a few steps but was reportedly very lame in his pelvic limbs. No other significant preceding history was reported.

Major body system examination

On presentation the cat was depressed and recumbent. Cardiovascular examination revealed a heart rate of 150 beats per minute and neither a gallop sound nor a heart murmur was detected. Both femoral pulses were palpable but very weak and dorsal pedal pulses were not identified. Mucous membranes were pale, dry and cold to touch, and capillary refill time was 2 seconds. The extremities were also cold.

Respiratory rate was 50 breaths per minute with a shallow, nonparadoxical and regular pattern. Lung sounds were diffusely harsh and bilaterally symmetrical. The pupils were equal and reactive and there was no external evidence of significant head trauma. No gait assessment was made at this stage. Abdominal palpation revealed a small soft bladder and was unremarkable. There was evidence of urine staining around the perineum and the cat was moderately hypothermic (rectal temperature 35.5°C).

Assessment

The cat was assessed as hypoperfused due to moderate hypovolaemia (presumably due to haemorrhage plus effects on vasomotor control). The degrees of hypothermia and bradycardia were not considered unusual for a moderately hypovolaemic cat (see Ch. 2), and his mentation was considered appropriate for the severity of hypoperfusion with a low index of suspicion for raised intracranial pressure. Some respiratory compromise was present and pulmonary contusions were considered the most likely cause of the harsh lung sounds.

Management discussion

There is no information in this cat's history prior to the traumatic incident that would contraindicate the use of aggressive fluid therapy. In addition, both the absence of any significant preceding history and the time scale in question do not support the likelihood of pre-existing dehydration.

The suspicion of pulmonary contusions (see Ch. 28) is a reason to be more conservative with resuscitative fluid therapy in this case. The aim of fluid therapy should be to restore acceptable tissue perfusion while avoiding excessive fluid administration. Commencing volume expansion using an isotonic replacement crystalloid solution is an appropriate choice in this cat but a conservative initial bolus of only 5–10 ml/kg may be most sensible. At the end of the bolus perfusion parameters and respiratory status should be reassessed. If significant hypovolaemia persists, another 5–10 ml/kg isotonic crystalloid bolus may be given and the cat reassessed.

If significant hypovolaemia still persists after the second crystalloid bolus, the next step may be to assess the cat's response to a conservative (e.g. 2–3 ml/kg) synthetic colloid bolus. This may reduce the risk of expanding the pulmonary interstitial space to the point of alveolar flooding, which would exacerbate the existing respiratory compromise from contusions. However, in some types of lung pathology, the pulmonary vasculature can become leakier to colloid molecules despite their large size. Once the colloid molecules move into the pulmonary interstitium they may worsen pulmonary oedema and may persist there for some time. Nevertheless, it is not possible to predict in advance whether this will occur and it is therefore recommended to assess the patient's response to a colloid bolus and discontinue this therapy if the respiratory status worsens as a result.

Given the concerns in this case regarding pulmonary contusions, intravenous fluid therapy should be discontinued as soon as the cat's perfusion is adequately restored. Conservative fluid therapy may need to be restarted for any procedures subsequently performed under general anaesthesia or sedation if hypotension becomes a concern. Maintenance fluids (including potassium supplementation) may be required if the cat is anorexic while hospitalized.

Intravenous fluids should be warmed to body temperature prior to administration. However, it is important to start fluid therapy before other warming measures are instituted. This is because warming a hypothermic (and therefore peripherally vasoconstricted) animal will cause cutaneous vasodilation that may exacerbate existing hypotension. Oxygen supplementation is recommended and opioid analgesia is mandatory in this cat.

Case example 2 – cardiac disease, intracranial hypertension

CLINICAL TIP

- Cardiac disease is a reason to be more conservative with resuscitative fluid therapy. Animals with diseased hearts are generally less able to cope with sudden increases in blood volume and are more likely to develop congestive heart failure (see Ch. 31).
- The majority of dogs with clinically significant heart disease will have a murmur on auscultation. However, failure to identify a murmur or gallop sound, especially in cats, does not rule out clinically significant heart disease.

CLINICAL TIP

- Raised intracranial pressure (ICP) is a reason to be more conservative with resuscitative fluid therapy. Causes of raised ICP include head trauma, severe seizuring and intracranial mass lesions. Overzealous intravenous fluid therapy can lead to cerebral oedema and thereby exacerbate existing raised intracranial pressure. However, the correction of hypovolaemia and consequence systemic hypoperfusion must take precedence over concerns regarding intracranial hypertension. This is because maintaining adequate cerebral perfusion is the priority and this is highly dependent on systemic arterial blood pressure (see Ch. 28).

PRESENTING SIGNS AND CASE HISTORY

A 10-year-old male neutered Cavalier King Charles spaniel presented 30 minutes after a motor vehicle accident witnessed by the owner. The dog fell over briefly as a result but no loss of consciousness was observed. He had been very subdued since the incident. The owner also reported that the dog had been less keen to exercise for a few weeks and was panting more during his walks. He had also been coughing intermittently although this had not become noticeably worse. His appetite had been variable but there had been no other clinical signs.

Major body system examination

On presentation the dog was markedly depressed. Cardiovascular examination revealed a heart rate of 140 beats per minute and a grade IV/VI systolic murmur with the point of maximal intensity over the mitral valve region. Femoral pulses were hyperdynamic and dorsal pedal pulses were readily palpable. Mucous membranes were mildly hyperaemic with a capillary refill time of 1 second and the dog's extremities were normal to the touch. Respiratory rate was 20 breaths per minute with normal pattern and effort, and lung field auscultation was unremarkable. Gait assessment was not made at this stage.

Anisocoria was present with slow but intact pupillary light reflexes (both direct and consensual); bilateral menace responses were identified. There was left-sided scleral haemorrhage but no blood in the left ear canal and no readily palpable skull fractures. Abdominal palpation was nonpainful with a moderate size bladder palpable and rectal temperature was mildly reduced (37.7°C).

Assessment

The dog was assessed as mildly hypovolaemic with an inappropriately depressed mentation, i.e. he was more depressed than would be expected from mild hypovolaemia/hypoperfusion alone. This finding, supported by the anisocoria and scleral haemorrhage, was suggestive of raised ICP secondary to head trauma. The tachycardia may have been compensatory for the hypovolaemia and/or secondary to pain. However, the possibility of pre-existing cardiac insufficiency could not be excluded and it was possible that the dog had had a resting tachycardia in the weeks prior to this incident.

Management discussion

This dog is of a breed that is predisposed to mitral valve disease and his reported history raises the suspicion of this becoming clinically significant. It is difficult to know how important the heart disease is in the dog's clinical presentation.

Commencing acute volume expansion using an isotonic crystalloid solution is an option in this dog. However, the benefits of restoring euvolaemia and thereby optimizing cerebral perfusion have to be balanced with the possibility of clinically significant cardiac disease. If the dog was suitably compliant, conscious thoracic radiography may help guide therapy by providing further information with respect to left atrial enlargement and pulmonary congestion and oedema. If facilities and expertise allow, echocardiography to evaluate left atrial size more accurately would be very useful.

In this case it may be more appropriate for example to administer an initial isotonic crystalloid rate of 3 ml/kg/hr rather than bolus therapy. This is especially true if blood pressure measurement was possible and the dog was found to be normotensive. Perfusion parameters and respiratory status should be reassessed regularly and the rate adjusted as appropriate. Given the greater concerns in this case with respect to fluid overload, intravenous fluid therapy should be discontinued as soon as possible. Although this dog does not have any pre-existing dehydration that requires replacement, maintenance fluids may be required if he remains depressed for an extended period of time. A conservative isotonic crystalloid rate of 1 ml/kg/hr should be considered and a hypotonic solution such as 0.45% sodium chloride may be more appropriate if available. Oxygen supplementation is recommended and opioid analgesia is mandatory.

Case example 3 – rehydration

PRESENTING SIGNS AND CASE HISTORY

A 3-month-old male entire Staffordshire bull terrier (4 kg) presented with a 2-day history of vomiting and diarrhoea. The puppy had not eaten anything at all for 12 hours and although continuing to drink was typically vomiting immediately afterwards. He had vomited approximately four times each day. The diarrhoea was occurring with increasing frequency and while watery initially had progressed to being bloody.

PRESENTING SIGNS AND CASE HISTORY—cont'd

The puppy had been in the owner's possession for 1 week and was acquired from a private family. He had been appropriately wormed but had not been vaccinated and the owner was unsure regarding the dam's vaccination status. The owner was unaware of any significant scavenging incidents and the puppy had been confined to the house.

Major body system examination

On presentation the puppy was ambulatory but markedly depressed. Cardiovascular examination revealed a heart rate of 130 beats per minute and no murmur, gallop sound or dysrhythmia was detected. Femoral and dorsal pedal pulses were unremarkable and mucous membranes were pink and dry with a normal capillary refill time. Respiratory rate was 30 breaths per minute, and respiratory pattern and effort and lung field auscultation were unremarkable.

The puppy's abdomen was diffusely painful on palpation and the intestines were fluid-filled with no normal faeces palpable. A focal lesion suggestive of surgical disease was not identified. Rectal temperature was 37.5°C and there was fresh blood on the thermometer.

Skin turgor was markedly reduced.

Assessment

The puppy was assessed on the basis of physical examination findings as being moderately dehydrated but still normovolaemic. Dehydration was estimated at 8% of body weight.

Management discussion

The puppy will have salt and water losses affecting both the extravascular and intravascular compartments and a replacement isotonic crystalloid solution is an appropriate initial choice. Additional potassium and glucose supplementation may be indicated once an emergency database has been obtained. The initial fluid rate for this puppy is calculated as follows:

$$\text{Fluid requirement} = \text{Replacement volume} + \text{Maintenance requirement} + \text{On-going losses}$$

Replacement volume

Fluid deficit (ml) = % dehydration × body weight (kg) × 10
= 8 × 4 × 10
= 320 ml.

It is decided to replace this deficit over 12 hr.

Maintenance requirement

Given this dog's age an estimated maintenance requirement of 4 ml/kg/hr is used:

= 16 ml/hr
= 192 ml/12 hr.

On-going losses

Given this dog's presenting history, an additional maintenance requirement is added initially to allow for on-going losses:

= 192 ml/12 hr.

The puppy's fluid requirement for the replacement period of 12 hours is therefore:

= (320 ml + 192 ml + 192 ml) over 12 hr
= 704 ml over 12 hr
= 58.7 ml/hr
= ~15 ml/kg/hr

At the end of the replacement period, the fluid rate should be reduced to meet maintenance and on-going loss requirements. The reader is reminded again that this type of calculation is helpful to provide an initial fluid rate but is derived using a number of assumptions and approximations. The rate should be adjusted as necessary in accordance with regular assessment of both physical and laboratory parameters.

5 Analgesia for the emergency patient

'An hour of pain is as long as a day of pleasure' (English proverb)

PAIN IN COMPANION ANIMALS

The advantages that the ability to feel pain confers with respect to survival are well recognized. However, on-going pain results in a number of physiological and psychological responses that are disadvantageous to any animal and especially one that is affected by illness or injury. These are summarized in Box 5.1.

Pain assessment

NURSING ASPECT

Nurses should be considered central to on-going pain assessment as they typically spend more time with and around hospitalized patients. They are therefore often better suited to detect changes in pain status, especially as most of the signs of pain in companion animals are subjective.

BOX 5.1 Disadvantages associated with on-going pain

- Unnecessary suffering
- Altered mentation: anxiety, agitation; dullness, depression
- Reduced food intake – may slow recovery
- Prolonged recumbency
- Self-mutilation
- Impaired respiration
- Sensitization to noxious stimuli
- Excessive sympathetic stimulation, enhanced catabolism, delayed wound healing, immune suppression
- Inability to monitor patients effectively due to aberrant physiological changes and consequent clinical findings

The assessment of pain in animals is more difficult and more subjective than in people and veterinary personnel have to rely much more on a combination of sign recognition, patient interaction, experience, and a degree of anthropomorphism. The signs that an animal in pain may exhibit depend on various factors, including:

- The source, severity and duration (acute, chronic) of pain
- Individual patient variability – age, species, breed, tolerance, temperament.

Signs consistent with pain are summarized in Box 5.2 in no particular order and it is important to realize that these signs are derived from both patient observation and interaction. Painful cats are often much less demonstrative than painful dogs, and sick animals in general may be unable to show expected behavioural signs of pain. In addition, physiological parameters are not consistently reliable as indicators of pain.

CLINICAL TIP

- There are certainly cases where it is not clear whether an animal is in pain. A liberal approach (i.e. if in doubt, treat for pain) is essential and carries minimal risk when based on good knowledge of the analgesics currently available. A low testing dose can be given and the patient monitored for a favourable response.
- The reader is also reminded that cats are not inherently at greater risk of adverse effects from analgesics and pain relief is as important in cats as it is in dogs.

BOX 5.2 Signs consistent with pain in dogs and cats

- Consistent response on palpation of painful area
- Poor appetite
- Restlessness (especially dogs); dullness, depression and lack of activity (especially cats)
- Looking, licking, biting or scratching at painful area; self-mutilation
- Vocalization: dogs – growling, whining, groaning; cats – purring, growling, hissing
- Reduced grooming behaviour
- Altered gait and reluctance to walk
- Abnormal posture (especially cats who often sit with a hunched sternal posture rather than lying curled in lateral recumbency)
- Reluctance to sleep
- Uncharacteristic behaviour (aggression or affection) towards humans
- Inappropriate urination and/or defecation
- (Unexplained tachycardia, tachypnoea/panting, hypertension, or pupillary dilation)

The pain pathway

A basic knowledge of the pain pathway is essential to understand the modes of action of available analgesics and the rationale behind multimodal therapy. The pain pathway essentially consists of the following.

- Peripheral component:
  - Tissue receptors that detect painful stimuli (nociceptors)
  - Primary afferent nerve fibres that conduct the subsequent signal to the spinal cord (dorsal horn) or cranial nerve nuclei
- Central component:
  - Processing of nociceptive signals (modulation) in the spinal cord
  - Further processing in higher centres resulting in conscious perception of pain.

Sensitization

Sensitization (or wind-up) refers to increased sensitivity to noxious stimuli following injury to either peripheral tissues (causes inflammatory pain) or the central nervous system (causes neuropathic pain). This increased sensitivity results in:

- Hyperalgesia: an exaggerated responsiveness to a given noxious stimulus
- Allodynia: stimuli that are normally innocuous become painful.

Sensitization can occur in either or both of the peripheral and central components of the pain pathway.

The clinical relevance of sensitization

In practical terms, once sensitization is underway, conscious perception of pain is greater, it is more difficult to control and higher drug doses are required. It is therefore preferable to try to prevent pain rather than merely to treat it once it is established. A significant proportion of emergency patients are already in pain at initial presentation. In order to minimize sensitization, pain management should be instituted as soon as possible and, once the pain is under control, the patient kept on a level pain-free plateau. All animals going on to have operative procedures performed will benefit from adequate preoperative analgesia, i.e. in advance of the significant noxious stimulation resulting from surgical intervention.

ANALGESIC AGENTS

Balanced analgesia involves the use of one or more appropriate analgesics (multimodal therapy) in an effective dosing regimen given by the appropriate route(s). Analgesic agents that are commonly available in emergency clinics include:

- Opioids
- Nonsteroidal antiinflammatory agents (NSAIAs)
- Local analgesic/anaesthetic agents
- Ketamine
- Medetomidine.

An intuitive approach to pain management is based on thorough initial evaluation followed by regular reassessment of the patient and adjustment of the treatment protocol as indicated. This is especially relevant to the use of full agonist opioids which may be used at highly variable dose rates and dosing frequencies. As described later in this chapter, nonpharmacological measures are also very important in pain management.

Opioids

CLINICAL TIP

- In the author's opinion, all veterinary practices that may see animals in moderate to severe pain should have a full (pure) opioid agonist available, ideally morphine or methadone. These agents are extremely affordable, highly effective, and allow dose titration to effect. Although they need to be stored and administered in accordance with regulations for controlled drugs, this should not be considered an impediment to their use.

Opioids (predominantly) act in the central component of the pain pathway. Most opioids used clinically are selective for the μ-receptor and are full (pure) agonists, partial agonists or agonists–antagonists. They are the mainstay of pain management in the emergency patient and block central sensitization. Opioids are also used in low doses for sedation or anxiolysis. High doses of pure opioids in particular may result in dysphoria (vocalization, anxiety, restlessness) that can be difficult to differentiate from on-going pain. Naloxone (or butorphanol) can be used to reverse the effects of full opioid agonists.

Both respiratory depression and bradycardia are rarely seen as side effects of concern during opioid administration in clinical veterinary patients that are not under anaesthesia. Furthermore, pain itself can cause respiratory compromise and appropriate opioid administration can normalize respiratory status in such cases. Until adequately treated, pain can also confuse assessment of other parameters such as heart rate and blood pressure. Dose rates, routes of administration and dosing frequencies of opioids in current use in emergency clinics are summarized in Table 5.1.

Morphine

Morphine is a full μ-agonist and remains the gold standard analgesic for moderate to severe pain. Onset of action is usually 10–15 minutes following intravenous administration. In addition to its analgesic effects, morphine is also extremely useful as an anxiolytic in respiratory distress. Vomiting is more likely than with other opioids and will further exacerbate raised intracranial or intraocular pressure. Morphine should therefore be avoided in patients where this is of concern. Rapid intravenous administration may cause signs associated with histamine release (transient vasodilation and hypotension)

Table 5.1 Clinical information on opioid analgesics

Drug	DOGS		CATS	
	Dose/routes of administration	**Dosing frequency**	**Dose/routes of administration**	**Dosing frequency**
Morphine	0.1–1.0 mg/kg slow i.v., i.m. or s.c. 0.1–0.5 mg/kg/hr CRI	prn, q 4 hr	0.1–0.5 mg/kg slow i.v., i.m. or s.c. 0.05–0.2 mg/kg/hr CRI	prn, q 6 hr
Methadone	0.1–1.0 mg/kg slow i.v., i.m. or s.c.	prn, q 4 hr	0.1–0.5 mg/kg slow i.v., i.m. or s.c.	prn, q 6 hr
Pethidine	2–10 mg/kg i.m. 5–15 mg/kg s.c.	prn, q 1–2 hr	5–10 mg/kg i.m. 8–15 mg/kg s.c.	prn, q 2 hr
Buprenorphine	0.01–0.02 mg/kg i.v., i.m. or s.c.	q 6–8 hr	0.01–0.02 mg/kg i.v., i.m., s.c. or o.t.m.	q 6–8 hr
Butorphanol	0.1–0.6 mg/kg i.v., i.m. or s.c. 0.05–0.2 mg/kg/hr CRI	prn, q 1–4 hr	0.1–0.6 mg/kg i.v., i.m. or s.c. 0.05–0.2 mg/kg/hr CRI	prn, q 1–4 hr
Naloxone (antagonist)	0.01–0.1 mg/kg slow i.v. to effect	prn	0.01–0.1 mg/kg slow i.v. to effect	prn

CRI, constant rate infusion; i.m., intramuscular; i.v., intravenous; o.t.m., oral transmucosal; prn, pro re nata (as needed); s.c., subcutaneous.

and slow intravenous boluses or a constant rate infusion are recommended.

Methadone

Methadone is a full μ-agonist that has the same or greater potency as morphine. Its sedative and dysphoric effects are reportedly less marked than with morphine and it does not typically induce emesis. Methadone does not cause histamine release following intravenous administration. In the author's experience, panting (due to effects on the thermoregulatory centre) occurs much more commonly following methadone administration in dogs than it does with morphine and this may complicate clinical assessment.

Buprenorphine

CLINICAL TIP

- Although buprenorphine may be effective for mild to moderate pain, it has a slow onset of action and is therefore not ideal as a first line analgesic for rapid pain relief. Full opioids are preferred in such cases.

Buprenorphine is a partial μ-agonist and a κ-antagonist. It has a slow onset of action that is typically up to 45 min and is therefore not useful for rapid management of pain. Buprenorphine is indicated for mild to moderate pain and appears to be especially effective as an analgesic in cats. The mixed agonist–antagonist actions of this opioid mean that doses above a certain level may be progressively less effective (i.e. buprenorphine has a bell-shaped dose–response curve with a ceiling effect). This means that in theory there is limited capacity to increase the administered dose of buprenorphine in an animal that remains painful. However, the ceiling may be higher than the typical clinical dose range used and this may therefore be more of a theoretical concern. Furthermore, buprenorphine is reported to have a strong receptor affinity and in theory clinical doses of alternative opioids are therefore unlikely to be effective for a variable but lengthy period of time, i.e. until the buprenorphine has detached from the receptors. However, clinical experience suggests that full agonists can be used effectively much sooner than traditionally thought possible.

Oral (orogastric) buprenorphine preparations are available for people but have not been widely used in veterinary medicine. However, oral transmucosal administration of injectable buprenorphine at standard clinical doses results in similar pharmacokinetics to intravenous administration. The solution is tasteless and does not typically cause salivation or nausea. Oral transmucosal administration of buprenorphine is therefore a useful option in cats requiring continued short-term analgesia at home, either in addition to an NSAIA or where the use of an NSAIA is inappropriate. The drug is administered under the tongue or in the side of the mouth.

Butorphanol

Butorphanol is both a μ–antagonist and a κ-agonist with an onset of action of 15–20 minutes. Like buprenorphine, its analgesic effect is likely to reach a ceiling as the dose increases. Clinically, butorphanol seems more useful for its sedative and antitussive effects than as a potent analgesic. It may also be used to reverse sedation and respiratory depression associated with full μ-agonist opioid use.

Tramadol

Tramadol is an entirely synthetic centrally acting analgesic that has been widely used in people and with which there is growing and encouraging veterinary experience. Its analgesic efficacy is derived from complex interactions between opiate (primarily μ), serotonin and adrenergic receptor systems. At least one metabolite (*O*-desmethyl-tramadol; M1) is significantly active and may be essential in tramadol's opioid effect. Tramadol is also reported to have antitussive activity.

While a range of adverse effects are theoretically possible, the main clinically relevant side effects are sedation and nausea. The potential for cardiovascular and respiratory depression may be greater following parenteral (intravenous) administration but is unlikely to be clinically relevant when used judiciously (the injectable preparation is not currently available in the USA). Naloxone will partially antagonize the effects of tramadol. The recommended dose range for dogs is 1–5 mg/kg q 6–12 hr a similar range is likely to be appropriate for cats; pharmacokinetic data suppoprts starting at the lower end of the dose range and upper end of the dosing interval.

An oral preparation of tramadol is available that also contains paracetamol (acetaminophen) – its use should therefore be avoided in cats.

Titration

CLINICAL TIP

- Pain management should be dynamic and based on regular reassessment. Full opioids – morphine, methadone – are typically the

CLINICAL TIP—cont'd

most appropriate analgesic agents for use in moderate to severe pain. The initial dose chosen should be guided by the severity of pain identified or suspected; intuitively, the same dose of the same drug cannot be appropriate in all situations.

- The patient should be reassessed once the drug has had enough time to take effect and additional analgesia administered if indicated.
- Clinically significant side effects of full opioids are rare in companion animals that are not under general anaesthesia and these concerns should not prevent administration of adequate analgesia.

Animals presenting in pain need to be constantly reassessed following initial treatment to ensure that treatment has been effective. Full opioids – morphine, methadone – are typically the most appropriate analgesic agents for use in moderate to severe pain. Their efficacy, rapid onset of action, linear dose–response curve and high index of safety make them highly suitable for titration in severe pain management.

Constant rate infusions

Constant rate infusions (CRI) of opioids (morphine in particular), as well as ketamine and lidocaine, are in widespread use in referral emergency centres as they offer clear advantages for pain management and most of the cases in question will have intravenous access available. CRIs avoid the peaks and troughs in plasma drug concentrations associated with intermittent boluses. They also provide more sensitive control over the degree of analgesia being provided, thereby avoiding both breakthrough pain and overdosing. There is no reason why this mode of drug administration cannot be employed in the first opinion setting as long as facilities allow and adequate monitoring is available.

CLINICAL TIP

- The author would only recommend the use of a constant rate opioid infusion if an infusion pump or syringe driver is available; without their use, it is very difficult to guarantee a constant rate of infusion and there are inherent risks of both under- and overdosing.

CLINICAL TIP—cont'd

- When a constant rate infusion is used, the author cannot stress enough the importance of ensuring that all calculations are double checked, clearly documented and legible to avoid confusion and potentially disastrous errors.

Although some institutions use standardized prepared stock solutions of morphine, lidocaine and ketamine (MLK) for convenience, the author prefers to make up the CRI solution on an individual patient basis with the initial concentrations being guided by the patient in question. An example of how to prepare an MLK solution is given in Box 5.3.

Nonsteroidal antiinflammatory agents

CLINICAL TIP

- The use of nonsteroidal antiinflammatory agents (NSAIAs) is contraindicated in patients with hypovolaemia, hypoperfusion from other causes, or dehydration. A large proportion of painful emergency patients fall into this category and NSAIAs should not be used in the initial management of such cases. Depending on the primary disorder, it may be appropriate to administer an NSAIA following correction of hypoperfusion and dehydration, for example 12–48 hours following initial presentation, as long as the patient is stable and there are no other contraindications.
- Other contraindications for NSAIA administration are renal or hepatic insufficiency, haemostatic abnormalities, evidence of or significant concern for gastroduodenal ulceration, and concurrent corticosteroid administration.

NSAIAs in general reduce the severity of the peripheral inflammatory response and minimize peripheral sensitization. They may be useful in moderate to severe pain and are especially effective as analgesics when used in combination with opioids – the overall analgesia achieved is greater when these agents are used together than when

BOX 5.3 *Preparation of a morphine, lidocaine and ketamine (MLK) solution for constant rate infusion*

Patient's name:
Patient's body weight: 20 kg
Initial infusion rate: 1 ml/kg/hr = 20 ml/hr

1. Select initial dose rates for analgesic agents:
   Morphine (10 mg/ml). Initial dose rate:
   0.2 mg/kg/hr = 4 mg/hr
   Lidocaine (20 mg/ml, i.e. 2%). Initial dose rate:
   50 μg/kg/min = 1000 μg/min = 1 mg/min = 60 mg/hr
   Ketamine (100 mg/ml). Initial dose rate:
   0.5 mg/kg/hr = 10 mg/hr.
2. Select volume of crystalloid to be used and calculate how long this volume will last for:
   Volume of crystalloid to be used: 500 ml bag
   ∴ 500 ml bag will last for 25 hr (i.e. 500 ml divided by 20 ml/hr).
3. Calculate volume of analgesic agents required for this period of time, i.e. in this example 25 hr:
   Morphine: 4 mg/hr × 25 hr = 100 mg = 10 ml (i.e. 100 mg divided by 10 mg/ml solution)
   Lidocaine: 60 mg/hr × 25 hr = 1500 mg = 75 ml (i.e. 1500 mg divided by 20 mg/mL solution)
   Ketamine: 10 mg/hr × 25 hr = 250 mg = 2.5 ml (i.e. 250 mg divided by 100 mg/ml solution).
4. Remove a volume of crystalloid from the bag that is equal to the total volume of analgesic agents to be added, i.e. in this example 10 + 75 + 2.5 = 87.5 ml.
5. Add analgesic agents to the crystalloid solution.
6. Label the MLK solution for infusion clearly with drug concentrations, date, time, name of person preparing the solution, and name of person double-checking preparation.

Note: it is extremely important to ensure that two individuals check all of the above calculations and all of the volumes of analgesic agents and crystalloid removed/added. This safeguard will hopefully prevent potentially serious errors from occurring.

either is used alone. Multimodal therapy may also allow lower doses of each agent to be used, thereby reducing the risk of side effects.

The effects of most NSAIAs are related to the impairment of prostaglandin production. This involves cyclooxygenase (COX) of which there are (at least) two types. COX-1 (constitutive, housekeeping) is variably found in all tissues of the body and is involved in the production of prostaglandins that are essential for a variety of normal functions. Levels of COX-2 (inducible) on the other hand are typically very low but increase during tissue injury. It is primarily responsible for the production of prostaglandins that mediate the inflammatory response and pain associated with tissue injury. Most NSAIAs are COX inhibitors. Newer agents (e.g. carprofen, meloxicam) have more selective inhibition of COX-2 versus COX-1 and may be associated with fewer side effects and a safer therapeutic index.

Side effects/contraindications

The two most commonly recognized side effects and/or contraindications of NSAIA use are gastroduodenal injury and renal injury.

Gastroduodenal injury

Prostaglandins are important for the integrity of the gastrointestinal mucosal barrier and their impaired production therefore increases the likelihood of mucosal injury (haemorrhage, erosions, ulceration) in an already compromised tissue. Intuitively therefore NSAIAs are contraindicated in animals with gastrointestinal abnormalities. However, there are patients with gastrointestinal signs in which the use of an NSAIA may be justified – examples include a dog that is heavily dependent on NSAIA therapy to manage discomfort associated with chronic osteoarthritis (for which opioids are less effective). Considerations in such cases include the following:

- Hypovolaemia or dehydration should be treated before NSAIA therapy.
- An agent reported to be COX-1 sparing should be chosen.
- The drug should be given at a low dose and systemically if possible (mucosal lesions are more likely to occur with oral dosing because there is a higher local concentration of the agent at the site of the tablet or liquid); oral administration should be accompanied by food.
- Gastroprotectants (e.g. omeprazole, ranitidine) should be used preemptively.

Renal injury

Prostaglandins are not critically involved in renal haemodynamics in normal healthy animals. However, in response to a decrease in renal blood flow, locally acting prostaglandins serve to protect renal perfusion. Their inhibition by NSAIA therapy can therefore result in renal ischaemia and insufficiency. This is applicable to both older NSAIAs and newer agents with more selective COX-2 inhibition as constitutive COX-2 is produced in the kidney. Emergency patients in whom renal blood flow may be decreased include those with hypovolaemia, cardiac insufficiency and pre-existing renal disease.

Other side effects of NSAIAs described include effects on the liver and interference with coagulation (see Ch. 30).

Paracetamol (acetaminophen)

CLINICAL TIP

- Paracetamol (acetaminophen) administration at any dose should never be recommended in cats due to the reduced capacity for glucuronidation in this species and therefore significantly increased risk of toxicity.

Paracetamol (acetaminophen) is not commonly used therapeutically in veterinary medicine due to the widespread availability of licensed veterinary products that are both effective and have been subjected to extensive clinical trialling. However, paracetamol is widely available from numerous outlets and frequently present within the home of many pet owners. It is therefore common in emergency practice either to receive enquiries about administering paracetamol to dogs and cats or to see animals to which this agent has been administered.

Paracetamol may be a useful (and possibly underused) analgesic in dogs but it should never be administered to cats at any dose. It is an NSAIA and interferes with prostaglandin synthesis but does not work via inhibition of COX-1 or COX-2. Although this makes it a poor anti-inflammatory agent, it does result in minimal gastrointestinal side effects. Paracetamol can therefore be used either in addition to conventional NSAIAs or alone in dogs in which these agents are contraindicated or poorly tolerated. As paracetamol interferes with prostaglandin production, it should be avoided in hypoperfused or dehydrated patients. Hepatotoxicity is a potential side effect of this drug. The recommended dose range in dogs is 10–15 mg/kg p.o. q 8–12 hr.

Local anaesthetic agents

Local anaesthetic agents work by blocking sensory input via afferent nerve fibres to the central nervous system and prevent central sensitization. Longer-acting agents in particular (e.g. bupivacaine, ropivacaine) are used extensively in referral centres in a number of ways, including:

- Epidural administration (often combined with morphine)
- Intrapleural administration via thoracostomy tubes following thoracotomy
- Local and regional nerve blocks
- CRI of 2% lidocaine solution without adrenaline (epinephrine) for analgesic purposes in dogs (see Box 5.3). Lidocaine infusion may result in significant cardiovascular depression in cats and is not recommended unless essential for controlling ventricular dysrhythmia.

While these uses may not be applicable to most nonreferral emergency patients, local anaesthetic agents can be employed to good effect in this setting.

Lidocaine

Lidocaine has a shorter duration of action (1–2 hr) than other agents but a rapid onset of action (can be as quick as 3–5 min). It is the most widely available local anaesthetic agent and may be used for emergency cases in a number of ways. For example:

1. Topical analgesia for wounds: while an emergency patient is undergoing initial stabilization, sterile gauze swabs can be soaked in a solution of 2% lidocaine mixed with normal saline (0.9% sodium chloride) and applied to wounds which are then wrapped in cling film pending management at the appropriate time (Figure 5.1). Lidocaine can also be mixed with the gel that is applied to the wound prior to clipping. Maximum recommended doses are 12 mg/kg in dogs and 6 mg/kg in cats. A 5% lidocaine patch (Lidoderm®, Endo Pharmaceuticals) is available and has been used for dogs and cats with severe skin abrasions, severe bruising and surgical wounds. However, the author has no experience with its use.
2. EMLA® cream 5% (AstraZeneca); contains 2.5% lidocaine and 2.5% prilocaine: can be applied to the skin prior to intravenous catheter placement or venepuncture. Depending on the site, a light occlusive dressing may be appropriate while anaesthesia

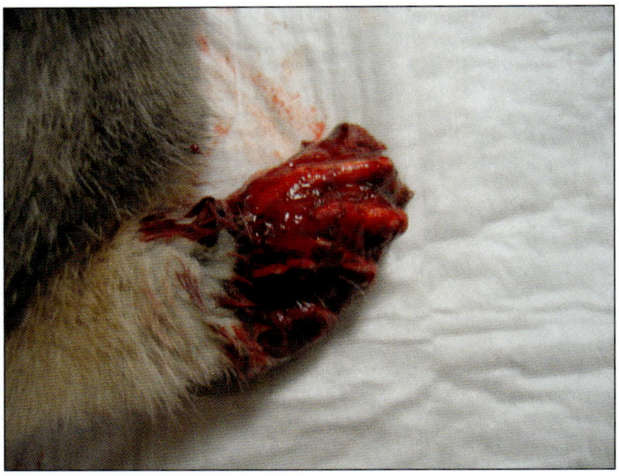

(a)

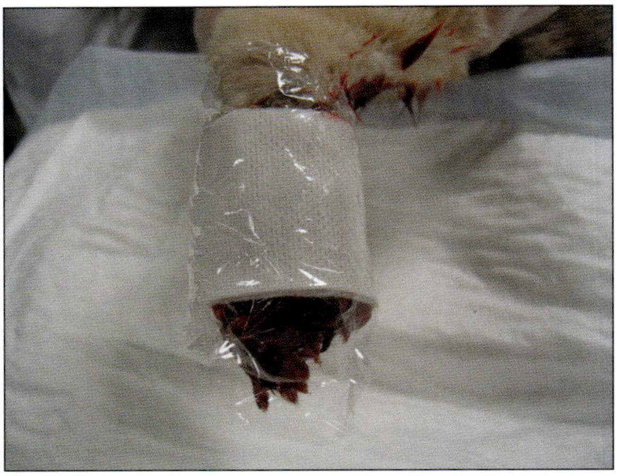

(b)

Figure 5.1 (a) Severe wound to the distal right pelvic limb of a cat. (b) Following application of sterile swabs soaked in a solution of 2% lidocaine and normal saline, the wound is wrapped in cling film.

takes effect. EMLA® cream is especially useful for example in puppies and kittens, in stressed animals and in rabbits. The author also tries to use this product as much as possible as a general rule in all cats. EMLA® cream can also be applied to wound edges to reduce irritation and thereby patient interference. Clinical experience suggests that onset of action in some cases is significantly shorter than the commonly reported 30–60 minutes. Minimal if any systemic drug absorption has been reported following topical application.

3. Lidocaine spray: in addition to facilitating endotracheal intubation of cats, proprietary lidocaine spray (e.g. Intubeaze®, Dechra Veterinary Products) may have diverse uses for mucosal desensitization, for example to facilitate nasal catheter placement or to examine the oropharyngeal region.
4. Lidocaine lubricant: a 2% lidocaine lubricant is commercially available; alternatively, it can be constituted by mixing 2% lidocaine solution, without adrenaline (epinephrine), for injection with a sterile lubricant. This is then used topically, for example prior to insertion of nasal catheters or urinary catheterization.

Ketamine

Ketamine is a dissociative anaesthetic agent that is used most commonly for sedation (see Ch. 39). However, it also has analgesic properties and blocks (and potentially reverses) central sensitization via its action as an *N*-methyl-D-aspartate (NMDA) receptor antagonist. It is especially effective in this respect when combined with a full opioid agonist and may be used as a CRI (see Box 5.3). The recommended dose for analgesic purposes is 0.1–1 mg/kg i.v. as needed (often every 30 minutes) or a single loading dose followed by a constant rate infusion of 0.1–1 mg/kg/hr.

Medetomidine

Medetomidine is an alpha$_2$-adrenergic agonist that is also used most commonly for its sedative properties (see Ch. 39). This agent does, however, also possess potent analgesic properties and can be a useful adjunctive analgesic in some cases. At the microdoses recommended here, cardiovascular and respiratory effects should be minimal and can be reversed by atipamezole if necessary. The sedative effects are likely to be advantageous for patient management in those cases in which this agent may be employed as an analgesic. Recommended doses for medetomidine when used for analgesic purposes are 2–5 μg/kg slow i.v. or i.m. as needed (often q 30–90 minutes but potentially much longer if an opioid is used concurrently); alternatively, a CRI of 1–3 μg/kg/hr may be used.

Sedation

Although sedation is not a substitute for pain relief, it can be invaluable in improving the welfare of animals that are especially anxious or distressed, allowing them to rest and to utilize their metabolic reserves for recovery rather than coping behaviour. In cases in which opioids being used for analgesia do not provide sufficient sedation, other agents such as acepromazine and benzodiazepines are options.

NON-PHARMACOLOGICAL MEASURES

NURSING ASPECT

Although analgesic agents are the mainstay of pain management, it is essential not to overlook the important contribution of good nursing care and other non-pharmacological measures. These measures reduce stress, improve patient wellbeing, and contribute significantly to pain management. Some of these measures are listed in Box 5.4.

BOX 5.4 Non-pharmacological measures of importance in pain management

- TLC, gentle handling (independent of interventions) and regular grooming
- Providing a suitable environment (some animals prefer a dimly lit quiet environment, others like to be distracted)
- Tempting to eat if appropriate
- Ensuring bedding is dry, clean and comfortable
- Providing a familiar blanket or toy from home
- Allowing or preventing visits by the owner depending on patient response
- Providing cats with a box or carrier to sleep in
- Helping dogs out to urinate/defecate
- Bladder management as necessary
- Coordinating interventions (e.g. venepuncture) to minimize the number of painful procedures performed
- Grouping treatments to allow undisturbed rest time
- Removing unnecessary catheters, tubing and bandages as soon as possible
- Using warm compresses or cold packs if appropriate

6 Oxygen supplementation

CLINICAL TIP

- Although there are some conditions that may not respond, the provision of oxygen supplementation initially to any patient with respiratory distress is intuitive. Oxygen supplementation may also be essential to animals presenting with disease processes affecting other major body systems as these can also impair oxygenation.
- The author would strongly encourage a liberal approach to the use of oxygen supplementation – if in doubt, provide supplemental oxygen.

INDICATIONS FOR OXYGEN SUPPLEMENTATION

Oxygenation may be impaired via a number of mechanisms (ventilation–perfusion mismatch, hypoventilation, diffusion impairment, intrapulmonary or cardiovascular shunt); more than one mechanism can, and often does, occur in the same patient at the same time. Oxygenation may be compromised in a large variety of disorders affecting the respiratory, cardiovascular and neuromuscular systems in particular. Oxygen supplementation is extremely unlikely to cause any harm (unless high concentrations are provided for a sustained period of at least 24 hours), and the author would strongly encourage a liberal approach to its use (bearing potential financial constraints in mind).

In essence, a positive response to oxygen supplementation confirms its requirement (i.e. trial therapy). However, animals in need of oxygen supplementation may be identified and monitored more objectively through the use of pulse oximetry (or preferably arterial blood gas analysis if available). Pulse oximetry measures saturation of arterial haemoglobin with oxygen (SpO_2) which should be more than 95% in normal dogs and cats on room air.

METHODS OF OXYGEN SUPPLEMENTATION

A number of oxygen supplementation techniques have been widely described that differ in terms of their cost, technical ease and efficiency. The method used is determined by both patient-related (level and duration of supplementation required, compliance, size) and non-patient-related (available facilities, clinical expertise, financial constraints) factors. Methods of supplementation include:

- Flow-by oxygen
- Mask
- Oxygen collar (using an Elizabethan collar)
- Nasal cannulae (prongs)
- Nasal/nasopharyngeal catheters
- Oxygen cage
- (Transtracheal oxygen)
- (Endotracheal intubation).

CLINICAL TIP

- Regardless of the method of supplementation used, oxygen should be humidified if possible prior to delivery if supplementation continues for more than a few hours

Flow-by oxygen

Flow-by oxygen supplementation is extremely easy to provide and is typically the first technique used in emergency patients while major body system examination is performed, an intravenous catheter is placed and other urgent interventions carried out. However, it is noteworthy that some animals, cats in particular, do better if placed in an oxygen cage first instead (depends on underlying disorder). Flow-by oxygen supplementation is usually only used short-term as it is wasteful. Some animals are intolerant of flow-by oxygen supplementation, even with minimal restraint, and it is clearly important not to stress these patients further.

Mask supplementation

Oxygen supplementation using a mask is another readily available technique that allows access to the patient. This technique is typically only used short-term and many of the same comments apply as for flow-by supplementation. In particular, some animals are very intolerant of having a mask placed over their muzzle and this should never be forced upon them. In addition, it must be remembered that panting is the major means of cooling in dogs. Placing a mask over a panting dog's mouth can result in a marked increase in humidity and lead to severe hyperthermia with potentially disastrous consequences. Although it reduces the inhaled oxygen concentration that can be achieved, masks may therefore need to be only loosely applied in some cases.

Oxygen collar

An oxygen collar is one means of providing more long-term oxygen supplementation, especially to cats and small dogs. A rigid Elizabethan collar is applied and the front of the collar is covered with cling film or a similar transparent wrap that is taped in place; it is important not to cover the whole of the front to allow the collar to vent and prevent the animal from overheating. Oxygen tubing is then passed into the collar from the rear and the tubing is taped to the inside of the collar to secure it in place.

Humidified oxygen is delivered at a higher flow rate initially (e.g. 2 l/min) and then reduced (e.g. to 1 l/min) once the collar has been filled. The author has achieved good results with this technique, which also allows on-going access to the patient.

Nasal cannulae (prongs)

Nasal cannulae (nasal prongs) for human use (e.g. Venticaire®, Flexicare Medical Ltd, Mountain Ash, UK) are available in a variety of sizes (Figure 6.1) that work well for some dogs. They are generally tolerated sufficiently well following application of local anaesthetic drops to the nostrils (Figure 6.2). Humidified oxygen is provided at an initial rate of 50–150 ml/kg/min. Nasal cannulae are less effective in dogs that are panting. Although easy to apply, nasal prongs must be checked regularly as they are very easily dislodged.

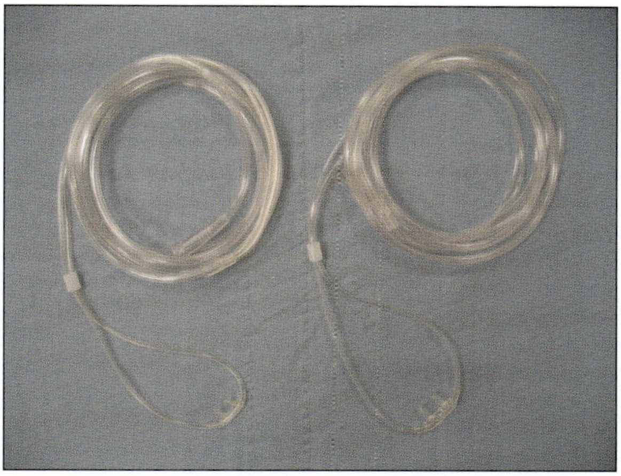

Figure 6.1 Human paediatric and adult nasal cannulae.

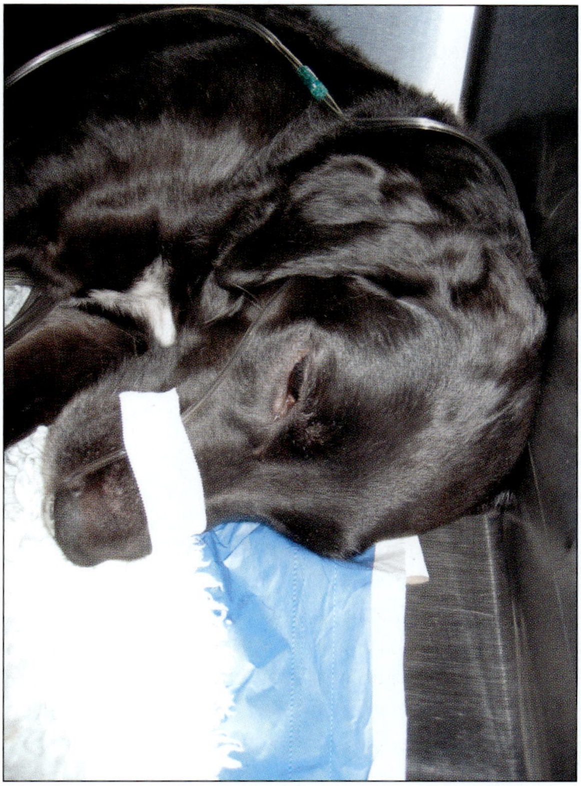

Figure 6.2 Labrador retriever with nasal cannulae in situ.

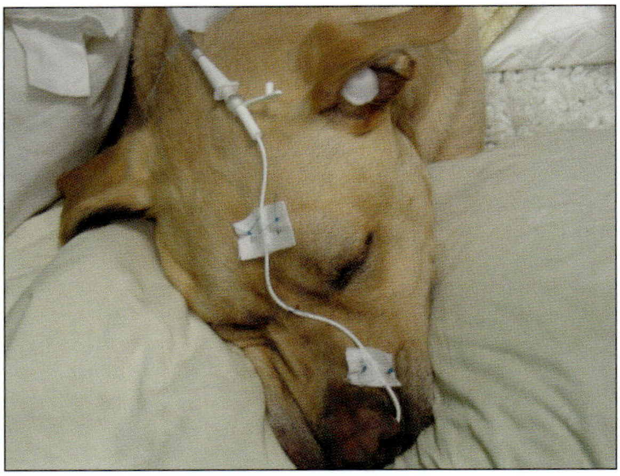

Figure 6.3 Labrador retriever with unilateral indwelling nasal catheter.

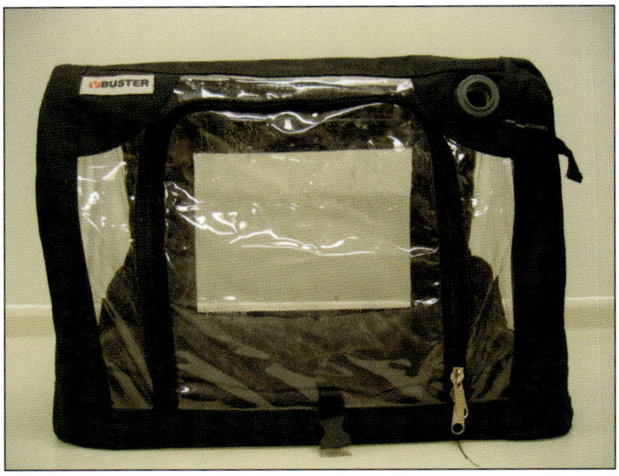

Figure 6.4 Buster ICU cage. (Kruuse UK Ltd, Leeds, UK)

Nasal/nasopharyngeal catheters

Unilateral or bilateral indwelling nasal catheters (Figure 6.3) are used less frequently nowadays with the availability of nasal cannulae but they remain invaluable in a proportion of patients. In general the author reserves nasal catheters for dogs that are poorly tolerant of nasal prongs and sometimes dogs in need of long-term supplementation that are being sedated or anaesthetized for another procedure (i.e. so as not to waste the episode of chemical restraint). Nasal catheter placement is a relatively simple procedure (see p. 291); some dogs are poorly compliant and mild sedation may be required.

Oxygen cage

Big sophisticated oxygen cages that allow the percentage of oxygen supplementation as well as environmental temperature and humidity to be controlled are found in a small number of referral centres. However, oxygen cages can be improvised and are used predominantly for long-term oxygen supplementation and to provide higher levels of inspired oxygen concentration than can be achieved with other methods. A potential disadvantage of oxygen cages is the inability to interact with and examine the patient regularly without causing repeated decreases in the environmental oxygen concentration. On the other hand, in some cases this lack of interaction is in fact desirable as long as the patient can be monitored closely by other means (e.g. observational, ideally using monitoring equipment as well). Oxygen cages are also not typically appropriate for larger dogs and hyperthermia is a potential complication in general.

Oxygen cages offer an ideal way of providing oxygen supplementation for initial stabilization to some animals presenting in respiratory distress without the need for manual restraint. This is especially the case for dyspnoeic cats and the author routinely leaves appropriate cases in an oxygen cage for 20–30 minutes following presentation prior to further intervention, with close monitoring throughout. It must be remembered that some causes of respiratory distress will be minimally or inadequately responsive to oxygen therapy and the above approach is not appropriate in all cases. The decision is made on an individual case basis and other interventions such as thoracocentesis or sedation may be more helpful.

Improvised oxygen cages can be created using a human neonatal incubator or by covering the front of a normal kennel with cling film and piping oxygen into the kennel; alternatively, a cat carrier or small puppy crate can be wrapped in cling film. Another technique is to place a cat carrier or small puppy crate inside a polythene or similar garbage bag, tie the bag, and pipe oxygen through a hole cut into the side. However, the author would not recommend the use of this technique unless a (relatively) transparent bag can be used as the patient is otherwise completely out of sight.

More recently the Buster ICU cage (Kruuse UK Ltd, Leeds, UK) has become available for cats and small dogs (Figure 6.4). Amongst other facilities, this cage allows oxygen supplementation with some degree of regulation, although overheating can be a problem.

CLINICAL TIP

- The provision of oxygen supplementation to panting dogs can be difficult. These dogs are predominantly breathing through their mouth and nasal oxygen supplementation may therefore be of limited use. Nasopharyngeal catheters may potentially be more effective as the oxygen is delivered closer to the site of communication between the oral and nasal cavities but this is debatable.
- Oxygen cages can be very useful as environmental oxygen concentration is increased and supplementation is not therefore dependent on whether the animal is breathing predominantly through the nose or mouth. However, hyperthermia can be a significant problem when panting dogs are confined in oxygen cages and most improvised oxygen cages are too small for bigger dogs.
- Transtracheal oxygen supplementation provides a possible effective solution as the oxygen is delivered lower down in the respiratory tract; however, it is technically more demanding to perform and more intensive to maintain.

Animals that remain severely dyspnoeic or have an SpO_2 of less than 90% despite aggressive oxygen supplementation are candidates for anaesthesia, endotracheal intubation and ventilation. However, in the absence of facilities to provide and maintain mechanical ventilation, the practical implications of this intervention need to be carefully considered. If affordable, referral should be considered but transportation should only be undertaken following as much stabilization as possible and preferably once arrangements to provide oxygen supplementation en route have been made.

SECTION 2

PROBLEM-ORIENTATED APPROACH

7 Abnormal urine or urination

A number of different terms are in use clinically to describe signs exhibited by animals with abnormal urine or urination and the following is the author's interpretation of these terms:

- Dysuria: painful urination
- Stranguria: straining to urinate (usually painful)
- Pollakiuria: passing small amounts of urine frequently (spotting)
- Macroscopic (gross, frank) haematuria: bloody urine (red blood cells)
- Pigmenturia: grossly discoloured urine
- Periuria: urination in inappropriate location
- Urinary incontinence: involuntary (unintentional) leakage of urine.

DYSURIA, STRANGURIA AND POLLAKIURIA

Dysuria, stranguria and pollakiuria are often seen in combination and are a relatively common cluster of signs in emergency patients, especially cats. These signs generally suggest inflammation or irritability of the lower urinary tract (see Ch. 36).

HAEMATURIA

Macroscopic haematuria may also occur as a result of an abnormality in the lower urinary tract but can be associated with a primary disorder of the kidneys or ureters. It is also important to remember that gross haematuria may also be the result of a systemic coagulopathy (e.g. immune-mediated thrombocytopenia, secondary to angiostrongylosis). Macroscopic haematuria may manifest simply as grossly discoloured urine or fresh blood may be more obviously visible, including as blood clots. The different appearances are variably associated with lesions lower down or higher up in the urinary tract. In addition, blood at the beginning of urination may indicate a disease process in the urethra or genital tract, while blood at the end of or throughout urination may signify a problem in either the bladder or the upper urinary tract (kidneys or ureters).

Haematuria may not always be grossly visible and dipstick analysis and urine sediment examination may be required to identify occult blood.

PIGMENTURIA

While it is not typically possible to make specific diagnoses on the basis of urine discoloration, the gross appearance may be suggestive of certain disorders. Haematuria, haemoglobinuria and myoglobinuria are variably associated with urine that is pink, red, red-brown or brown in appearance (see Box 3.3). Dipsticks are unable to differentiate haematuria, haemoglobinuria and myoglobinuria; haematuria and haemoglobinuria can be differentiated by sediment examination.

Methaemoglobinuria (e.g. paracetamol (acetaminophen) intoxication) is also associated with brown urine. Significant bilirubinuria is associated with orangey urine. Mild to moderate bilirubinuria may be normal in dogs, especially males, but is always considered an abnormal finding in cats. Causes of bilirubinuria include haemolysis, hepatobiliary disorders, pyrexia and starvation. Cloudy urine is typically the result of pyuria, crystalluria or mucus.

8 Acute abdomen

The term acute abdomen refers to a syndrome that involves the acute onset of clinical signs secondary to an intra-abdominal disorder which typically has the potential to be fatal. In a significant proportion of these cases, abdominal pain is a strong feature but may be harder to detect in cats. There are a large number of potential causes of acute abdomen, many of which require emergency surgical intervention following stabilization of major body system abnormalities. An important part of the early management of a patient with acute abdomen is to determine whether emergency surgical intervention is required. Some of the more common causes of acute abdomen are listed in Box 8.1.

BOX 8.1 Causes of acute abdomen

Surgical emergencies

- Gastric dilatation ± volvulus (GDV)
- Septic peritonitis, e.g. due to:
  - Gastrointestinal tract rupture/perforation
  - Dehiscence of surgical gastrointestinal tract wound
  - Uterine rupture
  - Prostatic abscess rupture
- Intestinal obstruction (complete or partial)
- Intussusception
- Penetrating abdominal wound
- Abdominal bite injury/crush injury
- Uroabdomen
- Urethral obstruction if catheterization is unsuccessful
- Pyometra – usually less urgent if open
- Dystocia if medical management ineffective or contraindicated
- Bile peritonitis
- Splenic torsion
- Strangulated hernia
- Intractable haemorrhage
- Mesenteric torsion

Nonsurgical disorders

- Pancreatitis
- Gastroenteritis, especially haemorrhagic gastroenteritis (HGE), parvoviral enteritis
- Gastrointestinal ulceration without perforation
- Ileus
- Acute hepatitis/cholangiohepatitis
- Pyelonephritis

ACUTE ABDOMEN LOOK-ALIKES

Acute abdomen can be mistaken for a small number of other conditions, most notably painful spinal disorders and hypoadrenocorticism (Addison's disease).

Spinal pain

In some animals, especially smaller ones, it can be difficult to differentiate abdominal pain from spinal (especially thoracolumbar) pain and the author is aware of animals with spinal disease that have undergone negative exploratory laparotomy following misdiagnosis.

Signalment, history, physical examination and diagnostic findings are often helpful in differentiating acute abdomen from spinal disease. In particular, animals with uncomplicated spinal disease are unlikely to show marked cardiovascular compromise that is a common feature of acute abdomen. Likewise animals with acute abdomen may be collapsed or weak but they are unlikely to show localized neurological signs.

CLINICAL TIP

- Although it may be difficult in smaller animals, it is important to try to palpate the abdomen without applying pressure over the spine with the thumbs.

Hypoadrenocorticism (Addison's disease)

Hypoadrenocorticism can be hard to differentiate from acute abdomen. Animals suffering from an acute Addisonian crisis may have a history of gastrointestinal signs, which is a common feature of acute abdomen. An acute Addisonian crisis almost by definition involves potentially marked cardiovascular compromise, and abdominal pain may also be a feature of this disease. Signalment, history and astute diagnostic investigations may be helpful here.

9 Acute diarrhoea

Acute diarrhoea is a frequently encountered clinical sign in emergency medicine. The majority of causes of acute diarrhoea relate primarily to the intestinal tract although small intestinal diarrhoea in particular may be associated with extraintestinal causes. There are a large number of causes of acute diarrhoea and some of the most important with respect to emergency cases are listed in Boxes 9.1 and 9.2. Clearly some of these conditions may also cause, or even be more frequently associated with, chronic diarrhoea.

Features used to distinguish small and large intestinal diarrhoea are listed in Box 9.3 but a definitive patient assessment should be made cautiously on the basis of the type of diarrhoea alone and both types may occur in the same patient (e.g. with diffuse inflammatory bowel disease). Animals with haemorrhagic watery diarrhoea are likely to be suffering from small intestinal disease (especially canine haemorrhagic gastroenteritis or parvovirus) but short transit time prevents the formation of melaena (i.e. as there is insufficient time for bacteria to break down haemoglobin).

BOX 9.1 Causes of acute small intestinal diarrhoea

Intestinal disease

- Dietary indiscretion
- Food intolerance
- Food allergy
- Infectious disorders (bacterial, viral, parasitic, protozoal)
- Foreign body ingestion
- Intoxication
- Inflammatory bowel disease (IBD)
- Canine haemorrhagic gastroenteritis (HGE)
- Intussusception
- Neoplasia

Extraintestinal disease

- Acute pancreatitis
- Hepatic disease
- Renal disease
- Hypoadrenocorticism (Addison's disease)
- Hyperthyroidism (cats)

BOX 9.2 Causes of acute large intestinal diarrhoea

- Dietary indiscretion
- Food intolerance
- Food allergy
- Infectious disorders (bacterial, parasitic)
- Foreign body ingestion
- Inflammatory bowel disease (IBD)
- Neoplasia

BOX 9.3 Distinguishing features of small versus large intestinal diarrhoea

Small intestinal diarrhoea

- Normal to slightly increased frequency of defecation
- Increased faecal volume
- Watery/fluid consistency
- Tenesmus rare
- Blood (melaena) and mucus rare/occasional
- Weight loss common

Large intestinal diarrhoea

- Increased frequency and urgency of defecation
- Small amount passed each time (overall volume may be normal)
- Soft consistency
- Tenesmus typical
- Blood (fresh) and mucus common
- Weight loss occasional

Possible iatrogenic causes of diarrhoea as a side effect of drug therapy must also be considered.

NURSING ASPECT

Owners quite commonly ring for advice with respect to cats and especially dogs that have diarrhoea and the duty nurse is often the person from whom this initial advice is obtained. Acute diarrhoea is often the result of dietary indiscretion or food intolerance and may be self-limiting without the need for veterinary intervention. The recommendation to examine the animal at the clinic should be guided by the owner's wishes but also after obtaining adequate information with respect to:

- The animal's current status
- The nature of the diarrhoea
- The duration, frequency and severity of diarrhoea
- Any known history of dietary indiscretion, especially with respect to foreign bodies and intoxication.

In the author's opinion it is reasonable to recommend withholding food for a short period (e.g. 12–24 hours) with continued monitoring at home if the animal remains relatively bright, is tolerant of water, and especially where there is a suspicion of dietary indiscretion not relating to a foreign body. An easily digestible food can then be introduced, feeding small amounts frequently. Owners should be advised to contact the clinic again should the animal's condition deteriorate, at which time examination can be arranged.

APPROACH TO DIARRHOEA

Signalment

Signalment may allow certain differential diagnoses to be viewed with a lesser or greater index of suspicion. For example, younger animals are more likely to present with dietary indiscretion, foreign body ingestion, or infectious diarrhoea including intestinal helminthiasis.

History

A thorough history is mandatory in all animals with diarrhoea, although the timing should be guided by the stability of the patient. It is important to try to determine from the owner's description whether small or large intestinal diarrhoea is present. The history may provide useful information with respect to the possible cause of the diarrhoea (e.g. witnessed scavenging, change of diet, other animals affected), and the nature, severity and duration of the diarrhoea will help establish the likelihood of clinically significant dehydration. In addition, the presence of other concurrent signs may raise the index of suspicion for systemic diseases. Worming and vaccination history should also be established as well as details of any recent drug therapy.

Major body system examination

Cardiovascular examination may be normal in animals with diarrhoea or may be consistent with variable degrees of hypovolaemia (see Ch. 2). Hypovolaemia may be secondary to severe dehydration and/or a consequence of the primary disorder. Signs of maldistributive shock (hypoperfusion with hyperaemic mucous membranes and a rapid capillary refill time) should raise the index of suspicion for severe acute pancreatitis or a septic focus. Respiratory examination may be unremarkable in animals with diarrhoea or may reflect pain, pyrexia or abnormalities in acid–base status. Neurological examination may also be unremarkable but abnormalities may be detected that reflect the underlying cause (e.g. seizuring from intoxication).

Abdominal palpation is very important but may be more or less rewarding depending on the size and demeanour of the patient in question. Abdominal pain may be identified and potentially characterized as diffuse or localized. Abdominal pain is not likely to be present with a number of the causes of diarrhoea and its presence may raise the index of suspicion for certain differential diagnoses (e.g. intestinal obstruction, foreign body ingestion, acute infectious enteritis, acute pancreatitis). In some cases focal abnormalities such as an intussusception, foreign body or mass may be identified.

Rectal temperature may be normal, increased or decreased depending on the underlying cause and clinical status of the patient. Digital rectal examination should also be performed and may allow visual examination of faeces, collection of faeces for analysis, and identification of local rectal lesions.

Complete physical examination performed at the appropriate time may reveal other significant findings that can help establish a diagnosis.

Emergency database

The need to perform an emergency database in a diarrhoeic patient should be guided by the animal's history and physical examination findings. The emergency database will allow the patient to be evaluated for dehydration (raised packed cell volume and serum total solids, prerenal azotaemia – see Ch. 3) as well as identify electrolyte and acid–base abnormalities. Some animals with diarrhoea will have a protein-losing enteropathy (PLE) and serum total solids may appear inappropriately low in comparison with packed cell volume in such cases. Dogs with hypoadrenocorticism (Addison's disease) may have hyponatraemia, hyperkalaemia and mild to moderate azotaemia. A faecal ELISA test for canine parvovirus may be appropriate in young dogs.

CLINICAL TIP

- As a general rule, diarrhoea is more likely to have clinically significant effects on hydration, perfusion, and electrolyte and acid–base status in puppies, kittens and toy breed dogs. Hypoglycaemia is a relatively common concurrent abnormality in such cases.

CLINICAL TIP

- Some dogs with diarrhoea due to primary intestinal disorders (e.g. salmonellosis, trichuriasis (whipworm infection)) may develop a very similar clinical picture to dogs with typical hypoadrenocorticism (Addison's disease), i.e. hyponatraemia, hyperkalaemia, and a mild to moderate prerenal azotaemia. This pseudo-Addisonian presentation must be kept in mind when considering the possibility of hypoadrenocorticism in such cases.

More extensive clinicopathological testing may be required in some diarrhoeic animals, especially in those with other systemic signs, but is generally not available in the emergency setting.

Diagnostic imaging

The need to perform diagnostic imaging in a diarrhoeic animal should be guided by the animal's history and physical examination findings. In the routine emergency setting, diagnostic imaging of the emergency patient is likely to consist of plain radiography and, if available, abdominal ultrasonography for the detection of free peritoneal fluid. Ideally orthogonal (right lateral and ventrodorsal views) abdominal radiographs should be taken and are most useful for identifying radioopaque intestinal foreign bodies and obstructions. Thoracic radiographs may be indicated to look for pulmonary metastases where neoplasia is considered a likely cause of diarrhoea.

Treatment

By collating all of the information obtained from the steps above, the clinician should be able to decide on the most appropriate management for the patient in question. This will depend not only on the underlying cause but also on the clinical status of the patient with respect to perfusion, hydration and electrolyte and acid–base abnormalities.

Acute diarrhoea is often self-limiting and may only require supportive care and short-term dietary management without a definitive diagnosis. Withholding food for a period of time (e.g. 12–24 hours) and then offering small amounts of an easily digestible diet may be all that is required. The use of specific antidiarrhoeal therapy is typically not necessary and may be contraindicated in some cases (especially diarrhoea of infectious origin).

Cases in which diarrhoea is severe or there are systemic signs such as pyrexia or neutropenia may require more aggressive therapy and investigations. Amongst the differential diagnoses for diarrhoea, the most severe clinical presentations are associated with infectious enteritides, intestinal obstruction, foreign body ingestion, canine haemorrhagic gastroenteritis, acute pancreatitis and hypoadrenocorticism. See Chapter 29 (The acute abdomen) and Chapter 34 (Endocrine emergencies) for further information on these conditions.

CLINICAL TIP

- Antibiotic therapy is typically not indicated in dogs and cats with acute diarrhoea and its routine use without confirmation of an infectious aetiology is not recommended.
- Antibiosis may have adverse effects on beneficial commensal intestinal flora and may also encourage bacterial antibiotic resistance. The author typically reserves antibiotic therapy

CLINICAL TIP—cont'd

for animals with severe haemorrhagic diarrhoea that are pyrexic or in which neutropenia is identified on peripheral blood smear examination.

- Metronidazole has been used extensively in the treatment of large intestinal diarrhoea for reported intestinal immunomodulatory effects rather than antimicrobial properties and the author has occasionally used this agent for this purpose.

HAEMATOCHEZIA

Haematochezia refers to bright red fresh blood either on the surface of or mixed in with faeces, and this must be differentiated from melaena (see below). The source of the blood is typically the anus, rectum or descending colon (see Box 9.4). Haematochezia often appears dramatic to owners but is typically not associated with significant morbidity and is rarely associated with mortality. In many cases, it is the only clinical sign present and conservative management using a diet containing fermentable fibre may be all that is needed. Empirical deworming using a broad-spectrum preparation may be appropriate as may a course of metronidazole. More intensive management and extensive investigations may be required in animals with systemic illness or persistent haematochezia.

BOX 9.4 Causes of haematochezia

Rectal and colonic disease

- Proctitis
- Rectal prolapse
- Colitis (e.g. idiopathic, inflammatory bowel disease (IBD), stress, infection)
- Parasitism (e.g. helminthiasis)
- Neoplasia (e.g. adenocarcinoma, lymphoma); rectal polyp
- Mucosal trauma

Anal or anal sac disease

- Anal sacculitis or abscess
- Perianal fistula
- Perianal hernia
- Stricture
- Trauma

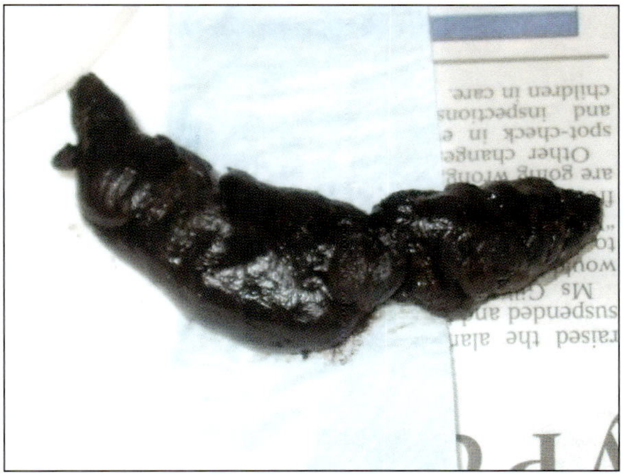

Figure 9.1 Dark tarry appearance of melaenic faeces.

MELAENA

CLINICAL TIP

- Not all dogs with dark stools have melaena; other causes of dark stools include diets high in iron, and ingestion of activated charcoal or proprietary veterinary treats/diets with a similar gross appearance if minimal digestion occurs.
- On occasion it may be unclear as to whether dark stools represent melaena or not; a high index of suspicion should be maintained in such cases and the uncertainty is typically resolved rapidly on the basis of clinical progression.

Melaena refers to dark tarry faeces that represents blood digested in the intestinal tract and is a much more serious clinical sign than haematochezia (Figure 9.1). Melaena may result from lesions in the gastrointestinal tract and is usually the result of gastric or proximal small intestinal haemorrhage. However, melaena may occur due to haemorrhage more distally in the intestinal tract. Importantly, melaena may also be the result of ingestion of blood or serious abnormalities in other organs or body systems (see Box 9.5).

Animals with melaena can suffer considerable blood loss resulting in mild to severe reduction in packed cell volume and serum total solids. Depending on the duration, anaemia due to acute melaena may be regenerative or preregenerative and peripheral blood smear

BOX 9.5 Causes of melaena

Primary gastrointestinal disease

- Ulceration/haemorrhagic erosion (e.g. secondary to nonsteroidal antiinflammatory agent or corticosteroid administration)
- Neoplasia (e.g. adenocarcinoma, lymphoma, mast cell tumour)
- Foreign body
- Intussusception
- Severe gastritis (e.g. inflammatory bowel disease (IBD))
- Parasitism (e.g. hookworms)

Ingested blood

- Nasal lesion (epistaxis)
- Oropharyngeal lesion
- Oesophageal lesion
- Pulmonary lesion (blood coughed up then ingested)
- (Dietary source)

Other organs/systems

- Coagulopathy (e.g. rodenticide intoxication, severe thrombocytopenia, hepatic failure)
- Uraemic gastritis due to renal failure
- Hypoadrenocorticism (Addison's disease)

examination is essential in these cases (see Ch. 3). Chronic melaena may result in hypochromic microcytic iron-deficiency anaemia. Peripheral blood smear examination is also essential to evaluate platelet numbers as melaena is relatively common in animals with sufficiently severe thrombocytopenia.

History and additional physical examination findings should help determine whether a primary gastrointestinal cause is more or less likely and therefore guide diagnostics. Treatment is ultimately aimed at the underlying cause but intensive supportive measures, including transfusion of appropriate blood products, may be required.

10 Acute red eye and pain

The majority of causes of acute red eye are also associated with varying degrees of pain. Ocular pain is typically associated with blepharospasm, excessive lacrimation and photophobia. These signs are likely to be more subtle in cats than in dogs, and enophthalmos may also be seen in the latter species.

The main causes of acute red eye, in particular in dogs, include:

- Traumatic injury
- Acute conjunctivitis
- Acute keratitis and corneal ulceration
- Acute anterior uveitis
- Acute glaucoma
- Haemorrhage, both externally and hyphaema
- Retrobulbar abscess and orbital cellulitis.

Most of these disorders are discussed in more detail in Chapter 35 (Ocular emergencies).

11 Acute vomiting

Acute vomiting is a frequently encountered clinical sign in emergency medicine. Causes of acute vomiting may broadly be divided into those that relate primarily to the alimentary tract and digestive system, and those that do not. There are a large number of causes of vomiting and some of the most important with respect to emergency cases are listed in Box 11.1.

> **NURSING ASPECT**
>
> Owners quite commonly ring for advice with respect to cats and especially dogs that have vomited and the duty nurse is often the person from whom this initial advice is obtained. In the author's opinion it is not necessary for all such cases to be seen at the clinic following initial contact. Acute vomiting is often the result of gastritis or gastroenteritis secondary to dietary indiscretion and may be self-limiting without the need for veterinary intervention. The recommendation to examine the animal at the clinic should be guided by the owner's wishes but also after obtaining adequate information with respect to:
>
> - The animal's current status
> - The duration, frequency and severity of vomiting
> - The nature of the vomitus
> - Any known history of dietary indiscretion, especially with respect to foreign bodies and intoxication
> - Previous medical and therapeutic history.
>
> In the author's opinion it is reasonable to recommend withholding food for a short period with continued monitoring at home for example for dogs that have vomited once or twice only, that remain relatively bright, that are tolerant of water, and especially where there is a suspicion of dietary indiscretion not relating to a foreign body.

> ***NURSING ASPECT—cont'd***
>
> Owners should be advised to contact the clinic again should the animal's condition deteriorate, at which time examination can be arranged.

APPROACH TO VOMITING

Signalment

Signalment may allow certain differential diagnoses to be viewed with a lesser or greater index of suspicion. For example, foreign body ingestion is more likely in a young Labrador retriever than acute pancreatitis, while the latter is more likely in a middle-aged overweight Miniature Schnauzer. Canine parvovirus infection is more likely in an unvaccinated 2-month-old male Rottweiler than in an elderly Great Dane.

History

A thorough history is mandatory in all animals with vomiting, although the timing should be guided by the stability of the patient. It is important to determine from the owner's description whether vomiting (active) as opposed to regurgitation (passive) or even retching, gagging or coughing is present (see Ch. 22). The history may provide useful information with respect to the possible cause of the vomiting (e.g. witnessed toxin ingestion), and the severity and duration of the vomiting will help establish the likelihood of clinically significant dehydration. A description of the vomitus may prove useful. For example, vomitus that contains fresh or digested ('coffee grounds') blood suggests gastric ulceration but may also occur for example in haemorrhagic gastroenteritis or canine parvovirus infection. In addition, the presence of other concurrent signs such as polyuria/polydipsia, weight loss or jaundice may raise the index of suspicion for systemic diseases.

BOX 11.1 Causes of acute vomiting

Alimentary tract/digestive system causes

- Acute gastritis/gastroenteritis, e.g.
  - Dietary indiscretion, including foreign body ingestion
  - Food intolerance
  - Intoxication
- Drug-induced (e.g. nonsteroidal antiinflammatory agents)
- Infectious diseases (e.g. leptospirosis, canine parvovirus infection)
- Haemorrhagic gastroenteritis (HGE)
- Gastric ulceration
- Small intestinal obstruction, e.g.
  - Foreign body
  - Intussusception
  - Neoplasm
- Acute pancreatitis

Other causes

- Acute hepatobiliary disease
- Urogenital:
  - Acute renal failure
  - Acute urethral obstruction
  - Pyelonephritis
  - Pyometra
  - Prostatitis/prostatic abscess
- Peritonitis: septic, urinary, biliary
- Endocrine:
  - Diabetic ketoacidosis (DKA)
  - Acute Addisonian crisis (hypoadrenocorticism)
- Central nervous system (CNS):
  - Acute vestibular disease
  - Raised intracranial pressure
  - Inflammatory CNS disease

CLINICAL TIP

- In general animals that are vomiting but lack other clinical signs (e.g. polyuria/polydipsia, weight loss, jaundice) are more likely to have a primary alimentary tract/digestive system cause of the vomiting.
- A primary cause outside the alimentary tract/ digestive system is more likely in animals with other clinical signs, in which vomiting may or may not be the most prominent feature.

Major body system examination

Cardiovascular examination may be normal in animals with vomiting or may be consistent with variable degrees of hypovolaemia (see Ch. 2). Hypovolaemia may be secondary to severe dehydration and/or a consequence of the primary disorder. Signs of maldistributive shock (hypoperfusion with hyperaemic mucous membranes and a rapid capillary refill time) should raise the index of suspicion for severe acute pancreatitis or a septic focus. Respiratory examination may be unremarkable in vomiting animals or may reflect pain, pyrexia or abnormalities in acid/base status. Vomiting animals are potentially at risk of aspiration pneumonia (although the risk is typically less than with regurgitation) that may cause dyspnoea. Neurological examination may also be unremarkable but abnormalities may be detected that reflect the underlying cause (e.g. seizuring from intoxication, vestibular signs).

Abdominal palpation is very important but may be more or less rewarding depending on the size and demeanour of the patient in question. Abdominal pain may be identified and potentially characterized as diffuse or localized. This may raise the index of suspicion for certain differential diagnoses (e.g. septic peritonitis with diffuse pain, acute pancreatitis with pain localized to the right cranial quadrant) but is by no means definitive. In some cases focal abnormalities such as an intussusception, foreign body or mass may be identified.

Rectal temperature may be normal, increased or decreased depending on the underlying cause and clinical status of the patient. Digital rectal examination should also be performed and may for example reveal melaena, foreign material or prostatomegaly.

Complete physical examination performed at the appropriate time may reveal other significant findings that can help establish a diagnosis. These include a linear foreign body trapped around the base of the tongue, oral ulceration following ingestion of a caustic intoxicant, vulval discharge in open-cervix pyometra, or goitre in a hyperthyroid cat.

Emergency database

The need to perform an emergency database in a vomiting animal should be guided by the animal's history and physical examination findings. The emergency database will allow the patient to be evaluated for dehydration (raised packed cell volume and serum total solids, prerenal azotaemia – see Ch. 3) as well as identify electrolyte (e.g. hypokalaemia) and acid/base abnormalities (e.g. hypochloraemic metabolic alkalosis with gastrointestinal foreign body). Dogs with hypoadrenocorticism (Addison's disease) may have hyponatraemia, hyperkalaemia and mild to moderate azotaemia. Severe azotaemia may be present with acute renal failure or urethral obstruction. A faecal ELISA test for canine parvovirus is recommended in young dogs as vomiting may precede haemorrhagic diarrhoea.

More extensive clinicopathological testing may be required in some vomiting animals, especially in those with other systemic signs, but is generally not available in the emergency setting.

Diagnostic imaging

The need to perform diagnostic imaging in a vomiting animal should be guided by the animal's history and physical examination findings. In the routine emergency setting, diagnostic imaging of the emergency patient is likely to consist of plain radiography and, if available, abdominal ultrasonography for the detection of free peritoneal fluid. Ideally orthogonal (right lateral and ventrodorsal views) abdominal radiographs should be taken and are most useful for identifying gastrointestinal foreign bodies and obstructions. Thoracic radiographs may be indicated for example where there is concern regarding aspiration or to look for pulmonary neoplastic metastases. In addition, they may uncover a megaoesophagus in animals in which regurgitation has been incorrectly described as vomiting.

Treatment

CLINICAL TIP

The two most important considerations in the evaluation of an animal with vomiting are:

- Does the animal need parenteral fluid therapy to correct hypovol-aemia, dehydration (and electrolyte or acid–base abnormalities), or both?
- Is surgical intervention indicated and if so, with what urgency?

By collating all of the information obtained from the steps above, the clinician should be able to decide on the most appropriate management for the patient in question. This will depend not only on the underlying cause, treatment of which is clearly essential, but also on the clinical status of the patient with respect to perfusion, hydration, and electrolyte and acid–base abnormalities. Appropriate management may range from sending the animal home on medical therapy for ongoing monitoring to hospitalization for aggressive fluid resuscitation and possible surgical intervention. Treatment of some of the specific causes of vomiting is covered in the discussion of those conditions elsewhere in this book.

Vomiting as a result of acute gastritis/gastroenteritis secondary to dietary indiscretion usually resolves over 24–48 hours. It is generally recommended to withhold food for 12–24 hours after the last episode of vomiting. Dehydration may develop in animals unable to tolerate water, necessitating parenteral fluid therapy. Small amounts of water and then of a low-fat bland diet are introduced gradually and offered frequently, and the patient is monitored closely for relapse. Antiemetics (e.g. maropitant, metoclopramide) are generally not administered until gastrointestinal obstruction has been excluded and may not be required in all cases depending on the severity of the vomiting.

12 Cardiac dysrhythmias

Cardiac dysrhythmias are a relatively common finding in emergency patients and are probably also underdiagnosed in general. Physical examination may generate the suspicion of a dysrhythmia (e.g. heart rate that is pathologically fast or slow, pulse deficits), but this can only be confirmed using electrocardiography. A wide variety of dysrhythmias exist and a full discussion is beyond the scope of this book. This chapter presents some of the most common dysrhythmias that the author sees, focusing on dogs, and summarizes the recommendations for their management.

NORMAL CARDIAC CONDUCTION

An impulse is normally generated at the sinoatrial (SA) node which is the dominant pacemaker. The impulse is conducted from there across the atria to the atrioventricular (AV) junction and into the AV node; it then passes down the bundle of His and bundle branches, on to the Purkinje fibres. The overall result is cardiac contraction. Impulse conduction is reflected as the normal sinus beat (P-QRS-T) and normal sinus rhythm results from impulses being generated at the SA node at a normal rate (Figure 12.1).

CLINICAL TIP

- Dysrhythmias can generally be classified into those that are due to primary cardiac disease, and those that are due to noncardiac systemic disease.
- As a general rule, dysrhythmias are not treated specifically with anti-dysrhythmic agents unless the rhythm disturbance itself is deemed to be clinically significant, i.e. associated with haemodynamic compromise. The emphasis is on treatment of the underlying disorder, and it must be remembered that anti-dysrhythmic agents are not benign and may have the potential to be pro-dysrhythmic.
- Haemodynamically significant dysrhythmias may need to be treated specifically prior to diagnosis of the underlying cause.

TACHYDYSRHYTHMIAS

Supraventricular tachycardia

Supraventricular tachycardia (SVT) may be atrial or junctional in origin and can be difficult to distinguish from ventricular tachycardia in some cases. On physical examination both may have rapid weak pulses with pulse deficits. Potential distinguishing features for SVT (Figure 12.2) on electrocardiography include:

- Tall and narrow QRS complexes in lead II
- Complexes typically uniform.

It is noteworthy that physiological or appropriate sinus tachycardia, including in response to severe hypovolaemia, rarely exceeds a rate of 220–240 beats per minute in dogs at rest (300 beats per minute in cats); heart rate may exceed this in dogs such as greyhounds during intense exercise. The finding of a heart rate above this level should prompt electrocardiography.

Causes

Supraventricular tachycardias most commonly occur as a result of primary cardiac disorders that result in atrial dilation (e.g. mitral or tricuspid regurgitation). Some animals present in congestive heart failure.

Indications for treatment

Supraventricular tachycardia should be treated with specific anti-dysrhythmic therapy if treatment of congestive

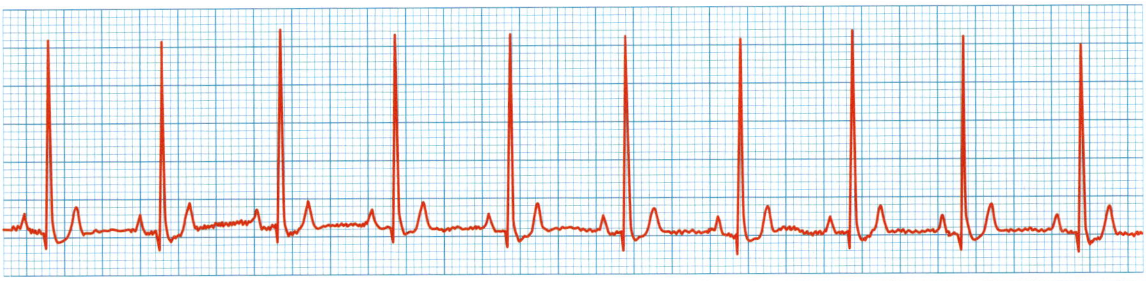

Figure 12.1 Normal sinus rhythm in a dog showing P-QRS-T complexes (lead II, 25 mm/s). (Courtesy of Simon Dennis)

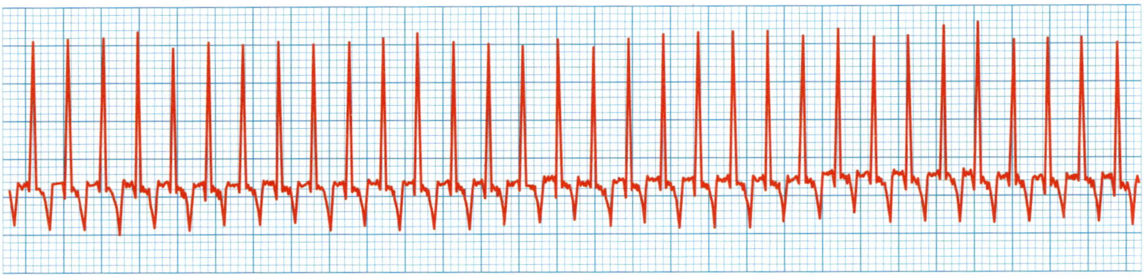

Figure 12.2 Supraventricular tachycardia in a dog at a rate of approximately 320 beats per minute (lead II, 25 mm/s). QRS complexes look relatively normal (tall, narrow, uniform) with a regular R-R interval. (Courtesy of Simon Dennis)

heart failure does not improve the dysrhythmia and it is deemed to be clinically significant.

Treatment

Although conversion to sinus rhythm is preferred, this is not always possible and the main aim of treatment is to slow the ventricular response rate such that the dysrhythmia no longer causes haemodynamic compromise. Oral digoxin and treatment for congestion are implemented in animals with congestive heart failure. The reader is referred to other sources for more information on the use of digoxin.

Vagal manoeuvres can be attempted and may be effective in some animals with SVT. This involves carotid sinus massage or applying pressure to the closed eyes. If vagal manoeuvres fail and treatment of congestion alone is ineffective, then additional medical therapy may be indicated. Diltiazem (a calcium channel blocker) is the most commonly used agent and may be given intravenously if available or orally. This agent must be used cautiously in animals with congestive heart failure if at all as it has negative inotropic effects that may cause clinical deterioration.

Atrial fibrillation

Atrial fibrillation (AF) (Figure 12.3) is characterized by a chaotic irregularly irregular heart rhythm on auscultation with marked pulse deficits. Electrocardiography shows:

- Absent P waves and irregular undulations of the baseline
- Normal-looking (tall and narrow) QRS complexes but an irregular R-R interval (this is an important diagnostic feature).

Causes

In emergency practice, AF is typically (although not always) seen in animals with severe primary structural heart disease, usually involving atrial dilation. The ventricular rate in such cases is typically fast (potentially over 200 beats per minute), and there is usually evidence of congestive heart failure (see Ch. 31). Lone AF is used to describe AF in dogs without evidence of structural heart disease (e.g. some Irish Wolfhounds). AF does occur in cats but less frequently than in dogs.

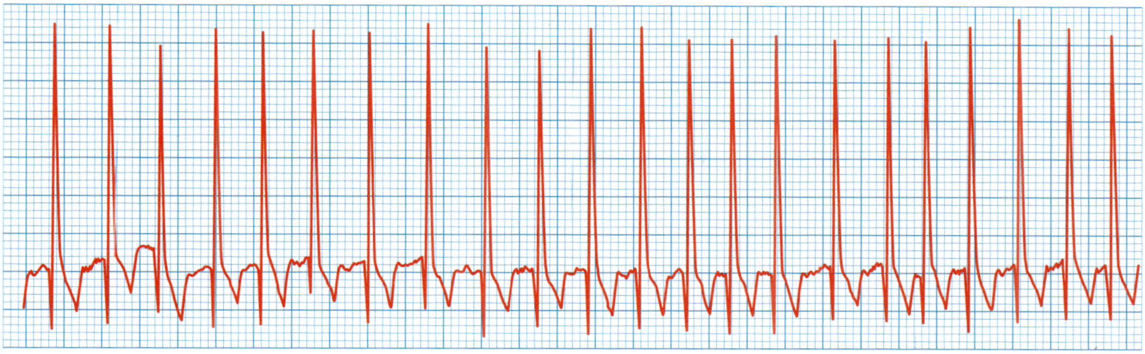

Figure 12.3 Atrial fibrillation in a dog at a rate of approximately 240 beats per min (lead II, 25 mm/s). QRS complexes look relatively normal (tall, narrow, uniform) but with an irregularly irregular R-R interval. (Courtesy of Simon Dennis)

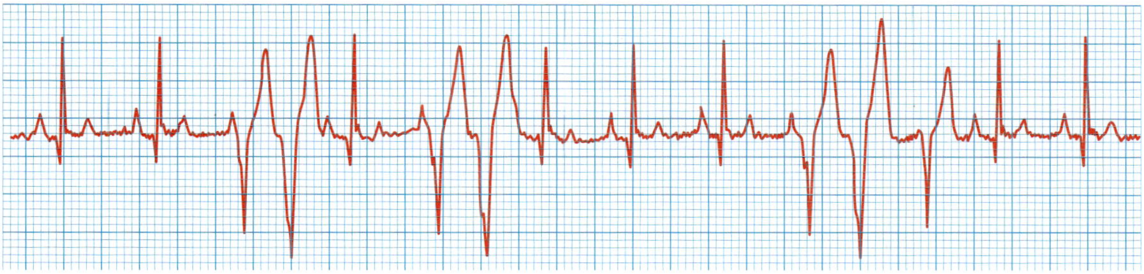

Figure 12.4 Ventricular premature complexes in a dog (lead II, 25 mm/s); two couplets and a triplet are present. The QRS complexes are wide and bizarre, and not related to the normal P waves. (Courtesy of Simon Dennis)

Indications for treatment

The approach to AF will depend on the rate, the underlying cause, and whether congestive heart failure is present. Stabilization of congestive heart failure is the priority, and treatment to control the ventricular response rate may then be included in subsequent therapy if still required.

Treatment

Treatment of AF is designed to slow the heart rate (typically to less than 160 beats per min in dogs) in order to improve cardiac output. However, as animals with severe heart failure may require some degree of heart rate elevation to maintain cardiac output, excessive reduction of ventricular response rate may not be desirable. Conversion to sinus rhythm is difficult and in fact not shown to be associated with any additional benefit.

Oral digoxin is the usual agent of choice for dogs with heart disease and the reader is referred to other sources for more information on the use of digoxin. Congestion should also be treated as required (see Ch. 31). Occasionally additional antidysrhythmic therapy (e.g. oral diltiazem) is indicated if treatment of congestion does not provide adequate ventricular rate control but care with dosing must be taken in animals with congestive heart failure.

Ventricular tachycardia

Ventricular premature complexes (VPCs) and ventricular tachycardia (VT) are commonly identified in emergency patients, especially dogs (Figures 12.4 and 12.5). VT is seven or more consecutive ventricular premature complexes. Complexes are usually wide and bizarre, and not associated with P waves.

Causes

These dysrhythmias may occur secondary to a large number of noncardiac disorders, but may also be the result of primary heart disease. Causes of VPCs and VT are summarized in Box 12.1.

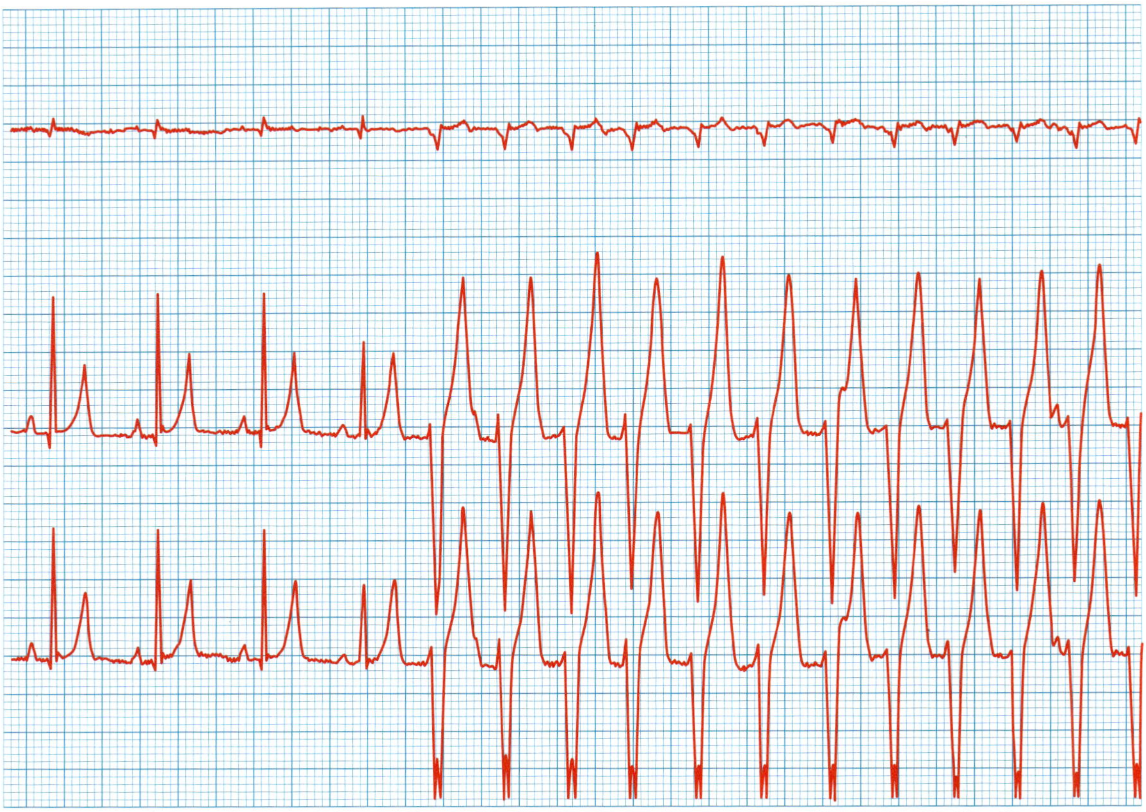

Figure 12.5 Ventricular tachycardia in a dog at a rate of approximately 180 beats per minute (leads I–III, 25 mm/s); QRS complexes appear uniform (monomorphic morphology) and R-on-T is not present. (Courtesy of Simon Dennis)

> **CLINICAL TIP**
>
> - It is very important to distinguish ventricular escape complexes (see Figure 12.9) from ventricular premature complexes and ventricular tachycardia.
> - Ventricular (or junctional) escape complexes typically occur in animals with a severe bradydysrhythmia and are responsible for maintaining cardiac output and essentially for keeping the animal alive.
> - A ventricular intrinsic escape rate (idioventricular rhythm) of less than 50 beats per minute is typical in dogs (less than 100 beats per minute in cats). The ventricular complexes in these cases must not be treated.

Indications for treatment

Ventricular premature complexes typically do not require specific intervention and treatment is aimed at the underlying disorder. VT is only treated when one of the following criteria is met:

- The dysrhythmia is thought to be causing significant clinical signs in the patient, e.g. lethargy, exercise intolerance, collapse
- The dysrhythmia is associated with evidence of sustained systemic hypoperfusion (pallor, poor peripheral pulses, slow capillary refill time, hypotension)
- VT is sustained (more than 30 seconds) at a rate above 180 beats per minute
- R-on-T phenomenon is identified (ectopic R wave superimposed on T wave of preceding complex; see Figure 12.6)
- VT includes (a significant number of) multiform complexes
- Structural heart disease, Boxer arrhythmogenic right ventricular cardiomyopathy or Doberman dilated cardiomyopathy is suspected and the rate exceeds 180 beats per minute, whether this is sustained or not.

An accelerated idioventricular rhythm refers to a ventricular rhythm occurring at a slower rate than VT,

BOX 12.1 Causes of ventricular premature complexes (VPCs) and ventricular tachycardia (VT) in companion animals

Primary noncardiac (systemic) causes

- Intra-abdominal disorders (e.g. splenic disease, GDV, canine HGE)
- Hypoxaemia and tissue hypoxia
- Systemic inflammation (e.g. SIRS/sepsis)
- CNS disease (brain disorders but also, e.g., inflammatory CNS disease)
- Variety of drug therapies
- (Electrolyte abnormalities)
- (Acid–base abnormalities)

Primary cardiac causes

- Variety of congenital and acquired heart diseases
- ARVC in the Boxer
- Dilated cardiomyopathy in the Doberman Pinscher
- Heart failure
- Myocardial trauma, inflammation, ischaemia, hypoxia, neoplasia
- Pericardial effusion

ARVC, arrhythmogenic right ventricular cardiomyopathy; CNS, central nervous system; GDV, gastric dilation/volvulus syndrome; HGE, haemorrhagic gastroenteritis syndrome; SIRS, systemic inflammatory response syndrome.

typically less than 100–140 beats per minute (definitions vary). QRS complexes are typically regular and uniform. Causes include major surgical procedures or other trauma, and systemic disease. Accelerated idioventricular rhythm does not typically cause haemodynamic compromise and therefore does not usually require treatment.

Treatment

CLINICAL TIP

- Treatment of ventricular tachycardia in emergency patients is unlikely to result in sustained conversion to sinus rhythm, at least in the short term; many animals remain in a predominantly ventricular rhythm or sinus rhythm with frequent ventricular premature complexes.
- Treatment can be considered successful, however, if there is sufficient improvement in terms of either the haemodynamic compromise resulting from the dysrhythmia or with respect to its malignancy.

Lidocaine is usually the first drug used for VT that is assessed to require treatment. In dogs, a bolus of 2 mg/kg is administered slowly intravenously; if there is no response to the first bolus after 2–3 minute, a further three boluses may be attempted (i.e. total dose of 8 mg/kg); if there is a positive response, a constant rate infusion is started (50–80 μg/kg/min). Lidocaine may be less effective in the presence of hypokalaemia.

If the dysrhythmia fails to respond to lidocaine, and the clinician is sure that the dysrhythmia is not in fact an SVT, then alternative agents may be tried; however, this may be constrained by what agents are available within the practice. Sotalol and procainamide may both be given intravenously and the former is usually the author's next choice after lidocaine.

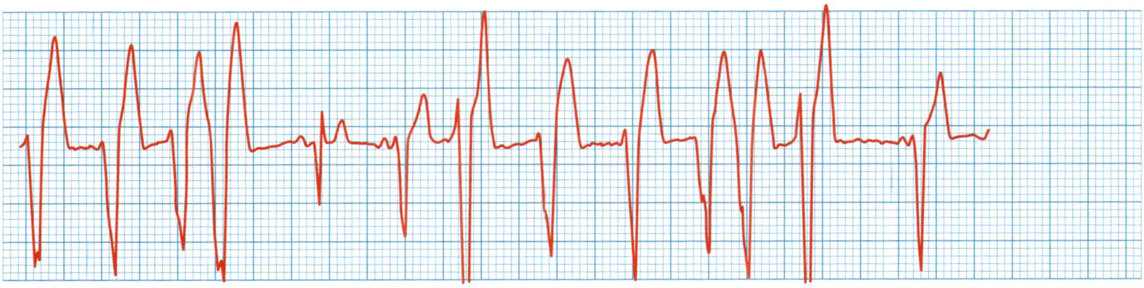

Figure 12.6 R-on-T phenomenon in a dog (lead II, 25 mm/s); the fourth ectopic R wave (from the left) is superimposed on the T wave of the preceding complex. This occurs again towards the end of the ECG strip. (Courtesy of Virginia Luis Fuentes)

In animals with VT as a result of primary cardiac disease, appropriate long-term medications are also started and these may include oral antidysrhythmic therapy (e.g. sotalol, mexiletine). In animals with secondary VT, it is very unusual to need to provide anything more than a lidocaine infusion for 24–72 hr while the primary disorder is treated or the animal is recovering following treatment.

BRADY-DYSRHYTHMIAS

CLINICAL TIP

- Some forms of brady-dysrhythmia (e.g. sinus bradycardia, first degree AV block) may occur in animals that have a physiological elevation in vagal tone either through high levels of fitness or for example when asleep. Clinical signs are typically not associated with the slow heart rate in such cases and treatment is not required.

Sinus brady-dysrhythmias

Sinus brady-dysrhythmias occur as a result of decreased impulse generation by the SA node or decreased conduction of the impulse through the atria. Sinus bradycardia, sinus arrest and SA block are types of sinus brady-dysrhythmia.

Causes

Sinus brady-dysrhythmias may occur as a result of primary cardiac or noncardiac causes. Systemic diseases (e.g. central nervous system disorders, gastrointestinal disorders) that result in high vagal tone are a relatively common cause in emergency patients, as are hypothermia and hypoglycaemia. Vagal involvement can potentially be confirmed by assessing response to vagolytic therapy (atropine, glycopyrrolate) although there may be some variation in individual patient response. Sinus brady-dysrhythmias may also occur secondary to administration of a variety of drugs, some of which are used commonly in emergency cases (e.g. opioids, sedatives); however, this is only likely to be clinically significant in excessive doses. Primary cardiac causes of sinus brady-dysrhythmias typically relate to disease of the SA node (e.g. idiopathic fibrosis, myocardial disease).

Sick sinus syndrome

Sick sinus syndrome (SSS) refers to a combination of dysrhythmias that typically include abnormalities in both impulse generation by the SA node and subsequent conduction. Sinus bradycardia, sinus arrest and SVT occur in variable combinations. This disorder is usually idiopathic and occurs most commonly in the West Highland White terrier and the Miniature Schnauzer amongst others. The syndrome has not been reported in cats thus far.

Indications for treatment

Treatment is typically indicated in all dogs that are symptomatic for SSS. Common clinical signs of low cardiac output include cardiac syncope as well as exercise intolerance and variable weakness.

Treatment

In less severe cases of SSS, it may be appropriate to attempt medical therapy (e.g. terbutaline, theophylline) and some clinical improvement may be observed, at least for a short while. In more severe cases, referral for pacemaker implantation is required and this may need to be arranged on an urgent emergency basis.

Atrioventricular block

AV block refers to delayed or failed impulse conduction through the AV node. There are three types of AV block – first degree, second degree and third degree (see Figures 12.7–12.9) – with some further subclassification.

Causes

High vagal tone is a relatively common cause of AV block, which may also result from hyperkalaemia and excessive doses of certain drugs. As with SA node disease, primary disease of the AV node (e.g. idiopathic fibrosis, myocardial disease) can also cause AV block. Third degree AV block is almost always due to heart disease.

Indications for treatment

Specific treatment of AV block is only indicated if the animal is deemed to be symptomatic from the dysrhythmia. Otherwise treatment is aimed at addressing the underlying cause. First degree AV block is unlikely to

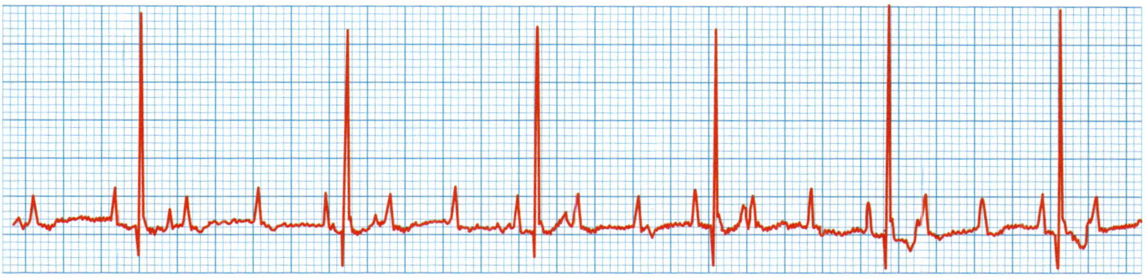

Figure 12.7 Second degree AV block in a dog (lead II, 25 mm/s); every third P wave is conducted and associated with a QRS complex (3 to 1 conduction). (Courtesy of Simon Dennis)

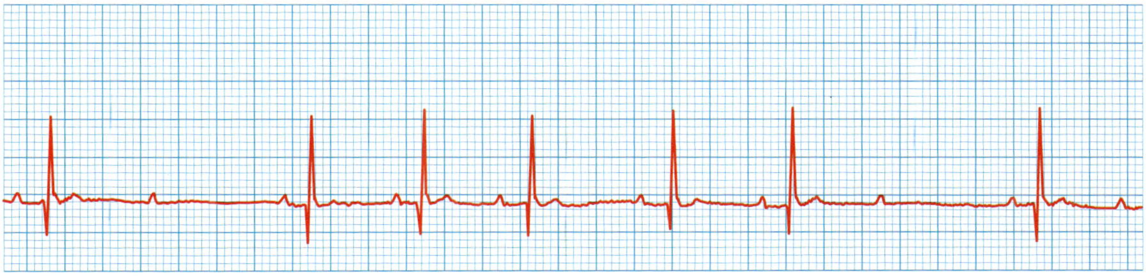

Figure 12.8 Low-grade second degree AV block in a dog (lead II, 25 mm/s); the majority of P waves are conducted and associated with a QRS complex. (Courtesy of Simon Dennis)

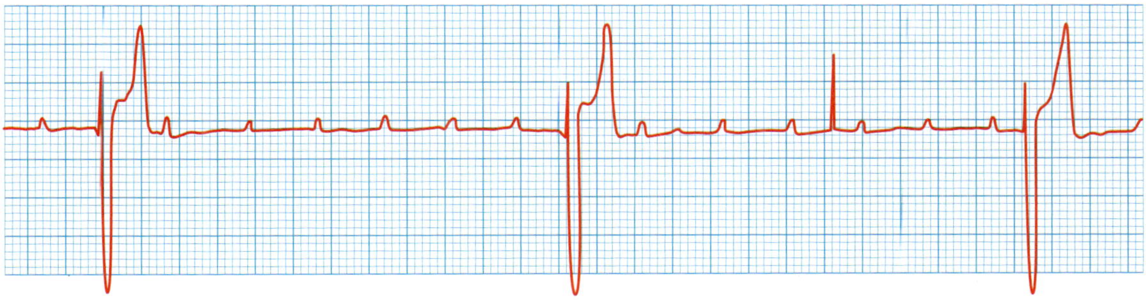

Figure 12.9 Third degree AV block in a dog (lead II, 25 mm/s). There is no P wave conduction and the QRS complexes are ventricular (wide and bizarre), occurring at a rate slower than the P waves; the ventricular escape rate is approximately 30 beats per minute. (Courtesy of Simon Dennis)

cause clinical signs, but second degree AV block may be clinically significant. Third degree AV block is almost always associated with haemodynamic compromise and causes signs such as exercise intolerance, variable weakness and cardiac syncope.

Treatment

Treatment of AV block is aimed at the underlying disorder if possible. Animals with irreversible cardiac damage and clinical signs of low cardiac output may require a permanent pacemaker to be implanted.

13 Collapse

The term 'collapse' is not specific to any one disorder or body system abnormality. All collapsed animals are recumbent but being able to classify them more specifically is important in order to allow appropriate emergency management to be instituted. In general, collapsed patients can be thought of in the following terms.

PRIMARY CARDIOVASCULAR DISORDERS CAUSING COLLAPSE

Cardiovascular causes of collapse centre on a lack of adequate tissue perfusion. This may be localized (e.g. feline aortic thromboembolism) but is typically generalized with the potential to cause inadequate perfusion of the brain, spinal cord and muscles. The majority of primary cardiovascular causes relate to primary cardiac dysfunction, for example:

- Congestive heart failure and cardiogenic shock
- Severe brady-dysrhythmia, e.g. sick sinus syndrome
- Severe tachy-dysrhythmia, e.g. ventricular tachycardia in Boxer arrhythmogenic right ventricular cardiomyopathy
- Congenital aortic stenosis in the German Shepherd dog.

PRIMARY NON-CARDIOVASCULAR DISORDERS CAUSING CARDIOVASCULAR COLLAPSE

A wide range of disorders may cause collapse due to severe secondary cardiovascular compromise. These may include:

- Hypovolaemic, maldistributive or obstructive shock (see Ch. 2)
- Severe dysrhythmias, e.g. vagally mediated brady-dysrhythmia due to an intrathoracic mass, severe ventricular tachycardia due to splenic neoplasia
- Hypoadrenocorticism (Addison's disease) – multifactorial causes of collapse (see Ch. 34).

NON-CARDIOVASCULAR PRIMARY DISORDER CAUSING NON-CARDIOVASCULAR COLLAPSE

This category includes a wide variety of disorders that may be classified as neurological, neuromuscular, muscular, orthopaedic, metabolic/electrolyte-related, endocrine and haematological. Depending on the nature of the primary disorder, cardiovascular abnormalities of varying degrees may or may not be expected. For example:

- An animal that is recumbent because of a cervical spinal cord lesion would not typically be expected to have significant cardiovascular abnormalities (unless the aetiology is traumatic for example).
- Seizures, unless severe or prolonged, are not expected to cause significant cardiovascular abnormalities.
- Significant cardiovascular abnormalities would not usually be expected with hypoglycaemic collapse (although severe hypoglycaemia can cause high vagal tone with consequent brady-dysrhythmia).
- Animals with severe acute haemolytic anaemia may collapse due to a lack of tissue oxygen delivery. These animals would be expected to show signs of cardiovascular (and respiratory) compensation for the anaemia.
- Generalized myasthenia gravis is not typically associated with significant cardiovascular abnormalities.

Clearly in any one collapsed patient, the cause may well overlap between these categories as the body works as a whole unit. For example, cats with aortic thromboembolism typically have marked neurological abnormalities that are the result of a lack of perfusion, i.e. a cardiovascular cause with neuromuscular manifestations. Animals that suffer severe blood loss are likely to be collapsed due to a combination of marked hypovolaemia and lack of oxygen-carrying capacity. Nevertheless, considering the causes of collapse in the way described is important as cardiovascular abnormalities are frequently the most life-threatening and generally require most urgent treatment.

14 Cyanosis

CLINICAL TIP

- In most animals, cyanosis indicates very severe hypoxaemia. However, it is essential to remember that animals can be markedly hypoxaemic and on the cusp of severe deterioration without manifesting cyanosis; this is especially true in anaemic animals. A false sense of security should not therefore be derived either from the absence of cyanosis or from normal arterial oxygen saturation by pulse oximetry. In addition, cyanosis when identified must be treated as an emergency.

Cyanosis is a bluish or purplish discoloration of the mucous membranes or skin and occurs as a result of an increase in the concentration of unoxygenated (reduced) haemoglobin. Reduced haemoglobin must rise above a certain level (5 g/dl) before cyanosis is detectable. Animals can therefore be markedly hypoxaemic and on the cusp of severe deterioration without manifesting cyanosis; this is especially true in anaemic animals. Causes of cyanosis are typically classified as central or peripheral.

Central cyanosis most commonly occurs when arterial blood fails to become adequately saturated with oxygen. It may also occur if there is an increase in the concentration of other types of haemoglobin that are unable to carry oxygen (e.g. methaemoglobinaemia in paracetamol (acetaminophen) intoxication). Inadequate oxygen saturation may occur for example due to:

- Congenital cardiovascular anomalies causing right-to-left shunting such that unoxygenated blood bypasses the lungs and flows straight into the systemic arterial circulation (e.g. tetralogy of Fallot, reverse patent ductus arteriosus (PDA)). Cyanosis may also occur as a result of severe congenital pulmonic stenosis.
- Severe lung disease: this may be due to primary lung disease (e.g. aspiration pneumonia, bronchopneumonia, pulmonary contusions, neoplastic infiltration) but also to severe cardiogenic pulmonary oedema. Obstructive lower airway disease (especially feline bronchial disease) may also cause central cyanosis.
- Upper respiratory tract obstruction (e.g. laryngeal paralysis, foreign body, tumour).
- Severe hypoventilation, for example due to severe pleural effusion or pneumothorax, central nervous system depression or injury, neuromuscular disease (e.g. myasthenia gravis, tetanus) or intoxication/drug overdose.

Right-to-left shunting PDA may be associated with so-called differential cyanosis, in which unoxygenated blood flows to the caudal parts of the body but oxygenated blood flows to the cranial parts. Cyanosis is therefore only detected caudally in such cases.

Peripheral cyanosis occurs as a result of a disturbance in peripheral circulation. Slow peripheral blood flow results in a relative increase in the amount of oxygen extracted by the tissues and therefore the amount of oxyhaemoglobin that is reduced. The arterial blood in such cases may have normal or reduced oxygen saturation. The most common causes are intense peripheral vasoconstriction (e.g. severe hypothermia), low cardiac output, and thrombosis/thromboembolism (e.g. cyanotic nail beds in cats with feline aortic thromboembolism).

APPROACH TO CYANOSIS

CLINICAL TIP

- Central cyanosis is typically associated with a potentially life-threatening disorder and affected animals should be considered highly

Continued

CLINICAL TIP—cont'd

unstable, requiring gentle handling and minimal intervention.

- Many of the causes of central cyanosis (with the particular exceptions of right-to-left cardiovascular shunts and increased concentrations of non-oxygen-carrying haemoglobin) are responsive to oxygen supplementation that should therefore be provided from the outset. A period of oxygen supplementation prior to further examination/intervention can be invaluable in many cases. In the author's experience, severe respiratory disease is the most commonly identified cause of cyanosis in companion animals presenting as emergencies.
- It is important to remember that both types of cyanosis – central and peripheral – may be present in the same animal at the same time.

Signalment, history

Signalment and history may allow certain differential diagnoses to be viewed with a greater or lesser index of suspicion. For example, cyanosis in a young animal is more likely to be due to a congenital cardiovascular abnormality. A chronic history of consistent signs in a breed predisposed to idiopathic pulmonary fibrosis (e.g. the West Highland White terrier) may point to this as the cause of the cyanosis.

Major body system examination

Physical examination should hopefully allow central versus peripheral cyanosis to be differentiated. Peripheral cyanosis is more likely to be localized, being confined for example to the extremities or skin of a single limb. With the exception of differential cyanosis, central cyanosis is more commonly identified in the oral mucous membranes and tongue.

As described above, many of the causes of central cyanosis relate to the respiratory, cardiovascular or neurological systems. In general, cardiovascular abnormalities in animals with cyanosis of respiratory origin are likely to be less marked than in animals with primary cardiac cyanosis. In some animals with primary respiratory cyanosis, the underlying cause will be readily apparent (e.g. upper respiratory tract obstruction). Potentially the hardest cases to distinguish are animals that are cyanotic as a result of severe lung compromise as this could be due to primary lung disease or severe cardiogenic pulmonary oedema. With the exception of right-sided heart failure (jugular venous distension, ascites, pleural effusion) secondary to *cor pulmonale*, findings consistent with poor perfusion (poor pulses, pale mucous membranes, hypothermia), as well as marked cardiac murmurs and severe suspected dysrhythmias, point to a primary cardiac cause being more likely.

Emergency database

An emergency database should be performed in all patients presenting with cyanosis but the timing should be determined by patient stability and response to oxygen supplementation. Manual packed cell volume may be increased as a compensatory secondary absolute polycythaemia in response to chronic hypoxaemia. Pulse oximetry to measure arterial haemoglobin saturation with oxygen (SpO_2) should also be attempted if tolerated; values less than 80% are common in animals with central cyanosis. If available, electrocardiography is indicated in animals with suspected dysrhythmias.

Diagnostic imaging

Thoracic radiographs are invaluable in the investigation of pulmonary disease, as well as for identifying cardiomegaly and evidence of pulmonary congestion or oedema. However, radiography must only be performed at the appropriate time and judicious appropriate sedation (e.g. low dose butorphanol or morphine) may be helpful in some cases. If available, thoracic ultrasonography should be performed first in animals with suspected significant pleural space disease and diagnostic and therapeutic thoracocentesis (see Ch. 23) may be required with a greater or lesser degree of urgency. Referral for echocardiography will be required in animals suspected of having a congenital cardiovascular anomaly.

Treatment

In all animals with cyanosis, successful treatment ultimately depends on whether the underlying cause can be addressed. Peripheral cyanosis in itself is not usually life-threatening although the underlying disorder may have a very poor prognosis.

Central cyanosis is typically associated with a potentially life-threatening disorder. Oxygen supplementation is appropriate in all cases although, as described above, some underlying disorders will not respond to any notable extent. Further emergency intervention will then depend to a large extent on the underlying cause (see

Table 14.1 Causes, notable comments and recommended interventions for central cyanosis

Cause	Notable comments	Intervention
Congenital right-to-left cardiovascular shunt	Emergency presentation uncommon Differential cyanosis may be present	Cage rest/restricted exercise Referral for echocardiography and possible treatment
Primary lung/airway disease	Severe respiratory distress likely Abnormal lung sounds common Perfusion parameters may be normal	Oxygen supplementation Medical therapy (e.g. antibiotic, bronchodilator, glucocorticoid, anthelminthic) as appropriate Cage rest
Cardiogenic cause, including severe pulmonary oedema and low cardiac output	Severe respiratory distress and abnormal lung sounds may be present (congestion versus low output) Perfusion parameters likely to be markedly abnormal Significant cardiac murmur or dysrhythmia likely	Oxygen supplementation Appropriately aggressive diuresis and other medical therapy as indicated (e.g. glyceryl trinitrate, pimobendan, antidysrhythmic treatment) Cage rest
Upper respiratory tract obstruction	Severe respiratory distress with inspiratory stridor Dogs in particular may be (severely) hyperthermic	Oxygen supplementation Sedation Emergency removal of obstruction (e.g. foreign body) or creation of temporary airway (endotracheal intubation, tracheostomy) may be needed (rare)
Hypoventilation due to severe pleural space disease	Dull lung ± heart sounds (pleural effusion, pneumothorax)	Oxygen supplementation Thoracocentesis (therapeutic and diagnostic)
Hypoventilation due to CNS or neuromuscular disease	Causes include drug-induced CNS depression, brainstem respiratory centre injury, cervical spinal cord or chest wall injury, severe respiratory muscle weakness or paralysis	Oxygen supplementation Treatment for primary disorder General anaesthesia and manual ventilation may be required (consider practical and financial implications)
Hypoventilation due to intoxication or drug overdose	History may be very helpful May be related to overdose of anaesthetic drugs	Oxygen supplementation Administer antidote/reversal agent if available Endotracheal intubation and manual ventilation may be required (consider practical and financial implications)
Methaemoglobinaemia	Paracetamol (acetaminophen) intoxication – dietary indiscretion or misguided administration by owner	*N*-acetylcysteine (ascorbic acid) Treatment of anaemia Supportive measures

CNS, central nervous system.

Table 14.1). In the author's experience most animals with congenital right-to-left cardiovascular shunts have a more chronic history of cyanosis and do not typically present as emergency cases. Although there are exceptions, the prognosis associated with primary lung disease that is sufficiently severe as to cause cyanosis is generally very poor, with response to medical therapy being variable and often short lived.

15 Head tilt and nystagmus

The vestibular system is responsible for balance and coordinating movements of the eyes, trunk and limbs with changes in head position. Head tilt and nystagmus are typically associated with unilateral vestibular disease and are relatively common presenting signs in canine emergency patients. Jerk nystagmus is typical of vestibular disease with the slow (pathological) phase towards the side of the lesion and the fast (corrective) phase away from the side of the lesion. Occasionally animals present with nystagmus due to cerebellar disease (paradoxical vestibular disease) or abnormalities in visual pathways. Other clinical signs associated with vestibular disease are listed in Box 15.1.

TYPES OF UNILATERAL VESTIBULAR DISEASE

Vestibular disease may be the result of a lesion affecting either the central or the peripheral component of the vestibular system.

Central vestibular disease

The central component of the vestibular system is located in the brainstem and cerebellum. Nystagmus in central vestibular disease can be horizontal, rotatory, vertical or positional, with the fast phase towards or away from the lesion. Affected animals may well have additional clinical signs that reflect brain involvement, such as reduced mentation from depression through to coma, or ipsilateral paresis and proprioceptive deficits.

Box 15.1 Clinical signs of unilateral vestibular disease

- Head tilt towards the side of the lesion
- Nystagmus
- Ataxia
- Wide-based stance
- Circling, leaning or falling towards the side of the lesion
- Vomiting

Peripheral vestibular disease

The peripheral components of the vestibular system are sensory receptors in the inner ear and the vestibular portion of vestibulocochlear nerve. Nystagmus in peripheral vestibular disease can be horizontal or rotatory, with the fast phase away from the side of the lesion. Affected animals may have normal mentation or they may be markedly disorientated; signs of brainstem abnormality are not expected unless there has been extension of inner ear disease. Paresis and proprioceptive deficits should not occur.

Horner's syndrome (third eyelid protrusion, pupillary constriction, drooping of upper eyelid, enophthalmos) and facial nerve deficits (including ipsilateral drooping of and inability to move ear and lip, widened palpebral fissure, absent blinking) may occur with peripheral vestibular disease but are typically not recognized in the idiopathic form.

Paradoxical vestibular disease

Paradoxical vestibular disease refers to a syndrome of nystagmus, head tilt and circling due to cerebellar disease. Head tilt and circling occur contralateral to the side of the lesion and there are usually other more typical signs of cerebellar disease (e.g. head tremor, ipsilateral dysmetria).

CAUSES OF UNILATERAL VESTIBULAR DISEASE

The most common causes of central vestibular disease are brain tumours and inflammation (infectious or non-infectious). Trauma and metronidazole intoxication are other causes.

The most common causes of peripheral vestibular disease are otitis media or interna, and idiopathic vestibular disease. Ototoxicity (e.g. due to topical medications), middle or inner ear trauma or tumours, and hypothyroidism are other possible causes. Nasopharyngeal polyps can cause peripheral vestibular disease in cats.

CLINICAL TIP

- In the author's experience, idiopathic peripheral vestibular disease is the form of vestibular disease seen most commonly in routine emergency practice. This disease is seen especially in older dogs but may also affect cats of any age. Diagnosis is made on the basis of compatible history and examination findings and by exclusion of other causes of peripheral disease. Although patients may present with really quite severe and often peracute clinical signs, they can improve remarkably over a period of several days (typically within 48–72 hours) with adequate supportive care. The prognosis is good with complete recovery common (may take up to 4 weeks and mild residual signs may persist), although recurrence may occur.
- As the disease often occurs in older dogs, the major differential diagnosis on presentation is central vestibular disease secondary to a brain tumour. A thorough neurological examination to differentiate peripheral versus central signs is therefore essential in order not to inadvertently condemn these animals to having a worse prognosis. Owners can then be counselled appropriately and reassured about the rationale of giving their dog some time to improve.
- It is noteworthy that animals with idiopathic peripheral vestibular disease do not usually have Horner's syndrome or facial nerve deficits. In addition, there is no evidence for a beneficial effect from corticosteroid administration.

APPROACH TO UNILATERAL VESTIBULAR DISEASE

Signalment

Signalment may help to raise or lower the index of suspicion for certain differential diagnoses. For example, idiopathic peripheral vestibular disease is seen most often in older dogs and congenital vestibular disease is most likely in very young animals.

History

As always, a thorough history should be taken in all cases. Important pieces of information include:

- Onset and progression – clinical signs are usually progressive with central disease
- History of ear disease
- Clinical signs consistent with ear disease
- Non-vestibular potentially multifocal neurological signs suggestive of brain involvement
- History of trauma
- Medical therapy (e.g. potentially ototoxic topical therapy, metronidazole)
- Clinical signs consistent with other diseases (e.g. hypothyroidism).

Major body system examination

In the majority of cases, the neurological system is the only system to be significantly affected. Animals with central vestibular disease due to a primary brain lesion may have potentially significant cardiovascular abnormalities and hyperthermia may be identified in some very disorientated dogs. A range of abnormalities may be identified following trauma.

Bilateral otoscopic examination should be performed in animals with peripheral vestibular signs. The tympanic membrane is often ruptured but if it remains intact it may not be possible to detect fluid in the middle ear. Myringotomy may need to be performed both for diagnostic purposes and to collect a fluid sample for cytology and microbiology. Most animals require heavy sedation or preferably general anaesthesia for a reliable otoscopic examination to be performed.

Emergency database

The emergency database is likely to be unremarkable in a lot of animals with vestibular disease. Dehydration may be identified in some animals and peripheral blood smear examination may reveal leucocytosis in some cases (e.g. otitis media or interna, inflammatory brain disease).

Diagnostic imaging

Central vestibular disease

Animals with signs of central vestibular disease require referral for advanced diagnostic imaging (computed tomography or magnetic resonance imaging) and cerebrospinal fluid analysis.

Peripheral vestibular disease

Well-positioned plain radiographs of the skull designed to highlight the tympanic bullae may provide evidence of infection or neoplasia of the middle or inner ear. However, general anaesthesia is required and this should therefore only be undertaken in cases with signs suggestive of peripheral disease. Advanced diagnostic imaging modalities are considerably more sensitive so referral may be appropriate.

Treatment

Treatment of vestibular disease centres on addressing the underlying disorder if this is possible. For example, administration of toxic drugs should be discontinued and bacterial otitis should be treated with several weeks of systemic antibiosis (preferably based on culture and sensitivity testing).

Supportive care is also required with respect to intravenous fluid therapy in animals that are unable or unwilling to drink. Some dogs may also require assistance for toileting purposes and other nursing measures including well-padded bedding. Symptomatic anti-emetic treatment (maropitant, metoclopramide, ondansetron) is indicated in animals that are vomiting and may also help with nausea.

Animals presenting with head trauma must be stabilized as required (see Ch. 28).

16 Hyperthermia and pyrexia

CLINICAL TIP

- Hyperthermia and pyrexia both manifest as elevated core body temperature but they have different causes, represent different pathophysiological processes, and require a different clinical approach. Appreciating this distinction is important so that the most appropriate management can be provided.

THERMOREGULATION

The thermoregulatory centre is located in the hypothalamus and controls core body temperature closely around the thermoregulatory set point. This is achieved through a balance between heat loss and heat gain. Heat loss occurs via evaporation, conduction, convection and radiation. In people, evaporative cooling is mainly by perspiration. In dogs, evaporative cooling is mainly through panting that brings large amounts of air into contact with the nasal and oral mucosa. Minimal perspiration occurs through the footpads. Heat dissipation also occurs via radiation and convection through the skin. Heat gain can be classified as endogenous production (from metabolic processes and exercise) or exogenous gain (from the environment). Thermoregulatory mechanisms are summarized in Box 16.1.

Marked elevations in core body temperature may have severe consequences, with cellular injury possible above 41.5°C. Multiple organs and body systems may be affected, and disseminated intravascular coagulation (DIC) and multiple organ dysfunction syndrome (MODS) are possible sequlae.

BOX 16.1 Thermoregulatory mechanisms in dogs and cats

Heat loss

- Panting
- Cutaneous vasodilation
- Postural changes (e.g. lying prostrate on cool floor)
- Seeking cool environment (e.g. lying out on patio)
- (Perspiration)

Heat gain

- Catecholamine and thyroxine production
- Shivering
- Increased muscle activity

Heat conservation

- Cutaneous vasoconstriction
- Postural changes
- Piloerection
- Seeking warm environment

HYPERTHERMIA VERSUS PYREXIA

In dogs and cats, normal core (rectal) temperature is approximately 38.0–39.0°C, although some normal fluctuation outside this range is likely during the day. This range reflects the normal thermoregulatory set point. Core temperature may become elevated due to hyperthermia and/or pyrexia. An important distinction exists between these two processes that has important implications in terms of appropriate management.

Hyperthermia

In hyperthermia the thermoregulatory set point is unchanged and the hypothalamus attempts to return core temperature to normal limits. Clinically significant consequences occur when physiological attempts to cool the body become overwhelmed and active cooling is therefore appropriate. The most common causes of hyperthermia are heat stress (see Ch. 38) and severe or sustained seizure activity (see Ch. 24). Other causes include malignant hyperthermia, primary brain lesions and drug reactions.

Hyperthermia is identified most commonly in dogs and is a rare presentation in cats. In most (but not all) hyperthermic animals, the history is suggestive of this being the cause of temperature elevation and the diagnosis is usually relatively straightforward.

Management

CLINICAL TIP

- Wetting the patient with cool water and then applying one or more fans is likely to be the most effective method of cooling. Placing towels on the patient will impede maximum heat loss and should be avoided. Applying alcohol to footpads is unlikely to be very effective given the small surface area involved. It is very important to cease active cooling when rectal temperature is less than 39.5°C to prevent rebound hypothermia.
- As the thermoregulatory set point is unchanged in hyperthermic animals, the use of antipyretic agents is contraindicated.

Wetting the patient with cool water and then applying one or more fans is likely to be the most effective method of cooling. This will promote heat loss predominantly via evaporation, convection and conduction. Excessively cold water should be avoided (see below under ice baths) and although common practice, placing towels on the patient will impede maximum heat loss and should be avoided. Clipping of fur may be helpful in some cases although the author has not found this to be necessary and the time delay in clipping bigger dogs in particular must be borne in mind. Conduction may be further promoted by keeping the patient on a cool surface (e.g. steel worktop). The common practice of applying alcohol to footpads is unlikely to be very effective given the small surface area involved and poses risks with respect to the patient subsequently licking the alcohol.

It is very important to cease active cooling when rectal temperature is less than 39.5°C to prevent rebound hypothermia that may persist for a period of several hours or longer. Rebound hypothermia may occur as a result of hyperthermia-induced dysfunction of the thermoregulatory centre that is therefore unable to stimulate heat production as core temperature declines.

Other methods of active cooling reported include ice water baths, various forms of lavage and cold water enemas. Ice water may cause intense peripheral vasoconstriction, thereby impairing heat loss. Shivering may also occur that will increase heat production and ice water is likely to be uncomfortable to the patient. The use of ice water baths is not recommended. Gastric lavage, peritoneal lavage, bladder lavage and cold water enemas are labour intensive, carry risks and may affect monitoring of temperature in the case of enemas. In addition, their use makes it more difficult to avoid rebound hypothermia and they are only recommended in the most severe of cases where other measures fail to reduce core temperature satisfactorily. The author has thus far never needed to resort to one of these methods.

Intravenous isotonic crystalloid therapy should also be implemented in all hyperthermic patients with the rate and volume used being determined by each patient's individual circumstances (see Ch. 4). Occasionally colloids may need to be employed. Intravenous fluids administered at room temperature will help to lower core temperature directly as well as increase peripheral blood flow, thereby encouraging heat dissipation. Intravenous fluids should not be cooled to lower than room temperature prior to administration. As the thermoregulatory set point is unchanged in hyperthermic animals, the use of antipyretic agents is contraindicated because these agents reduce the set point. Animals that have suffered heat-induced hypothalamic injury may temporarily lose the ability to compensate for changes in their thermoregulatory set point induced by exogenous factors such as antipyretic drugs.

Judicious sedation, using butorphanol and/or acepromazine, can prove useful in the treatment of hyperthermia, in particular in brachycephalic animals, by reducing heat production from breathing and by calming the patient.

Pyrexia

CLINICAL TIP

- Although bacterial infection is a common cause of pyrexia, it is not the only cause and others include noninfectious inflammatory conditions and neoplasia. The automatic use of antibiotics in pyrexic animals is therefore discouraged due to the ever-increasing problem of bacterial antibiotic resistance. Antibiosis should be

CLINICAL TIP—cont'd

reserved for animals in which bacterial infection is either confirmed or at least highly suspected on the basis of additional findings (i.e. beyond pyrexia alone). Antibiosis is also recommended in pyrexic animals with neutropenia.

- The reader is also reminded that neutrophilia may occur as a result of noninfectious processes and its presence in a pyrexic animal is not unexpected regardless of the presence or absence of infection. Again, neutrophilia alone is not an indication for antimicrobial administration.

Pyrexia occurs as a result of pyrogens acting on the hypothalamus, causing the thermoregulatory set point to be raised. The hypothalamus therefore stimulates heat production and heat conservation. Pyrogens may be exogenous or endogenous, although the majority of exogenous pyrogens cause pyrexia by stimulating the release of endogenous pyrogens. Exogenous pyrogens may be involved in infectious disorders (e.g. bacteria, bacterial endotoxins, viruses) as well as for example with intoxication or neoplasia, while endogenous pyrogens (e.g. cytokines, prostaglandins) may be generated for example in inflammation or with neoplasia.

Management

CLINICAL TIP

- Pyrexia is a physiological defensive mechanism and active cooling is inappropriate unless temperature elevation is severe enough to potentially cause tissue injury (>41.5°C). Treatment of pyrexia should be aimed at identifying and addressing the underlying cause.

Pyrexia is a physiological defensive mechanism and active cooling is inappropriate unless temperature elevation is severe enough to potentially cause tissue injury (>41.5°C). Cooling pyrexic animals may reduce body temperature but this will most likely cause the thermoregulatory centre to stimulate heat production and conservation further (i.e. to return body temperature to the raised set point) which is counterproductive. Treatment of pyrexia should therefore be aimed at identifying and addressing the underlying cause.

Antipyretic agents, typically nonsteroidal antiinflammatory agents (NSAIAs), have a role in the treatment of pyrexia and may contribute to improving patient morbidity. However, the potentially beneficial effect of pyrexia must not be discarded and the use of NSAIA therapy is not necessarily indicated in all cases. In those animals in which the primary underlying cause can be directly addressed (e.g. appropriate antibiosis for bacterial infection), or in which clinical signs are not too severe or prolonged, there is an argument for withholding NSAIA therapy to allow the beneficial effects of pyrexia to occur. In addition, withholding NSAIA therapy will allow resolution of pyrexia to be interpreted more reliably as a positive response to treatment of the primary disorder. In the author's experience, pyrexia resolves satisfactorily in a large proportion of patients in which the primary disorder is addressed, often with temporary provision of intravenous fluid therapy. If NSAIA therapy is considered, due attention must be paid to other possible contraindications (especially hypovolaemia, hypoperfusion from other causes, dehydration, renal insufficiency and gastrointestinal abnormalities).

17 Hypothermia

Hypothermia is a condition in which an animal's core body temperature falls below the normal physiological range for that species (approximately less than 37.5°C in dogs and cats). This may occur as a result of decreased heat production, increased heat loss or thermoregulatory dysfunction. Some causes of hypothermia are listed in Box 17.1.

Hypothermia is common in emergency patients and may have a variety of adverse effects. The severity of these adverse effects is likely to be correlated with the severity of hypothermia and they are summarized in Box 17.2. Peripheral vasoconstriction occurs and some animals show a cold diuresis. Hypothermia is particularly common in puppies and kittens, toy canine breeds, geriatric animals, cachectic animals and cats in general.

BOX 17.1 Causes of hypothermia

- Inadequate thermoregulation – young puppies and kittens
- Prolonged general anaesthesia, especially with open cavity surgery
- Exposure to cold environment
- Immersion in cold water
- Trauma
- Systemic disease (e.g. hypothyroidism, uraemia)

BOX 17.2 Potential adverse effects of hypothermia

- Cardiovascular system: initial tachycardia then bradycardia, hypotension, dysrhythmias
- Respiratory system: reduced respiratory rate and depth (hypoxaemia, tissue hypoxia; pulmonary tissue injury)
- Neurological system: depressed mentation (mild through to coma)
- Acid–base abnormalities: respiratory and/or metabolic acidosis
- Coagulation abnormalities
- Cold-induced gastrointestinal, renal and hepatic dysfunction

MANAGEMENT

CLINICAL TIP

- Hypothermic animals that present with hypovolaemia should not be actively warmed until volume resuscitation is underway. This is because warming will lead to cutaneous vasodilation that may exacerbate hypotension. Hypovolaemic cats in particular are often hypothermic. Preventing further heat loss (e.g. by wrapping in a blanket) is however appropriate.
- Animals that present with hypothermia as a result of cardiac dysfunction typically should not be warmed because the same concerns apply as for hypovolaemic patients. An increase in temperature in these cases may be supportive of a positive response to appropriate treatment of the heart disease.
- Although hypothermia is especially common in young animals, feeding is not recommended until temperature has been improved.

Management of hypothermia centres on intravenous fluid therapy and rewarming prior to addressing the primary disorder as appropriate. Appropriate warming measures depend on the severity and duration of hypothermia as well as the primary disorder. Passive external rewarming (i.e. wrapping the animal in blankets and allowing him/her to generate his/her own heat) is likely to be all that is required for mildly hypothermic patients (36.0–37°C). Active external rewarming is indicated for animals with moderate to severe hypothermia (32.0–36.0°C) and measures include the use of a forced-air warming blanket (e.g. Bair Hugger®, Arizant UK), an

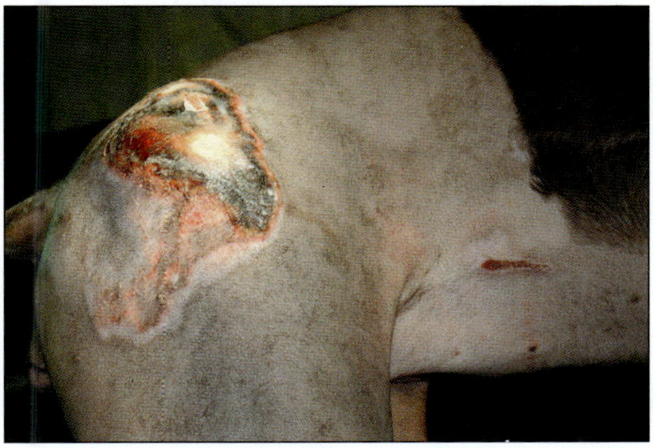

Figure 17.1 Severe cutaneous thermal injury in a dog as a result of a hot intravenous fluid bag being placed in direct contact with the skin. (Photograph courtesy of Arthur House)

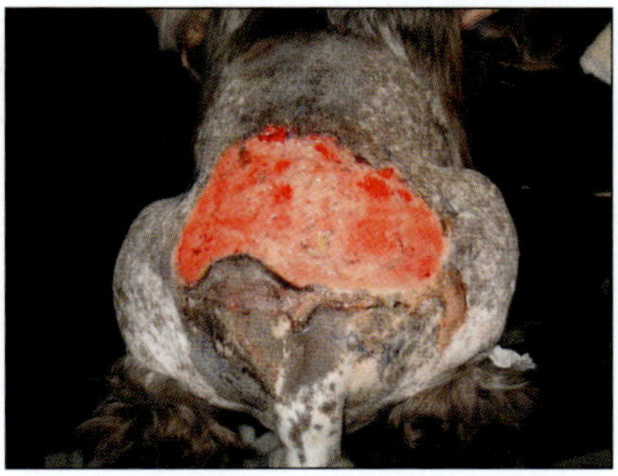

Figure 17.2 Severe burn injury in a dog from a heat pad. (Photograph courtesy of Stephen Baines)

incubator, or warm blankets. If a forced-air warming product is not available, the patient can be covered with a blanket and a hair dryer used to blow hot air under the blanket.

Active internal or core rewarming may be required in animals with severe (less than 32°C) hypothermia. This typically takes the form of warm (not hot) intravenous fluids but occasionally more aggressive intervention in the form of pleural or peritoneal lavage may be required. Administering warmed humidified air or oxygen may also help with rewarming. Hypothermia-induced bradycardia is nonresponsive to atropine but will resolve as rewarming progresses.

CLINICAL TIP

- Warmed intravenous fluid bags or gloves filled with warm water can be placed next to the patient. However, in order to avoid potentially severe thermal injury, it is extremely important to ensure that these are not too hot and that some insulation is provided between the patient and the bag or glove (Figure 17.1).
- Caution is also essential when using heat pads and heat lamps to avoid iatrogenic burn injuries that can have disastrous consequences (Figure 17.2).

18 Jaundice

Jaundice (icterus) is a relatively common presenting complaint or finding in dogs and cats. This syndrome is characterized by hyperbilirubinaemia and deposition of bile pigment in tissues. Clinically, jaundice is most readily identified in the sclera, mucous membranes and nonpigmented hairless skin. A rational approach to the investigation of jaundice relies on classification of the type of jaundice and then more specific diagnostic tests to establish a definitive diagnosis. Clearly more than one type may occur in the same patient at the same time and this is especially true in the case of intrahepatic and posthepatic jaundice.

TYPES OF JAUNDICE

Prehepatic jaundice

Prehepatic jaundice typically occurs due to haemolytic anaemia. Under normal circumstances, the majority of plasma bilirubin is derived from the catabolism of haemoglobin released from ageing or damaged red blood cells that are phagocytosed by macrophages in the liver and spleen. Acute haemolysis, especially intravascular haemolysis, may result in hyperbilirubinaemia due to overwhelming of normal metabolic pathways.

Intrahepatic (hepatocellular) jaundice

Hepatocytes take up albumin-bound unconjugated (free, indirect) bilirubin from the circulation and then excrete conjugated (direct) bilirubin into the bile canaliculi. The bilirubin then travels via the bile duct into the gut lumen. Hepatic diseases may cause intrahepatic impairment of bile flow (cholestasis). Causes of intrahepatic jaundice typically involve inflammation of the hepatobiliary system, both acute and chronic. Examples are listed in Box 18.1.

BOX 18.1 Some causes of hepatic (hepatocellular) jaundice

Dogs

- Cholangiohepatitis
- Chronic active hepatitis
- Cirrhosis/fibrosis
- Leptospirosis
- Neoplasia (primary, secondary)
- Copper-associated hepatitis in Bedlington terriers (and other breeds)
- Drug-induced or toxic hepatitis (e.g. anticonvulsants; paracetamol (acetaminophen))

Cats

- Feline cholangitis/cholangiohepatitis complex
- Hepatic lipidosis
- Neoplasia, especially lymphoma
- Feline infectious peritonitis (FIP)
- Drug-induced or toxic hepatitis (e.g. diazepam and other anticonvulsants; paracetamol (acetaminophen))
- Cirrhosis/fibrosis

Posthepatic jaundice

Posthepatic jaundice typically occurs due to obstruction of the larger bile ducts. This obstruction may be intraluminal or due to extraluminal compression and a combination may occur in any one case. The most common causes of posthepatic jaundice are pancreatitis and pancreatic neoplasia causing bile duct compression. Other causes include inflammatory disorders of the biliary system, and obstruction of bile flow due to inspissated bile or cholelithiasis. Biliary tract rupture may also cause posthepatic jaundice.

Case example 1

PRESENTING SIGNS AND CASE HISTORY

A 5-year-old female neutered English springer spaniel presented with a 24-hour history of progressive lethargy, weakness and inappetence. Her owner had also noted her to be jaundiced. No other significant history was reported. The dog had a complete vaccination history but had not been vaccinated recently, and she was not receiving any drug therapy.

Major body system examination

On presentation the dog was depressed but ambulatory and responsive. Cardiovascular examination revealed tachycardia (heart rate 190 beats per minute) but no murmur and femoral pulses were hyperdynamic (snappy) with no deficits. Mucous membranes were very pale and yellow with a capillary refill time of 1 second. The dog was tachypnoeic (respiratory rate 48 breaths per minute) but lung auscultation was appropriate for the rate and effort. Neurological examination and abdominal palpation were unremarkable and rectal temperature was within normal limits (38.4°C). The rest of the physical examination was unremarkable.

Assessment

The dog's marked pallor and tachycardia may have been due to severe anaemia and/or hypovolaemia. However, in severe hypovolaemia peripheral pulse quality would be expected to be much worse and capillary refill time much slower than detected. It was therefore suspected that the dog was severely anaemic and showing signs of cardiovascular compensation. The jaundice was therefore likely to be due predominantly to haemolysis (i.e. prehepatic) and the dog's breed raised the suspicion for immune-mediated haemolytic anaemia (IMHA).

Case management

An intravenous catheter was placed into a cephalic vein and blood taken via the catheter for an emergency database and in-house biochemistry profile. This showed severe anaemia (manual packed cell volume (PCV) 9%, reference range 37–55%) which was markedly regenerative on blood smear examination (marked polychromasia and anisocytosis; see Ch. 3). Moderate spherocytosis was also present and in-saline agglutination was strongly positive for auto-agglutination. Serum total solids (TS) were within normal limits, supporting haemolysis (as opposed to haemorrhage) as the cause of the regenerative anaemia. The biochemistry profile revealed severe hyperbilirubinaemia but was otherwise unremarkable, thereby reducing the likelihood of a hepatic or posthepatic component to the jaundice.

A diagnosis of IMHA and prehepatic jaundice was made and the dog went on to receive appropriate further investigations and management (see Ch. 33).

Case example 2

PRESENTING SIGNS AND CASE HISTORY

A 2-year-old female neutered Cocker Spaniel presented for severe vomiting. The dog had a 2-week history of occasional vomiting, reduced appetite, mild lethargy and weight loss, but the frequency of vomiting had worsened on the day of presentation. The vomitus consisted of dark brown liquid and undigested food. The dog was on a prescription diet for chronic intermittent diarrhoea but no other significant history was reported.

Major body system examination

On presentation the dog was bright and alert. Physical examination was unremarkable except for the presence of jaundice and the suspicion of mild dehydration.

Case management

The lack of pallor and the history in this case were suggestive of a hepatic or posthepatic cause of the jaundice. An intravenous catheter was placed into a cephalic vein and blood taken via the catheter for an emergency database and biochemistry profile. The emergency database showed high-normal PCV and TS suggestive of some dehydration but was otherwise unremarkable. The biochemistry profile revealed hyperbilirubinaemia (80 μmol/l, reference range 0–2.4 μmol/l), marked elevation in serum alanine aminotransferase (ALT) (2400 U/l, reference range 13–88 U/l) and moderate elevation in serum alkaline phosphatase (ALP) (1100 U/l, reference range 19–285 U/l).

A working diagnosis of hepatic jaundice with a possible posthepatic component was made and the dog was started on intravenous isotonic crystalloid therapy at 4 ml/kg/hr (this rate was calculated to achieve replacement of an estimated 5% dehydration over 24 hours; see Ch. 4). The dog was subsequently referred for further investigations that resulted in a diagnosis of acute idiopathic hepatitis.

CLINICAL TIP

- There are two main groups of serum enzymes that can be assessed in the evaluation of jaundice: one group (alanine aminotransferase (ALT), aspartate aminotransferase (AST)) reflects hepatocellular damage and consequent enzyme leakage, while release of the other group (alkaline phosphatase (ALP), gamma-glutamyl transferase (GGT)) into the bloodstream is increased by cholestasis.
- It is important to remember that the serum activities of these enzymes are not a reflection of liver function for which other parameters must be assessed (bilirubin, urea, glucose, albumin, cholesterol).

Case example 3

PRESENTING SIGNS AND CASE HISTORY

A 10-year-old female neutered Miniature Schnauzer presented with a several day history of vomiting, lethargy, depression and inappetence. The dog had a history of similar episodes that were milder and self-limiting. No other significant history was reported.

Major body system examination

On presentation the dog was depressed but responsive and ambulatory. Cardiovascular examination revealed tachycardia (heart rate 132 beats per minute) but was otherwise unremarkable. Mucous membranes and sclera were obviously jaundiced. The dog was panting incessantly and abdominal palpation was painful, especially in the mid-cranial region. Mild pyrexia was detected (rectal temperature 39.5°C).

Case management

The lack of pallor and the history in this case were suggestive of a hepatic or posthepatic cause of the jaundice. An intravenous catheter was placed into a cephalic vein and blood taken via the catheter for an emergency database and biochemistry profile. Given the dog's history, signalment, and the presence and location of abdominal pain, a sample was also submitted for measurement of canine pancreatic lipase (cPLI) concentration (in-house test not available).

The emergency database showed high-normal PCV and TS suggestive of some dehydration but was otherwise unremarkable. The biochemistry profile revealed marked hyperbilirubinaemia (250 μmol/l, reference range 0–2.4 μmol/l), and marked elevations in serum ALT (2200 U/l, reference range 13–88 U/l) and ALP (2900 U/l, reference range 19–285 U/l). Hypercholesterolaemia (20 mmol/l, reference range 3.3–8.9 mmol/l) was also identified.

Given the degree of elevation in ALP, it was suspected that there was a significant posthepatic component to the jaundice in this case. The dog was managed symptomatically and referred for abdominal ultrasonography that was compatible with acute pancreatitis with common and intrahepatic bile duct dilation secondary to obstruction. Secondary hepatitis was suspected. Pancreatitis was subsequently confirmed by significantly elevated cPLI concentration (600 μg/l, reference range less than 200 μg/l).

19 Pallor and approach to anaemia

PALLOR

Pallor of the mucous membranes is a common finding during major body system examination of dogs presenting as emergency patients. Pallor is harder to detect in cats but many of the points that follow are equally applicable. Pallor is most commonly the result of anaemia or vasoconstriction secondary to hypovolaemia and both processes may be present within the same patient. In addition, hypoperfusion due to cardiogenic or obstructive shock may also cause mucous membranes to appear pale, as can thermoregulatory vasoconstriction in hypothermia.

In many cases it will be possible on the basis of historical and physical examination findings to determine whether anaemia or hypovolaemia may be present. Concomitant hypovolaemia and anaemia are typically seen where anaemia is secondary to acute blood loss and the degree of pallor may be more severe than would otherwise be expected for the degree of hypovolaemia. It is important to remember that the packed cell volume may be normal for several hours following acute blood loss in dogs (but serum total solids should be low) (see Ch. 3).

Euvolaemic dogs with anaemia of sufficient severity are likely to show compensatory cardiovascular changes that may be distinguishable from hypovolaemia. In particular, capillary refill time (if detectable) is usually normal in euvolaemic anaemia. Euvolaemic dogs with acute anaemia may be distinguishable from chronically anaemic dogs as the former tend to be depressed or moribund while the latter are often remarkably bright (until a critical end-point is reached), having had time to adapt to the anaemia. In some cases anaemia is not identified until packed cell volume/haematocrit is measured.

ANAEMIA

A rational approach to the investigation of anaemia starts with classification of the anaemia as regenerative (due to red blood cell loss or destruction) or nonregenerative (due to reduced red blood cell production). In the emergency setting, this is done on the basis of peripheral blood smear examination, with regenerative anaemia being manifested as polychromasia, anisocytosis and a possible increase in nucleated red blood cells (see Figures 3.3 and 3.5). Regenerative anaemia occurs as a result of haemolysis or haemorrhage, and additional findings are used to determine which of these two processes is the likely cause (Figure 19.1).

> **CLINICAL TIP**
>
> - There is a lag phase following red blood cell loss/destruction such that a regenerative erythrocyte response can take 3–5 (or even 7) days to be detectable on peripheral blood smear examination. Thus an apparently nonregenerative anaemia may in fact be preregenerative, i.e. if insufficient time has passed since the inciting event for the regenerative response to be detectable.

Regenerative anaemia

Causes of regenerative anaemia are listed in Box 19.1.

Case example 1

> **PRESENTING SIGNS AND CASE HISTORY**
>
> An 8-year-old female neutered cross-bred dog presented for acute collapse. The owners reported a several week history of intermittent self-limiting lethargy.

Major body system examination

Major body system examination revealed the dog to be recumbent and depressed. Heart rate was 150 beats per

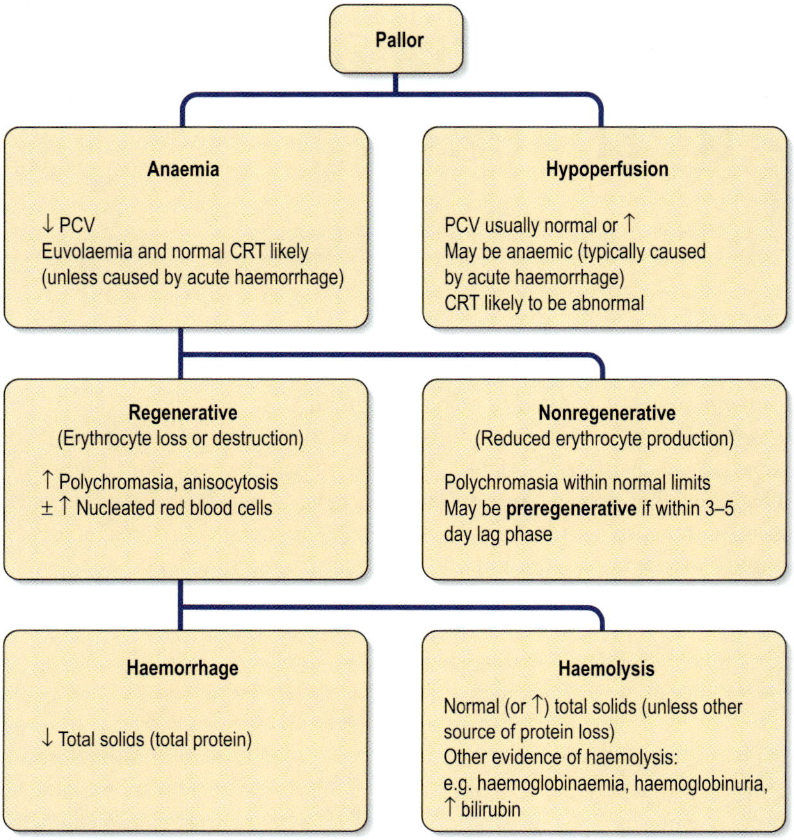

Figure 19.1 Algorithm for pallor and approach to anaemia. CRT, capillary refill time; PCV, packed cell volume.

minute with no murmur or gallop sound audible. Femoral pulse was (inappropriately) normal and no pulse deficits were detected; however, dorsal pedal pulse was only just palpable. Mucous membranes were markedly pale; capillary refill could only just be detected and took approximately 2 seconds. Respiratory rate was 36 breaths per minute with appropriate effort and auscultation. The abdomen was tense on palpation with a detectable fluid thrill. Rectal temperature was 38.5°C.

Assessment The cardiovascular assessment of this patient was consistent with moderate hypovolaemia in which mucous membranes are expected to appear inappropriately normal (i.e. pink) or perhaps mildly pale. The marked pallor in this case was therefore inconsistent with uncomplicated hypovolaemia and anaemia was therefore also suspected.

Case management

An intravenous catheter was placed in a cephalic vein and an emergency database performed that showed a manual packed cell volume (PCV) of 25% (normal range 37–55%). Serum total solids (TS) were also reduced (34 g/l, normal range 49–71 g/l) and anaemia secondary to blood loss was therefore suspected. Peripheral blood smear examination demonstrated a regenerative anaemia (moderate polychromasia and anisocytosis).

The dog was subsequently found to have a haemoabdomen that was the result of splenic rupture secondary to haemangiosarcoma (see Ch. 29).

Case example 2

PRESENTING SIGNS AND CASE HISTORY

A 6-year-old male neutered Cocker Spaniel presented with a 2-day history of progressive lethargy and inappetence. The dog had vomited twice the day before presentation.

BOX 19.1 *Causes of regenerative anaemia*

Haemorrhage

- Trauma (e.g. haemoabdomen, bleeding in/around pelvis, external blood loss)
- Surgery
- Neoplastic rupture (e.g. splenic haemangiosarcoma)
- Coagulopathy (e.g. anticoagulant rodenticide intoxication, immune-mediated thrombocytopenia, angiostrongylosis, congenital disorders)
- Gastrointestinal haemorrhage (e.g. gastric/duodenal ulceration, chronic occult haemorrhage from intestinal tumour, endoparasites)
- Severe flea (or lice) infestation

Haemolysis

Dogs

- Immune-mediated haemolytic anaemia (IMHA) – most common cause (especially primary IMHA)
- Infectious diseases (e.g. ehrlichiosis, babesiosis, mycoplasmosis, dirofilariasis)
- Intoxication (e.g. paracetamol (acetaminophen); members of *Allium* genus (e.g. onion, garlic); some heavy metals (e.g. zinc, lead, copper))
- Red blood cell membrane or enzyme defects (e.g. phosphofructokinase (PFK) deficiency (e.g. English springer spaniels); pyruvate kinase (PK) deficiency (e.g. Beagle, Basenji, West Highland White terrier, Abyssinian cats))
- Neonatal isoerythrolysis
- Blood transfusion reaction

Cats

- Infectious diseases: especially *Mycoplasma haemofelis,* feline leukaemia virus (FeLV), feline immunodeficiency virus (FIV)
- Intoxication (e.g. paracetamol (acetaminophen); members of *Allium* genus (e.g. onion, garlic))
- Immune-mediated haemolytic anaemia (IMHA) – less common than in dogs

Major body system examination

Major body system examination revealed the dog to be recumbent and depressed. Heart rate was 110 beats per minute with no murmur or gallop sound audible. Both femoral and dorsal pedal pulses were readily palpable and hyperdynamic with no deficits. Mucous membranes were pale and jaundiced with a normal capillary refill time. The rest of the major body system examination was unremarkable.

Assessment The dog was assessed as being euvolaemic and it was suspected that mucous membrane pallor was due to anaemia.

Case management

An intravenous catheter was placed in a cephalic vein and an emergency database performed that showed PCV 18% (37–55%) with normal serum TS 66 g/l (49–71 g/l) and icteric serum. Blood smear examination revealed a strongly regenerative anaemia (marked polychromasia, moderate anisocytosis) with moderate spherocytosis (see Figure 3.4) and in-saline agglutination testing was strongly positive. A diagnosis of immune-mediated haemolytic anaemia (IMHA) and prehepatic jaundice was made.

Nonregenerative anaemia

Causes of nonregenerative anaemia are listed in Box 19.2.

BOX 19.2 *Causes of nonregenerative anaemia*

- Anaemia of chronic disease/inflammation
- Chronic renal failure
- Endocrine disease (e.g. hypothyroidism, hypoadrenocorticism)
- Feline leukaemia virus-associated anaemia
- Bone marrow disorders
  - Pure red cell aplasia/erythroid hypoplasia
  - Aplastic anaemia
  - Myelodysplasia
  - Myeloproliferative disorders
  - Lymphoproliferative disorders
  - Myelofibrosis

Case example 3

PRESENTING SIGNS AND CASE HISTORY

A 6-year-old female neutered Boxer dog presented for self-limiting ataxia following a period of short exercise. This had occurred on two previous occasions in the preceding 2 weeks. The owners also reported progressive exercise intolerance over several weeks and that pallor of the mucous membranes had been present for some time.

Major body system examination

Major body system examination revealed the dog to be ambulatory and bright. Heart rate was 140 beats per minute and a grade II/VI systolic murmur was audible. Both femoral and dorsal pedal pulses were readily palpable and hyperdynamic with no deficits. Mucous membranes were pale with a normal capillary refill time. The rest of the major body system examination was unremarkable.

Assessment The dog was assessed as being euvolaemic and it was suspected that mucous membrane pallor was due to anaemia.

Case management

An intravenous catheter was placed in a cephalic vein and an emergency database performed that showed PCV 16% (37–55%), serum TS 60 g/l (49–71 g/l) and nonregenerative anaemia on blood smear examination. Subsequently a diagnosis of pure red cell aplasia was made on bone marrow sampling.

20 Pelvic limb paresis and paralysis

CAUSES OF ACUTE NONAMBULATORY PARAPARESIS/PARAPLEGIA

Paraparesis and paraplegia most commonly occur as a result of a spinal cord lesion caudal to the C6–T2 segment (cervicothoracic intumescence). Spinal cord disorders that commonly cause paraparesis or paraplegia are listed in Box 20.1. In some cases spinal cord injury is due to a cause with an acute onset (e.g. traumatic disc injury, fibrocartilaginous embolism) while in others it occurs due to acute deterioration of a more chronic disease (e.g. neoplasia).

APPROACH TO ACUTE NONAMBULATORY PARAPARESIS/PARAPLEGIA

Signalment

Signalment may allow certain differential diagnoses to be viewed with a lesser or greater index of suspicion. For example, chondrodystrophic dog breeds (e.g. Dachshunds, Pekingese) are classically affected by Hansen type I intervertebral disc disease, inflammatory disease is more common in younger dogs and neoplasia is more common in older dogs. Spinal lymphoma is always a differential diagnosis in cats.

> ***BOX 20.1 Common causes of acute pelvic limb paresis and paralysis***
>
> - Type I intervertebral disc protrusion
> - Trauma: vertebral fracture, vertebral luxation/subluxation
> - Fibrocartilaginous embolism (FCE)
> - Inflammatory central nervous system diseases (e.g. granulomatous meningoencephalomyelitis (GME))
> - Discospondylitis
> - Neoplasia
> - Aortic thromboembolism (typically cats)
> - Spontaneous spinal cord haemorrhage (e.g. canine angiostrongylosis)

History

History may be useful with respect to establishing the likely differential diagnoses, in particular for traumatic causes. A chronic history of intermittent pelvic limb neurological abnormalities prior to acute deterioration may be more suggestive for example of neoplasia.

The owner should also be asked about urination following onset of clinical signs as this may help to localize the lesion more accurately.

Major body system examination

> ***CLINICAL TIP***
>
> - The pelvic limbs are intuitively the focus of the physical examination in animals with paraparesis or paraplegia. However, it is important to remember that paraparesis and paraplegia in themselves are not life-threatening conditions and assessment of cardiovascular status, respiratory status, mentation and pain should be prioritized. Life-threatening abnormalities, typically the result of trauma in these cases, should be addressed first.

In the absence of traumatic injury, physical examination findings may help to raise the index of suspicion for certain differential diagnoses. For example, pyrexia may be more suggestive of an inflammatory cause rather than intervertebral disc disease. Gait assessment and testing of postural reactions are clearly not applicable to animals with nonambulatory paraparesis or paraplegia.

Neurological examination of the pelvic limbs in such cases incorporates the following:

- Assessment of deep pain perception: this is a useful prognostic indicator in spinal cord disease. Deep pain perception is confirmed as a conscious response (e.g. head turning, trying to bite, growling) to a painful stimulus and must be differentiated from limb withdrawal which only requires an intact local flexor reflex. The withdrawal reflex assesses the integrity of the L4–S2 spinal cord segments and their associated nerve roots, as well as the femoral and sciatic nerves.
- Spinal reflexes, typically patellar reflex: may be normal, hyperreflexive (upper motor neuron) or hyporeflexive (lower motor neuron).
- Spinal palpation: normal or painful depending on lesion; intervertebral disc disease, inflammatory causes and traumatic injuries are often painful, while fibrocartilaginous embolism is typically considered nonpainful. Neoplasia may or may not cause spinal hyperaesthesia.
- Urinary bladder palpation/expression: may be large and difficult to express (upper motor neuron) or easy to express (lower motor neuron).
- Perineal reflex: present (upper motor neuron) or reduced to absent (lower motor neuron).
- Muscle tone: normal, spasticity (increased extensor tone; upper motor neuron) or flaccidity (absence of normal tone; lower motor neuron).

CLINICAL TIP

- Assessment of pelvic limb deep pain perception is essential. Deep pain perception is confirmed as a conscious response to a painful stimulus (e.g. head turning, trying to bite, growling) and must be differentiated from limb withdrawal which only requires an intact local flexor reflex. It is crucial to remember this distinction as deep pain perception is the most important prognostic indicator available on the basis of physical examination.
- The prognosis in animals that lack deep pain perception varies depending on the underlying cause but is often poor. Rapid surgical intervention in animals with intervertebral disc disease may, however, result in a successful outcome. These cases require immediate referral.

Potentially the most important decision that needs to be made by the primary clinician following neurological examination is whether the animal requires immediate referral for advanced diagnostic imaging and surgical intervention if indicated, or whether referral can be delayed for a short period (e.g. overnight). Absent or severely reduced deep pain perception is typically interpreted as an indication for immediate referral.

CLINICAL TIP

- Following initial stabilization of life-threatening abnormalities if present, animals with paraparesis/paraplegia typically require referral for advanced diagnostic imaging and then surgical intervention or conservative management.
- The primary clinician seeing the case as an emergency must to be able to differentiate between those cases that require immediate referral – typically animals that have absent or severely reduced deep pain perception – from those that may be able to wait for a short period of time prior to referral. An incorrect decision in this respect can have potentially disastrous consequences.

Emergency database

The need to perform an emergency database in an animal with nonambulatory paraparesis or paraplegia should be guided by the historical and examination findings in each individual case. Indications for performing an emergency database would include animals presenting with cardiovascular compromise, typically as a result of trauma, or those with a more protracted history of illness. Manual packed cell volume, serum total solids and peripheral blood smear examination are important in animals suspected to have suffered haemorrhage.

Diagnostic imaging

Animals presenting following external trauma require emergency diagnostic imaging of the thoracic and peritoneal cavities at the appropriate time. Plain lateral spinal radiographs performed under sedation may help to identify obvious vertebral luxations/subluxations or fractures (Figure 20.1). However, these abnormalities can sometimes be subtle and may not be detected unless orthogonal views are obtained. Lateral views should always be obtained first. If a fracture or luxation is identified on

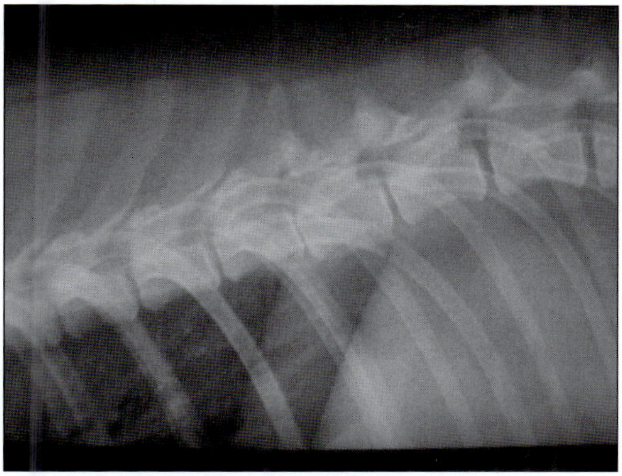

Figure 20.1 Right lateral spinal radiograph of a dog showing subluxation of the T10–T11 intervertebral joint. (Photograph courtesy of Holger Volk)

the lateral view, an orthogonal view should not be taken; the animal should be immobilized as quickly as possible and prepared for referral.

CLINICAL TIP

- All animals presenting with nonambulatory paraparesis or paraplegia following trauma should be handled very carefully until a diagnosis can be obtained in order to minimize the risk of further displacing possible vertebral luxations or fractures.

Myelography is the only additional diagnostic imaging modality that may be available in some nonreferral practices for investigations of spinal cord disorders. In general, however, the author does not believe that animals should be anaesthetized for myelography unless surgical intervention can be offered under the same episode of anaesthesia if required.

CLINICAL TIP

- The author does not believe that in general it is appropriate to anaesthetize animals for investigation of nonambulatory paraparesis or paraplegia unless it is possible to offer surgical intervention if required under the same episode of anaesthesia. Such cases should be referred

CLINICAL TIP—cont'd

instead to a hospital able to offer both investigations and intervention.

- In particular, the author has seen a number of cases that have been anaesthetized for myelography in practices that were unable to offer surgical intervention. Aside from the additional episode of general anaesthesia that could be avoided, it must also be remembered that myelography is not a benign investigation (possible complications include seizures, cardiorespiratory abnormalities and deterioration of neurological signs) and is also no longer considered the gold standard imaging modality for investigation of spinal disorders; financial constraints may, however, clearly influence decision-making.

Treatment

As always the priority in animals presenting following trauma is to address life-threatening injuries that may exist alongside the spinal cord disorder. Correction of systemic hypoperfusion (see Ch. 2) and ensuring adequate oxygenation (see Ch. 6) will also serve to minimize secondary spinal cord injury. Following injury, the spinal cord is even more dependent on adequate systemic perfusion and oxygen delivery. Many of the principles are the same as those described for traumatic brain injury (see Ch. 28).

In the absence of a definitive diagnosis, treatment of paraparesis or paraplegia thereafter centres on analgesia if indicated and other stabilization measures as appropriate prior to referral. Pure opioids (see Ch. 5) are the analgesic agents indicated initially and nonsteroidal anti-inflammatory agents should not be administered to hypovolaemic or dehydrated animals, or those suspected of having a coagulation defect. The use of methylprednisolone succinate (or any other corticosteroid) is no longer recommended in spinal cord injury and is to be strongly discouraged. Nonsteroidal anti-inflammatory agents should definitely not be administered to animals that have been treated with a corticosteroid due to a significant risk of gastrointestinal injury and haemorrhage.

Animals that have suffered traumatic spinal injury should be transported under controlled conditions, ideally strapped on to a rigid flat surface (e.g. purpose-built stretcher, large plank of wood, suitcase). Adequate chemical restraint in the form of opioid analgesia with or without additional sedation should be provided to ensure the animal remains calm en route.

Subsequent treatment of nonambulatory paraparesis or paraplegia following diagnosis may include surgical intervention or conservative management, with or without long-term analgesia and other medical therapies.

CLINICAL TIP

- The use of methylprednisolone succinate for spinal cord injury was a longstanding practice in both human and veterinary medicine. However, it was not based on robust clinical evidence and is no longer recommended as the standard of care in human medicine.

CLINICAL TIP—cont'd

  Considering the potential adverse effects (e.g. gastrointestinal ulceration, increased risk of infection, hyperglycaemia), current recommendations are that methylprednisolone succinate (or any other exogenous corticosteroid) should not be used for spinal cord injury.
- The reader is alerted to the fact that some popular drug formularies and texts continue erroneously to recommend the use of corticosteroids for spinal cord injury, mainly because some of these agents remain licensed for this purpose despite current recommendations.

21 Petechiae and ecchymoses

Petechiae and ecchymoses represent superficial bleeding into the skin or mucous membranes. Petechiae are small pinpoint haemorrhages and ecchymoses are larger areas. Petechiae are more commonly identified in mucous membranes, especially the buccal and gingival mucosa, the prepuce and the vulva. Ecchymoses may be more evident following venepuncture. Ecchymoses are sometimes difficult to distinguish from cutaneous erythema on inspection; however, this is readily achieved by pressing a glass slide on to the affected area – an erythematous lesion will blanch but an ecchymosis will not. Petechiae and ecchymoses are rare in cats.

CAUSES OF PETECHIAE AND ECCHYMOSES

Petechiae and ecchymoses are typically the result of severe thrombocytopenia, platelet function disorders, or a localized or systemic vasculopathy. Thrombocytopenia is the most common cause in companion animals, and there may be other signs of haemorrhage such as epistaxis, melaena (see Figure 9.1), haematuria and active gingival bleeding.

CLINICAL TIP

- Traditionally petechiae and ecchymoses were said to be the result of disorders affecting so-called primary haemostasis, while conditions involving coagulation factor deficiencies (e.g. anticoagulant rodenticide intoxication, liver failure) were said to cause disorders in secondary haemostasis.
- Coagulation factor disorders typically present differently from platelet or vascular disorders, with bleeding occurring more commonly into body cavities or as haematomas rather than as mucosal or cutaneous haemorrhage; these animals are also more likely to bleed excessively following venepuncture.
- Although in recent years it has been shown that the traditional classification of coagulation is too simplistic in vivo, the distinction remains very important to avoid misdiagnosis and inappropriate investigation. In particular, the author is aware of many dogs with petechiae that have been erroneously investigated or treated for anticoagulant rodenticide intoxication that is extremely unlikely to present in this way.

Thrombocytopenia

The possibility of spontaneous haemorrhage is said to arise when total platelet count falls below 30×10^9 platelets/litre. On peripheral blood smear examination, this equates approximately to two platelets per high power (×1000) field. However, it must be remembered firstly that this is only a guideline, and secondly that not all animals with this level of thrombocytopenia will necessarily suffer bleeding.

In the author's experience, clinically significant haemorrhage associated with thrombocytopenia is most commonly the result of primary (idiopathic) immune-mediated thrombocytopenia (ITP) (see Ch. 33). It is also noteworthy that thrombocytopenia secondary to haemorrhage is extremely unlikely to be sufficiently severe as to induce further bleeding.

Platelet function disorders

Platelet function disorders may be inherited or acquired. Inherited thrombopathies have been identified in several dog breeds (e.g. the Bassett hound, the Otter hound, the American Cocker Spaniel) and also a small number of cats. Acquired disorders may potentially occur for example due to uraemia, liver disease or various drug therapies.

Von Willebrand disease (vWD) is the most common inherited bleeding disorder in dogs. This disease most commonly presents with bleeding from mucosal surfaces (e.g. epistaxis, melaena and haematuria) and excessive bleeding following surgery or other trauma. However, ecchymoses (and petechiae) may occasionally occur. Type I vWD (reduced but measurable levels of vWF) is the most common and is seen especially in the Doberman Pinscher.

Vasculopathy

Vasculitis may occur as part of the syndrome associated with a number of infections, tumours, immune-mediated disorders and drug reactions. Pyrexia, oedema and multiorgan signs are likely.

APPROACH TO PETECHIAE AND ECCHYMOSES

Signalment

Signalment may help to raise or lower the index of suspicion for certain differential diagnoses. In particular, ITP is seen most commonly in female dogs and an increased incidence is reported in a number of breeds (e.g. the Cocker Spaniel, poodles, the Old English Sheepdog); this disorder is relatively rare in cats.

History

The history in animals with petechiae and ecchymoses is variable depending on the underlying cause. Some animals have nonspecific signs such as lethargy and inappetence, and present primarily for investigation of bleeding. In other cases, other clinical signs associated with the primary disorder are more significant (e.g. jaundice with leptospirosis) and petechiae or ecchymoses are identified almost incidentally.

A complete medical history, with particular focus on vaccination, drug administration and travel, is essential, and all current or previous medical problems should be explored. In particular, the owner should be asked about any previous episodes potentially consistent with coagulopathy, as well as whether there is a history of excessive bleeding following surgical or nonsurgical trauma.

Major body system examination

Physical examination findings vary in animals with petechiae or ecchymoses, depending on the extent and sites of the bleeding and the underlying disorder. In some cases, evidence of external haemorrhage is the most remarkable finding; in addition to petechiae or ecchymoses, there may also be epistaxis, gingival haemorrhage, subcutaneous haematomas and melaena on rectal examination (see Figure 9.1). Animals with gastrointestinal haemorrhage may suffer severe blood loss and may present with findings consistent with clinically significant anaemia (tachycardia, hyperdynamic pulses, tachypnoea; lethargy, depression). In a multisystemic disorder such as leptospirosis, evidence of bleeding is likely to be only one of the significant abnormal findings on physical examination.

Emergency database

CLINICAL TIP

- Extra care with venepuncture is required in animals with petechiae or ecchymoses where a systemic coagulopathy is suspected. These findings are not an absolute contraindication to the use of the jugular vein but it is recommended to use a peripheral vein as much as possible.
- Venepuncture should be performed by experienced personnel, using a small needle, and with prolonged pressure over the site following sampling. Subcutaneous and intramuscular injections should be minimized.

An emergency database should be performed in all animals presenting with petechiae or ecchymoses. An indwelling intravenous catheter is likely to be required in most of these cases and the emergency database is therefore usually performed on blood obtained via the catheter at the time of placement. The emergency database must include peripheral blood smear examination as this is the most reliable means of identifying severe thrombocytopenia (see Ch. 3). Reduced serum total solids and manual packed cell volume are suggestive of anaemia secondary to haemorrhage, and a regenerative anaemia (anisocytosis, polychromasia, increase in nucleated red blood cells) may be seen on smear examination in such cases.

Animals with petechiae or ecchymoses primarily as a result of platelet dysfunction may have a normal platelet count or only mild thrombocytopenia. Platelet function is very difficult to assess reliably in routine practice but measurement of buccal mucosal bleeding time (BMBT) is typically used. The results of this test can be quite discrepant depending on the individual performing the test, the technique (including restraint) used, and the patient's haematocrit. Nevertheless, a severely prolonged BMBT in an animal without severe thrombocytopenia is likely to suggest a clinically significant platelet function disorder, vWD or vasculopathy. Normal BMBT in dogs and cats is generally considered to be less than 4 minutes and less than 2 minutes, respectively.

CLINICAL TIP

- There is no rationale for performing a buccal mucosal bleeding time (BMBT) in an animal with (severe) thrombocytopenia and excessive haemorrhage may occur in such cases.

Treatment

Treatment in animals with petechiae or ecchymoses is aimed at the underlying cause.

22 Regurgitation

Regurgitation is the passive expulsion of oesophageal or gastric contents from the oral cavity, and is most commonly the result of oesophageal disease. Regurgitation is the most common sign of, but not pathognomonic for, oesophageal disease, and other differential diagnoses, in particular pharyngeal disorders, must be considered. There are a large number of possible causes of regurgitation; some of the more common are listed in Box 22.1. In the author's experience, megaoesophagus and oesophageal foreign bodies are the most common reasons for regurgitation in emergency patients.

CLINICAL TIP

- Regurgitation must be differentiated from vomiting in particular by careful history-taking and sometimes actually observing the behaviour. A comparison of the main distinguishing features is presented in Table 22.1. Occasionally an animal may demonstrate both regurgitation and vomiting (e.g. with a sliding hiatal hernia).
- Signs consistent with possible oesophageal discomfort (e.g. pain on swallowing, repeated swallowing, arching of neck) are more suggestive of oesophagitis or foreign body obstruction rather than megaoesophagus.

CLINICAL TIP

- The airway is unprotected by the epiglottis during regurgitation and therefore there is a risk of inhalation. Aspiration pneumonia is a common and potentially life-threatening complication.

APPROACH TO REGURGITATION

Signalment

Signalment may help to raise or lower the index of suspicion for certain differential diagnoses. Puppies with

BOX 22.1 Causes of regurgitation related to the oesophagus

Oesophageal obstruction

- Especially foreign body
- Stricture
- Congenital vascular ring anomaly
- Neoplasia
- Extraluminal compression (e.g. mediastinal or cervical mass)
- Hiatal hernia

Oesophagitis

- Gastro-oesophageal reflux (e.g. general anaesthesia, hiatal hernia)
- Drug-related (especially doxycycline)
- Dietary indiscretion (e.g. ingestion of caustic or corrosive substance)
- Secondary to oesophageal disease (e.g. foreign body, megaoesophagus)

Idiopathic (primary) megaoesophagus, congenital or acquired

Secondary megaoesophagus

- Myasthenia gravis, especially focal but also generalized
- Generalized neuromuscular disease
- Neuropathy, peripheral or central
- Hypothyroidism
- Hypoadrenocorticism

Table 22.1 Comparison of regurgitation and vomiting

Regurgitation	Vomiting
No prodromal signs; signs associated with pain may mimic nausea	Prodromal signs of nausea (e.g. hypersalivation, restlessness)
Passive (no abdominal contractions); postural changes associated with pain possible (e.g. stretching neck)	Active with abdominal contractions
No consistent relationship with feeding	No consistent relationship with feeding
Undigested (or digested) food, or liquid; undigested food often tubular in shape	Digested food
No bile but may contain frothy saliva	Bile may be present

regurgitation are most likely to be suffering from congenital abnormalities, especially vascular ring anomaly (often present soon after weaning) and idiopathic megaoesophagus. Oesophageal foreign bodies are more common in smaller dogs, while some breeds (e.g. Golden Retrievers, German Shepherd dogs) are at increased risk of megaoesophagus (see below).

History

It is important to question the owner carefully for a good description of the animal's behaviour in order to differentiate regurgitation from vomiting and even retching or gagging (see Table 22.1). Other signs consistent with oesophageal disease may also be present and include hypersalivation, pain on eating and dysphagia. A history of coughing or respiratory abnormalities may suggest aspiration pneumonia.

In addition, the animal may be exhibiting other clinical signs that will help to raise the index of suspicion for localized versus generalized causes. There may also be a history of recent general anaesthesia or drug administration, or a witnessed or suspected episode of ingestion of an irritant substance.

Major body system examination

Physical examination findings are largely dependent on the underlying cause and may be completely normal in animals with localized oesophageal disease. Respiratory examination may be abnormal in animals with aspiration pneumonia (e.g. dyspnoea, harsh lung sounds, crackles); in severe cases there may be evidence of systemic cardiovascular compromise (sepsis) and possibly pyrexia. Signs of systemic disease, in particular neuromuscular, may be present in some cases, and weight loss occurs with chronic regurgitation. Puppies with congenital abnormalities are often thin and stunted.

Emergency database

The emergency database may well be unremarkable in a number of animals with regurgitation. Manual packed cell volume and serum total solids may be consistent with dehydration in some cases. Peripheral blood smear examination may demonstrate leucocytosis consistent with inflammatory disease, including moderate to severe oesophagitis, and neutrophils may show toxic changes and band forms with aspiration pneumonia (see Ch. 3). Megaoesophagus is occasionally identified in animals with hypoadrenocorticism (Addison's disease, see Ch. 34) and consistent abnormalities may be identified (hyponatraemia, hyperkalaemia, hypoglycaemia, azotaemia; lack of stress leucogram).

Diagnostic imaging

Plain thoracic radiographs (typically right lateral and dorsoventral (or left lateral) views) are useful in animals with regurgitation and may help to identify megaoesophagus, radiopaque oesophageal foreign bodies, aspiration pneumonia and mediastinal masses (Figures 22.1–22.3).

If megaoesophagus is considered a significant possibility, radiographs should be taken without sedation or general anaesthesia. Aspiration pneumonia is most commonly identified as an alveolar pattern with air bronchograms in the right middle lung lobe and ventral parts of the other lobes, especially cranioventrally (Figure 22.3). Radiographs must not be prioritized over oxygen therapy and cardiovascular stabilization in animals with severe dyspnoea at presentation and these animals should be subjected to minimum stress.

Most oesophageal foreign bodies diagnosed in dogs are radiopaque (e.g. bones, fish hooks). Occasionally a lodged foreign body causes oesophageal perforation or rupture that may be identified radiographically as pneumomediastinum (possibly with pneumothorax) (Figure 22.4). Small volume pneumomediastinum is most often identified as gas lucency within the mediastinum that outlines the tracheal wall.

If plain radiographs do not provide a diagnosis, contrast radiography may be employed. A water-soluble

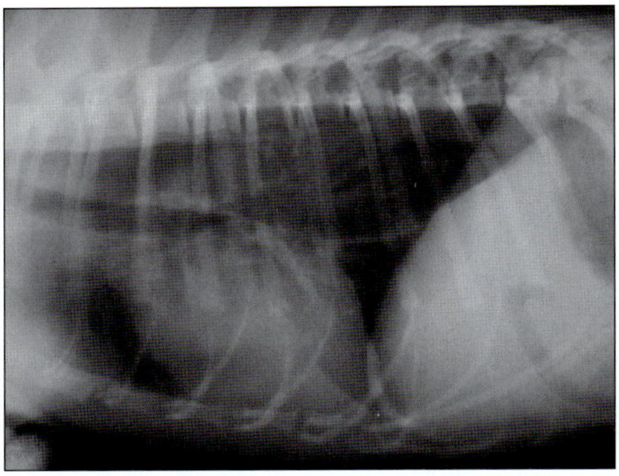

Figure 22.1 Right lateral thoracic radiograph in a dog showing megaoesophagus secondary to myasthenia gravis.

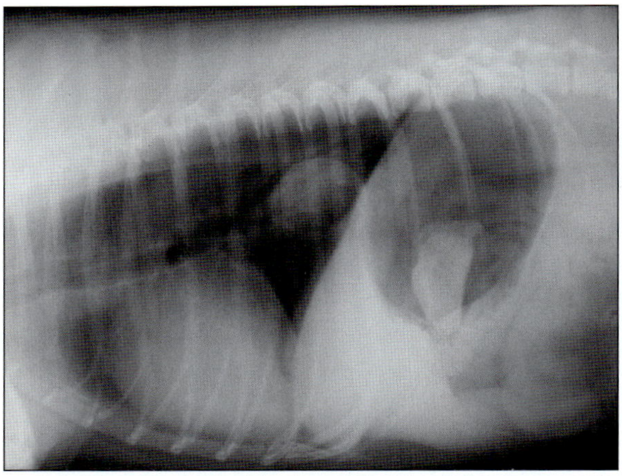

Figure 22.2 Right lateral thoracic radiograph in a dog showing a distal oesophageal foreign body (bone). Oesophageal dilation is present and a bone is also visible in the stomach.

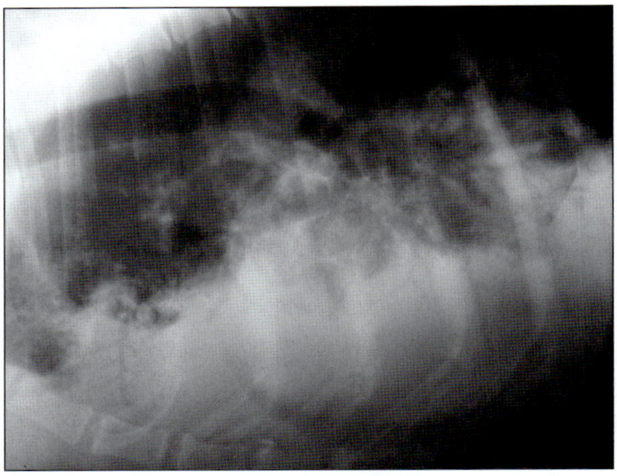

(a)

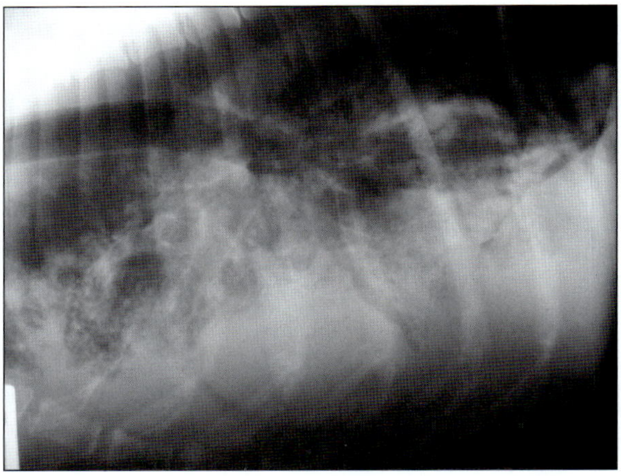

(b)

Figure 22.3 (a) Right lateral and (b) left lateral thoracic radiographs in a dog with severe aspiration pneumonia. Multiple air bronchograms are clearly visible in the ventral lung fields.

contrast medium should be used in animals in which oesophageal rupture or aspiration is considered likely as the presence of barium in the lungs or mediastinum can induce marked chronic inflammation. Liquid contrast medium may delineate the oesophagus or confirm the presence of a radiolucent foreign body. A barium meal can be helpful to identify megaoesophagus or vascular ring anomalies, strictures and extraluminal compression. Barium meals should not be attempted in animals that may have compromised swallowing, either due to dysphagia or severe morbidity.

Some animals require referral for more advanced imaging, fluoroscopy in particular.

Endoscopy

Endoscopy can be extremely useful in oesophageal diseases allowing diagnosis of mural and intraluminal lesions as well as sites of extraluminal compression. It also allows therapeutic interventions, especially foreign body removal (Figure 22.5).

Treatment

Treatment of regurgitation centres on addressing the underlying disorder if possible and an extensive discussion is beyond the scope of this book. Successful management of the primary disorder may or may not resolve clinical signs of oesophageal disease, especially if

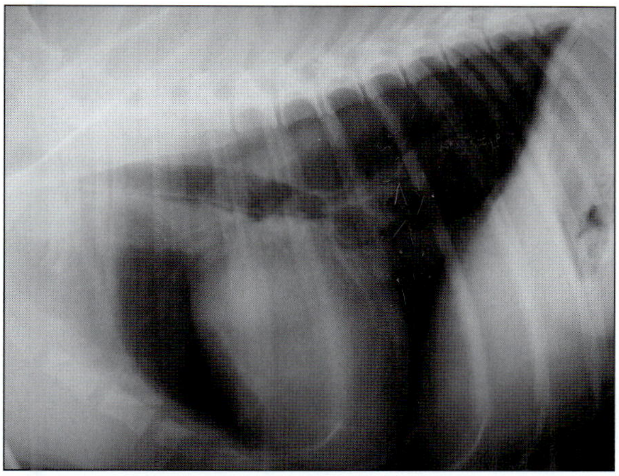

Figure 22.4 Right lateral thoracic radiograph in a dog showing air in the mediastinum highlighting the tracheal wall.

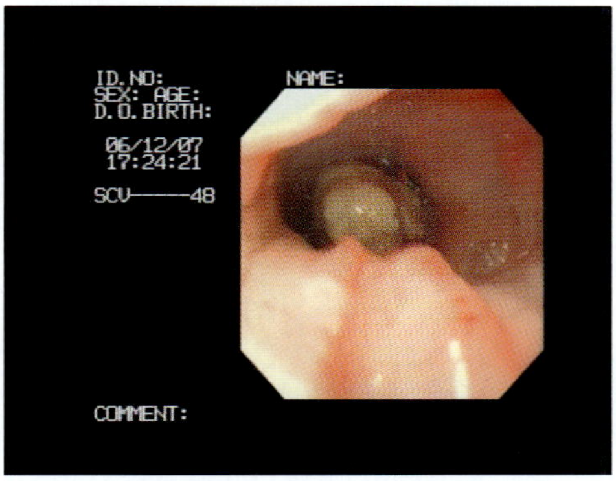

Figure 22.5 Endoscopic appearance of an oesophageal bone in a dog.

severe oesophagitis is present. Treatment of oesophagitis may include administration of sucralfate and reducing gastric acidity. The latter is ideally achieved through the use of a proton pump inhibitor such as omeprazole; however, a histamine (H_2) receptor antagonist (e.g. ranitidine, famotidine) may be used if omeprazole is not available.

Aspiration pneumonia

Aspiration pneumonia typically requires aggressive intervention that is tailored to the circumstances of the individual patient. Broad-spectrum antibiosis is essential and is typically given intravenously initially; subsequent enteral antibiosis may need to be continued for several weeks. Appropriate choices initially include amoxicillin/clavulanic acid or a cephalosporin; ideally this should be reassessed on the basis of culture and sensitivity results obtained from samples collected via transtracheal aspiration, tracheal wash or bronchoalveolar lavage. Fluid therapy may be required to address systemic hypoperfusion in severe cases, as well as for rehydration and maintenance purposes. The need for oxygen therapy should be decided on the basis of the severity of respiratory compromise and pulse oximetry (or arterial blood gas analysis). Regular nebulization (without coupage) and gentle exercise are also important.

MEGAOESOPHAGUS

Megaoesophagus is characterized by generalized dilation of the oesophagus with lack of peristalsis. Both congenital and acquired forms are recognized. Congenital megaoesophagus is most commonly idiopathic or due to a vascular ring anomaly. Animals with vascular ring anomalies often present shortly after being weaned on to solid food, at which time the oesophageal obstruction becomes more obvious. Megaoesophagus in older animals is most commonly idiopathic but may be acquired as a secondary abnormality of a number of disorders; focal myasthenia gravis is the most common.

A number of dog breeds appear predisposed to vascular ring anomalies; for example the German Shepherd dog and the Irish Setter are predisposed to persistent right aortic arch. Vascular ring anomalies are less common in cats. A number of canine breeds are predisposed to congenital idiopathic megaoesophagus, including the Great Dane, the German Shepherd dog, the Irish Setter, the Labrador retriever and the Shar-pei. Congenital idiopathic megaoesophagus is rare in cats but the Siamese may be predisposed. Idiopathic megaoesophagus in adult dogs is seen more commonly in certain breeds, including the golden retriever and the German shepherd dog.

Megaoesophagus is usually readily diagnosed by plain radiography although occasionally a contrast study may be required (see Figure 22.1). The dilated oesophagus may be filled with air, fluid or ingesta. As described above, aspiration pneumonia is the most common complication of megaoesophagus and may be detected radiographically. Once the diagnosis is made, additional tests are indicated to screen for a primary underlying cause.

> **CLINICAL TIP**
>
> - Sedation and general anaesthesia can both cause oesophageal relaxation that may be misdiagnosed as megaoesophagus on plain thoracic radiographs. If megaoesophagus is considered a significant possibility, radiographs should be taken without sedation.

Treatment of megaoesophagus centres on addressing an underlying cause if one is identified. Animals with idiopathic megaoesophagus or in which megaoesophagus does not resolve despite treatment of the underlying disorder require long-term symptomatic and supportive care. Controlled feeding is often the mainstay of management and usually involves feeding small frequent meals (e.g. four to six meals per day) of a high calorie diet from a height and then maintaining the animal in an erect posture for 10–15 minutes if possible. It is noteworthy that some animals do better with food moulded into balls while gruel works better in others; dietary consistency must therefore be tailored to the individual patient. Treatment of aspiration pneumonia may be required as described above and in some animals long-term feeding via gastrostomy tube may be the only option.

OESOPHAGEAL FOREIGN BODIES

A variety of objects may become lodged in the oesophagus. Bones (especially lamb and chicken) are undoubtedly the most common culprits but others include fishing hooks, balls, toys and dental chews.

Signalment

Oesophageal foreign bodies appear to be a more common problem in certain dog breeds and the majority of affected dogs are small. In the author's experience in the United Kingdom, terriers appear at increased risk and in particular the West Highland White terrier. Oesophageal foreign body obstruction is rare in cats. Most dogs with oesophageal foreign body obstruction are young to middle-aged.

History

In the author's experience, in most cases there is a reported history of the dog either having been fed or having scavenged a foreign body. However, not all cases present acutely and clinical signs may have been present for several days or even 2–3 weeks before dogs are presented. Sometimes it is only following diagnosis that owners remember the exact episode when the foreign body was ingested.

Clinical signs of oesophageal foreign body obstruction include regurgitation or vomiting, retching, gagging and hypersalivation. Dogs may be anorexic, may approach the food and then turn away, or may attempt to eat with subsequent pain on swallowing and/or dysphagia. Repeated gulping or swallowing, restlessness, distress, coughing and increased respiratory effort may also be reported.

Major body system examination, emergency database

Physical examination and the emergency database may be unremarkable in dogs with oesophageal foreign body obstruction. In some cases there is evidence of nonspecific pain on examination and the author has also occasionally identified respiratory abnormalities. Very occasionally it is possible to palpate foreign bodies lodged in the cervical oesophagus from the outside. Fishing line may be identified trapped around the tongue base in dogs that have ingested a fishing hook. Dehydration may be identified on examination and emergency database.

Diagnostic imaging

In the author's experience, the vast majority of oesophageal foreign bodies are radiopaque enough to be detected on plain radiographs; however, occasionally contrast radiography or endoscopy is required. The most common site of foreign body entrapment is the caudal oesophagus between the heart base and the cardiac sphincter (see Figure 22.2). In addition to the foreign body itself, plain radiographs often demonstrate increased soft tissue density around the foreign body and air in the oesophagus.

Plain radiographs are also useful to exclude pneumomediastinum (and possible pneumothorax) as a result of oesophageal rupture, and to identify evidence of aspiration pneumonia.

Treatment

> **CLINICAL TIP**
>
> - In the author's experience, the incidence of oesophageal perforation or rupture in dogs with foreign body obstructions is very small, either as a result of the foreign body or due to

CLINICAL TIP—cont'd

iatrogenic injury during removal. The potential consequences can, however, be rapidly disastrous and there is therefore perhaps an argument for referral of all dogs with oesophageal foreign body obstruction to a hospital where immediate surgical intervention can be offered if required. However, there are clear financial and practical considerations in this respect and the decision should therefore be made on an individual case basis in discussion with the owner.

Oesophageal foreign body obstruction should be treated as an emergency and removal should be undertaken as soon as any initial stabilization that may be required has been performed. On-going obstruction is associated with an increased risk of oesophageal rupture, stricture formation and aspiration pneumonia. Damage to the wall of the oesophagus depends on the type, size and sharpness of the foreign body, and the duration of obstruction. If facilities or expertise are not available to perform removal in-house, immediate referral should be arranged. It is essential to ensure that animals that have been anaesthetized for radiography are adequately recovered before being transported.

Treatment of oesophageal foreign body obstruction involves removal of the foreign body from the oesophagus. The author uses flexible endoscopy for this purpose but some clinicians prefer to use fluoroscopic guidance. The foreign body is removed orally, typically using large rigid grasping forceps but occasionally other types of forceps are required. The oesophageal mucosa is evaluated at the time of removal for the severity of injury that will both help to guide the length of any subsequent medical therapy and potentially inform on the risk of possible stricture formation.

CLINICAL TIP

- Insufflation with air is usually required to facilitate endoscopic oesophageal foreign body removal and results in gastric distension that may compromise respiratory function under anaesthesia. It is essential to monitor this closely (including using pulse oximetry if available) and decompress the stomach via endoscopic suction or external manual pressure as necessary.

Occasionally it is not possible to remove the foreign body orally, even in little pieces, and it has to be pushed into the stomach. Many foreign objects will then either dissolve over time or go on to be passed in the faeces; occasionally, however, surgical removal via gastrotomy is required. Very occasionally oesophagotomy (or gastrotomy for very distal oesophageal foreign bodies) is required as the foreign body cannot be dislodged in either direction; however, in the author's experience, this is rare.

The author typically takes plain radiographs following removal to check for the presence of pneumomediastinum suggestive of oesophageal rupture during removal. If there is any doubt, a positive contrast oesophagram using water-soluble contrast medium may be helpful although interpretation may be difficult. Surgical repair via thoracotomy is traditionally required if rupture occurs given the risks of mediastinitis and pleuritis. However, if financial constraints preclude this intervention, some dogs may recover fully with prolonged antibiosis; prognosis for recovery is likely to be related to the extent of leakage.

Management following removal is guided by the findings in each individual case. In some cases, no additional medical therapy is required and the dogs can be discharged once they have fully recovered from the procedure and demonstrated an interest in food. In other cases, hospitalization for on-going analgesia (typically buprenorphine) and intravenous fluid therapy may be indicated for 24–48 hr. Medical therapy for oesophageal mucosal injury and oesophagitis may include sucralfate, omeprazole and/or a histamine (H_2) receptor antagonist, with the extent and duration of treatment depending on the individual case. Occasionally some dogs continue to regurgitate for several days following removal due to moderate-to-severe oesophagitis necessitating lengthier hospitalization.

The author typically recommends feeding of a soft food for a few days following discharge. Owners should be warned of the possibility of stricture formation that may lead to recurrence of clinical signs of oesophageal disease 1–4 weeks later.

23 Respiratory distress

Dogs and cats with respiratory distress are a relatively common presentation to emergency clinics. These patients are often extremely unstable and a rational approach to their management can make the difference between life and death in the initial period following presentation. This is especially true of cats and the bulk of this chapter will therefore focus on this species. However, many of the principles discussed are equally applicable to dogs, about which some information is provided at the end.

APPROACH TO FELINE RESPIRATORY DISTRESS

Respiratory distress can occur as a result of an abnormality affecting any one or more of the following areas:

- Upper respiratory tract (URT) (e.g. laryngeal neoplasia)
- Lower respiratory tract (e.g. feline bronchial disease)
- Lung parenchyma (e.g. pulmonary contusions, pulmonary oedema)
- Pleural space (e.g. pleural effusion, pneumothorax)
- Thoracic wall and diaphragm (e.g. traumatic diaphragmatic rupture).

Being able to identify the area affected is extremely important with respect to patient management.

> **CLINICAL TIP**
>
> - Abnormal respiratory behaviour can also occur as a result of changes affecting other systems, in particular the central nervous system and alterations in acid–base physiology.

Signalment, history

It is often possible to make sensible judgements as to the most likely causes of a cat's respiratory distress on the basis of its signalment and a very brief history. For example:

- A 1-year-old male domestic short hair with no significant preceding history returns home with difficulty breathing, pelvic limb lameness and blood on the face. The most likely cause of this cat's respiratory distress is traumatic injury resulting in pneumothorax and/or pulmonary contusions (haemothorax and diaphragmatic rupture also possible).
- A 4-year-old female neutered Abyssinian with no outdoor access is found with severe difficulty breathing on the owner's bed, where she has been all evening. The most likely causes of this cat's respiratory distress are feline bronchial disease and pleural effusion due to neoplasia or heart disease. The owner goes on to report that the cat has had intermittent self-limiting episodes of coughing over the preceding 3 months. This extra information makes feline bronchial disease the most likely diagnosis.

Following presentation

> **CLINICAL TIP**
>
> - A cat with respiratory distress is likely to be at its most unstable on presentation. The stress of being in the carrier, of travelling and of a strange environment is much more significant in a cat with potentially life-threatening respiratory embarrassment. Even gentle restraint at initial presentation can be enough to cause some cats to fully decompensate, and a hands-off approach with an initial period of oxygen therapy is most prudent.
> - The degree of handling is a judgement to be made on an individual case basis but where there is any doubt at all, the reader is encouraged to adopt the principle of first doing

CLINICAL TIP—cont'd

no harm. The majority of cats with respiratory distress will benefit from a period of oxygen therapy before thorough evaluation and intervention.

- There is no rational justification for excessive manual restraint of a cat with respiratory distress.

The author's initial approach to a cat that presents with moderate or severe respiratory distress is as follows.

Observation

The cat is first briefly observed in its carrier as much information can often be obtained from this approach (see Table 23.1).

Brief examination

An extremely brief examination is then performed. This is done with the cat in its carrier, if that is the cat's preferred option and the carrier design allows. Otherwise, it is done in close proximity to a prepared oxygen cage and only if the cat has not been distressed in any noticeable way by removal from its carrier. Attention is paid to the following:

- Sternal cardiac auscultation:
  - Is the heart rate subjectively fast or slow? Is there a gallop sound or a murmur? (Bradycardia in a cat with respiratory distress may be an ominous finding; marked tachycardia with a gallop sound or murmur may point to a cardiogenic cause but it is noteworthy that the lack of a murmur or a gallop sound does not rule out heart disease.)
  - Are the heart sounds muffled?
  - Are the heart sounds in a normal position?
- Lung field auscultation:
  - Are lung sounds audible ventrally? Dorsally?
  - Are lung sounds loud or quiet? Harsh? Crackles?
  - Is the loudness of the lung sounds appropriate for the respiratory rate and degree of effort? (Apparently normal lung sounds in a cat with marked respiratory effort may in fact be inappropriately quiet.)
  - Are lung sounds symmetrical?
- Chest compliance:
  - An intrathoracic mass may reduce the compliance of the chest wall (as may pleural effusion and the presence of abdominal contents).

Table 23.1 Observations and their interpretation in cats with respiratory distress

Observation	Interpretation
Mental alertness and pupil size	An anxious cat is likely to be more severely affected Marked pupil dilation can be an ominous sign indicating impending respiratory arrest and should prompt rapid intervention
Respiratory rate, effort and pattern	Observing respiratory patterns can be difficult but may yield very useful information. Reported associations include: mixed (inspiratory and expiratory) dyspnoea with a fixed upper respiratory tract obstruction (e.g. laryngeal mass); mixed dyspnoea, in particular with prolonged expiration and an expiratory push, in feline bronchial disease Increased abdominal effort may be seen Paradoxical abdominal movement (where the thorax and abdomen move in opposite directions) may occur with severe dyspnoea
Mucous membranes	Unless severe, pallor of mucous membranes may be difficult to identify from afar Cyanosis is indicative of severely compromised oxygenation and should prompt rapid intervention An animal with pink mucous membranes may still be severely hypoxaemic and the clinician should not be lulled into a false sense of security
Position and posture	Cats in respiratory distress will usually sit in sternal recumbency or show orthopnoea Lateral recumbency is often an ominous sign indicating impending respiratory arrest and should prompt rapid intervention Neck extension and open mouth breathing may be seen
External evidence of trauma	Raises the index of suspicion for common traumatic causes of respiratory distress (e.g. pulmonary contusions, pneumothorax)

Table 23.2 Some causes of respiratory distress in cats and possible associated findings on auscultation

Cause of respiratory distress	Possible findings on auscultation
URT obstruction	Increased URT noise with possible stridor/stertor
Feline bronchial disease	Harsh lung sounds, wheezes, (crackles)
Pulmonary oedema	Harsh lung sounds, crackles
Pulmonary contusions	Loud/harsh lung sounds (crackles)
Pleural effusion	Lung sounds quieter ventrally (harsh dorsally); heart sounds may be muffled
Pneumothorax	Lung sounds quieter dorsally (or diffusely)
Intrathoracic mass	Lung sounds dull (heart sounds displaced)
Diaphragmatic rupture	Lung sounds dull, gut sounds in thorax

URT, upper respiratory tract.

- Laryngeal auscultation if appropriate:
  - Is it louder than normal?
  - Is there stridor?
- Femoral pulse palpation:
  - Difficulty breathing *per se* should not reduce pulse quality.
  - The presence of weak or absent femoral pulses may suggest a primary or concurrent cause of hypoperfusion, such as cardiac disease or hypovolaemic shock.

Table 23.2 presents some of the more common causes of respiratory distress in cats and possible associated findings on auscultation. The reader is reminded that normal lung sounds are quieter caudodorsally and louder cranioventrally.

Oxygenation and client discussion

Following brief examination, the cat is placed in an oxygen cage and kept under close observation. The author uses this time to have a discussion with the owner. The combination of the cat's signalment, history, observation and brief examination may well have identified the anatomical location and possibly the specific cause of the cat's respiratory distress. It may therefore be possible at this stage to discuss the treatment plan, prognosis and costs with the owner before the cat is subjected to further management. For example:

- It is often possible to identify marked pleural effusion by auscultation. The two most common causes of this in cats are neoplasia and congestive heart failure. The owner must therefore be made aware that while it is usually possible to improve the animal's quality of life in the short term, its long-term prognosis is guarded. Pyothorax is another cause of pleural effusion. Although the prognosis with this condition is much better, it is expensive to treat.
- Harsh lung sounds following suspected or confirmed traumatic injury are most likely due to pulmonary contusions from which the vast majority of cats recover. The owner must be made aware of the possible need for short- to medium-term oxygen therapy and the costs involved. The possibility of discovering other significant injuries when the cat is able to be examined more thoroughly should also be discussed.

Further management

CLINICAL TIP

Given the often unstable and precarious status of dyspnoeic cats, it is more important than ever to subject each proposed intervention to a risk–benefit analysis.

- What is the benefit to the patient?
- What is the stress involved to the patient?
- Will the results of diagnostic testing alter the patient's initial management in any significant way?

The clinician should not be afraid to leave a cat in oxygen for an extended period of stabilization without performing any interventions (other than possibly drug therapy).

The next step in the patient's management is dependent on the suspected diagnosis, on the cat's response to oxygen therapy and on the owner's position with respect to the costs involved. It is not therefore possible to be too prescriptive here and what follows is a general discussion of the interventions that may be indicated.

A more comprehensive physical examination is required but this is often delayed until intravenous access has been established.

Intravenous catheter placement

There are a number of benefits of establishing intravenous access as soon as possible, including more rapid drug administration in a subsequent crisis. Nevertheless, there is no rational justification for excessive manual restraint of a cat with respiratory distress and an intravenous catheter should only be placed if the patient is sufficiently compliant. If a catheter is placed, blood should be obtained for an emergency database (see Ch. 3).

Venepuncture for in-house laboratory analysis

The results of standard haematology and biochemistry screening are extremely unlikely to affect the management of a cat with respiratory distress in the initial period. If blood sampling is deemed to be important in the patient's management, the reader is encouraged to delay venepuncture until the cat is much more stable and to make use of topical local anaesthesia (EMLA® cream 5%, AstraZeneca – see Ch. 5).

Drug therapy

A number of different drugs may be indicated in the early management of a cat with respiratory distress and these are summarized in Table 23.3. If a diagnosis is not immediately forthcoming when presented with a cat in severe respiratory distress, and the cat is in extremis or response to oxygen therapy alone is poor, it is reasonable to administer an empirical combination of agents via the intramuscular route. The author administers furosemide, dexamethasone and terbutaline by intramuscular injection in such cases and this is usually accompanied

Table 23.3 Drugs that may be indicated in the early management of cats with respiratory distress

Drug	Dose/route	Indications/comments
Furosemide	1–4 mg/kg i.v., i.m. q 1–2 hr until clinical improvement; then q 12 hr	Initial dose may need to be given i.m. depending on patient stability Indicated for suspected cardiogenic pulmonary oedema; unlikely to help with pulmonary contusions Contraindicated in hypovolaemia or dehydration Excessive administration can cause severe dehydration, electrolyte abnormalities and renal failure
Glyceryl trinitrate 2% ointment	Apply 6 mm q 6–8 hr topically	Indicated for congestive heart failure Wear gloves when applying, avoid contact with site, rotate application sites, highlight treatment on kennel/chart
Morphine	0.1 mg/kg slow i.v., s.c., q 6 hr	Indicated for anxiolysis and as a venodilator in congestive heart failure May be given prior to thoracocentesis Higher doses indicated in trauma
Butorphanol	0.1 mg/kg i.v., s.c.	Indicated for anxiolysis or prior to thoracocentesis
Dexamethasone	0.25 mg/kg i.v., i.m, s.c. q 24 hr	Indicated for feline lower airway disease and upper respiratory tract dyspnoea Initial dose may be given i.m. depending on patient stability Can repeat dose if insufficient response
Terbutaline	0.01 mg/kg slow i.v., s.c. q 4 hr	Beta$_2$-agonist bronchodilator indicated for feline bronchial disease i.m. injection may be painful
Midazolam	0.1–0.2 mg/kg i.m. or i.v.	May be required for thoracocentesis
Ketamine	1–2 mg/kg i.m. or i.v.	May be required for thoracocentesis Use judiciously if congestive heart failure is suspected as relatively contraindicated in hypertrophic cardiomyopathy

i.m., intramuscular; i.v., intravenous; s.c., subcutaneous.

by morphine at a dose rate of 0.1 mg/kg (estimated body weight).

Pulse oximetry

Although there are potential pitfalls with relying solely on pulse oximetry, it does provide an easy and non-invasive technique for monitoring compliant cats with respiratory distress. The probe may be fixed in place (e.g. on the pinna, paw or tail) and the monitor left in or out of the oxygen cage as appropriate.

Ultrasonography

Ultrasonography is extremely useful for respiratory distress in cats, where it is used to identify pleural effusion in particular. Even in the most novice hands, it may also be possible to detect gross abnormalities in cardiac morphology and fractional shortening, and diaphragmatic rupture can also be identified. Following an initial period of stabilization, it is the author's experience that the vast majority of cats tolerate this procedure very well. If facilities allow, scanning can be done without removing the cat from the oxygen cage. Pleural fluid is identified as a predominantly anechoic or hypoechoic area between the hyperechoic lung margin and the chest wall. The edges of the lung lobes may be seen to be flapping about in the fluid.

Thoracocentesis

Thoracocentesis is a relatively simple procedure to perform (see pp. 291–293). It readily allows pleural space disease to be identified, and can markedly improve a patient's respiratory status by evacuating the pleural cavity and allowing the lungs to expand more fully. If pleural effusion is present, samples can also be collected for laboratory analysis. If pleural space disease is suspected, thoracocentesis should be performed before radiography to improve patient stability and to produce radiographs that are likely to yield more useful information.

In non-compliant cats with confirmed pleural space disease, it is preferable to use judicious cardiovascular-sparing sedation in order to allow the procedure to be performed successfully. This is likely to be safer for the patient than repeated attempts, with the extra potential for complications and greater stress to the cat. If circumstances allow, the author prefers to administer a low dose of an opioid (e.g. 0.1 mg/kg morphine slow i.v. or i.m.) to all cats prior to thoracocentesis. If this is inadequate alone, midazolam (0.1–0.2 mg/kg i.v. or i.m.) is administered in addition. If yet more sedation is required, ketamine (1–2 mg/kg i.v. or i.m.) is administered and topped up as necessary; however, ketamine must be used judiciously in cats with suspected heart disease as it is relatively contraindicated in hypertrophic cardiomyopathy.

It is neither possible nor indeed necessary to evacuate the pleural space entirely. That said, the removal of less than 15–20 ml/kg of pleural space-occupying material is unlikely to produce significant improvement in the patient's respiratory status.

Radiography

CLINICAL TIP

- Thoracic radiography is both typically not required for the initial stabilization of cats with respiratory distress and extremely risky in these critical and highly vulnerable patients. Radiography performed prior to adequate stabilization is a high-risk test which is likely to have little benefit early on and the author would strongly discourage its use in all but the most exceptional circumstances.

Thoracic radiography is usually indicated at some point in cats with respiratory distress that does not emanate from the upper respiratory tract. However, it is hopefully clear from this discussion that much information can be obtained through a combination of the patient's history, signalment, observation, brief examination and response to medical therapy. Thoracic radiography straight after presentation is not typically necessary.

The approach advocated throughout this chapter of subjecting the patient to minimum stress is no more applicable than in the context of radiography. If radiography is performed, everything should be prepared before bringing the cat to the radiography room and minimal restraint should be used. If tolerated, oxygen supplementation is provided by mask or flow-by. The intention here is to produce an image that allows the anatomical area affected to be identified and not to produce the perfect thoracic radiograph. Even a rotated dorsoventral radiograph can provide more than enough information for the cat's initial management. A dyspnoeic cat should never be restrained in dorsal recumbency and it is typically best to minimize the amount of time spent in lateral recumbency.

APPROACH TO CANINE RESPIRATORY DISTRESS

The approach to canine respiratory distress is very similar to that in cats as described above. In general, dogs are less precariously poised and less vulnerable to stress but nevertheless minimal stress, gentle handling and strict rest are paramount. In the author's experience, dogs presenting with severe respiratory distress are most commonly suffering from:

- Upper respiratory tract disease, especially laryngeal paralysis or brachycephalic airway obstruction syndrome (BAOS) (see Ch. 32)
- Disorders of the lung parenchyma, especially cardiogenic oedema (see Ch. 31), aspiration pneumonia (see Ch. 22), and pulmonary contusions (see Ch. 28).

24 Seizures

Seizure disorders represent a relatively common reason for emergency consultation and presentation. Seizures are classified as generalized or partial/focal, and the tonic–clonic form of generalized seizures forms the basis of the following discussion. In some animals with generalized seizures, the inciting cause is transient or rapidly reversible (e.g. intoxication, hypoglycaemia), while in others seizures occur due to a more long-term abnormality (e.g. chronic brain disorder resulting in epilepsy). The causes of seizures are typically divided into primary intracranial or extracranial causes and are summarized in Box 24.1.

NURSING ASPECT

Owners quite commonly ring for advice with respect to cats and especially dogs that have suffered one or more seizures and the duty nurse is often the person from whom this initial advice is obtained. In the author's opinion, not all animals that have suffered a seizure need to be examined. The recommendation to examine the animal at the clinic should be guided by the owner's wishes but also after obtaining adequate information with respect to:

- Current status with respect to postictal abnormalities and recovery
- Number of seizures and their timing
- Nature and duration of the seizure(s)
- Any known history of exposure to possible inciting factors (e.g. toxins, trauma)
- Previous seizure history
- Previous medical and therapeutic history.

In animals that have suffered only one self-limiting (isolated) seizure, that appear to have recovered satisfactorily, and in which an obvious inciting

NURSING ASPECT—cont'd

cause has not been identified, it may be appropriate for the animal to remain at home for close monitoring. However, owners must be advised to ensure that the animal is not able to harm him/herself should another seizure occur. They should also contact the practice again either if another seizure occurs or if behavioural signs suggestive of prodrome or aura (pre-seizure behaviour) are observed.

It is recommended that animals with cluster seizures (two or more seizures within 24 hours) are examined as soon as possible, and animals in status epilepticus must be presented to the clinic immediately.

APPROACH TO SEIZURES

Signalment

Signalment is important when considering the possible aetiology of a seizure disorder. For example, young animals are more likely to suffer intoxication from dietary indiscretion or to seizure as a result of congenital anomalies. Hypoglycaemia-induced seizures are more common in puppies, especially of toy breeds, while older animals are more likely to seizure as a result of intracranial neoplasia. Idiopathic epilepsy is more common in certain breeds (e.g. German shepherd dogs) and affected animals usually seizure for the first time at 1–5 years of age. Intracranial tumours are more common in certain breeds (e.g. Boxers), as are the range of inflammatory central nervous system diseases (e.g. Maltese terriers, Yorkshire terriers, Pugs). True idiopathic epilepsy is much less common in cats than it is in dogs.

BOX 24.1 Causes of seizures

Primary intracranial

- Idiopathic epilepsy (especially purebred and large dogs, first onset 1–5 years old)
- Intracranial neoplasia, primary or metastatic (especially older animals)
- Noninfectious inflammatory central nervous system (CNS) disease
- Infectious causes
- Cerebrovascular abnormalities
- Developmental abnormalities, especially younger animals (e.g. hydrocephalus)
- Degenerative disorders (e.g. storage diseases)
- Traumatic brain injury
- Intracranial haemorrhage (e.g. due to systemic hypertension, coagulopathy)

Extracranial

- Hypoglycaemia
- Intoxication (e.g. metaldehyde)
- Hepatic encephalopathy (e.g. portosystemic shunt)
- Hyper- or hyponatraemia
- Hypocalcaemia
- (Uraemic encephalopathy – rare cause of seizures)

History

CLINICAL TIP

- It is important to remember that owners may mistake other episodes of abnormal behaviour for seizures and this distinction may be crucial in some cases. In particular, animals suffering from syncope of cardiac origin may temporarily lose consciousness and demonstrate involuntary urination while recumbent. However, these animals typically return to complete normality within seconds to a minute of the onset of the episode and this provides a useful distinguishing feature from the postictal period associated with seizures. Severe acute vestibular signs may also be mistaken for seizures (see Ch. 15).

A thorough history is mandatory for all animals with seizures, although the timing should be governed by the patient's clinical status on presentation. Owners should be asked to describe the seizure episode(s) as thoroughly as possible, including pre-, intra- and postictal phases. It is important to establish the number of seizures that have occurred and their timing, the nature and duration of the seizure(s), any known or possible exposure to inciting factors (e.g. intoxication; recent feeding with portosystemic shunt), previous seizure history and previous medical history. If the patient is already on anticonvulsive therapy, the drugs, dosages and timing of last administration should be established. Details of any monitoring of serum anticonvulsant levels should be obtained if the owner knows this information.

Major body system examination

Major body system examination may need to be delayed in an animal that presents actively seizuring. Neurological examination may be normal or severely abnormal in animals with seizure disorders. Some animals present in the middle of a seizure, some with postictal abnormalities, while others have fully recovered. A full neurological examination is warranted in any animal with a seizure history but it is sometimes necessary to wait for postictal abnormalities to resolve before a reliable examination can be performed. In addition, anticonvulsive medications that may need to be administered in an emergency will also potentially alter the findings of a neurological examination.

Cardiovascular examination may be abnormal in animals that have seizured. True seizures are unlikely to occur as a result of a primary cardiovascular disorder although cerebrovascular abnormalities may cause other neurological signs. Cardiovascular abnormalities that may occur secondary to seizures include tachycardia, hyperaemic mucous membranes and rapid capillary refill time. Furthermore, in some cases the cause of the seizure may also have direct effects on the cardiovascular system; this is especially common with certain poisons. In general, seizures should not cause systemic hypoperfusion but perfusion abnormalities may be seen following severe sustained seizure activity. In addition, the author has anecdotally noted a variety of cardiovascular abnormalities in animals with primary brain disease that have been presumed to be a direct result of the cerebral disorder (a brain–heart connection has been documented in people). Finally, depending on the cause of the seizures and their severity and duration, some animals may present with intracranial hypertension that may be detectable clinically as bradycardia and systemic hypertension (Cushing's reflex – see Ch. 28). If facilities allow, systemic blood pressure should be measured in all animals presenting with active seizures or marked postictal abnormalities.

Respiratory examination may or may not be normal in animals with seizures. Seizures are unlikely to occur as a result of a primary respiratory disorder and the most common respiratory abnormalities identified are panting and tachypnoea. Aspiration may occur as a consequence of seizuring and other abnormal respiratory findings are possible in such cases. Neurogenic (noncardiogenic) pulmonary oedema may also cause respiratory abnormalities.

Rectal temperature may be normal, decreased or increased in animals with seizures depending on the timing of presentation. Severe seizure activity, in particular status epilepticus (see below), may result in marked hyperthermia which may need to be managed specifically (see Ch. 16).

Emergency database

CLINICAL TIP

- Blood glucose should be checked as a minimum in all animals that present either seizuring or with marked neurological abnormalities. If blood glucose cannot be checked, it may be appropriate in some cases to administer conservative empirical glucose therapy where there is a high index of suspicion for clinically significant hypoglycaemia. Such cases include puppies and kittens, especially with diarrhoea, and adult dogs with a history that is consistent with a possible insulinoma (e.g. intermittent self-resolving collapse, generalized weakness or neuromuscular signs, especially during exercise).
- More extensive clinicopathological testing may be appropriate in some cases but is unlikely to be available and of use during initial stabilization of a seizuring patient. Such investigations must not be prioritized at the expense of emergency treatment.

The need to perform an emergency database in an animal with a seizure disorder should be governed by the patient's clinical status at the time of presentation. Blood glucose should be checked as a minimum in all animals that present either seizuring or with marked neurological abnormalities. In middle-aged to older dogs that present with clinically significant hypoglycaemia, a blood sample should be collected for measurement of serum insulin concentration prior to therapeutic administration of intravenous glucose if possible. Insulinomas are seen most commonly in medium to large breed dogs and have been identified in dogs as young as 3 years old.

Checking for hyper- or hyponatraemia and hypocalcaemia is also recommended if possible although these abnormalities are much less frequently implicated than hypoglycaemia as a cause of seizures in small animals.

In animals that are already receiving anticonvulsive therapy, it is recommended to obtain samples as early on as possible for measurement of serum drug concentrations.

CLINICAL TIP

- Animals presenting during or after a seizure may have intracranial hypertension. This may be the result of a primary intracranial cause but also as a consequence of severe seizure activity. Jugular vein occlusion should be avoided in such cases and a peripheral vein used for early blood sampling if required.

Diagnostic imaging

Routine diagnostic imaging is rarely a priority in patients with seizures but may be required following initial stabilization. For example, respiratory abnormalities may need to be investigated with thoracic radiography that may show evidence of aspiration pneumonia (alveolar pattern in right middle lung lobe and ventral parts of other lobes) or neurogenic (noncardiogenic) oedema (caudodorsal interstitial to alveolar lung pattern). Abdominal radiography may occasionally be of use for example in some types of intoxication. Referral for more specialist and/or advanced diagnostic imaging may be indicated in patients thought to be suffering from an on-going seizure disorder (e.g. abdominal ultrasonography for portosystemic shunt, cerebral magnetic resonance imaging (MRI) for primary brain disorder).

Treatment

Animals presenting in the postictal phase of a generalized seizure do not require any treatment if physical examination is normal. Patients with persistent postictal abnormalities may need to be hospitalized for on-going monitoring. This is often determined as much by owner preference as it is by the patient's clinical status.

Diazepam should be administered per rectum (1 mg/kg; 2 mg/kg if receiving concurrent phenobarbital) in an animal that presents actively seizuring to facilitate intravenous catheter placement. Proprietary rectal diazepam tubes may be used, or injectable diazepam may be diluted with water or saline to increase the volume to be administered and then infused per rectum. Using injectable diazepam allows more accurate dosing but involves a greater time delay in preparation. Depending on the size of the animal, the use of a well-lubricated long intravenous catheter (with stylet removed), urinary catheter or nasooesophageal feeding tube will allow the diazepam to be administered more proximally in the rectum. This should minimize spillage from the anus and maximize drug absorption. The rectal mucosa has an extensive blood supply and drug absorption should occur readily so long as the solution is in contact with the mucosa and not mixed into faecal material. Flow-by oxygen supplementation should also be provided initially.

An intravenous catheter should be placed into a peripheral vein and a sample obtained via the catheter for blood glucose and serum electrolyte measurement and potentially a more extensive emergency database. Additional diazepam (0.5 mg/kg i.v.) should then be administered and additional anticonvulsive therapy employed (see Status epilepticus, below) if necessary. On-going maintenance fluid therapy (see Ch. 4) and close monitoring should be provided; glucose supplementation may be required in some cases.

The decision to start oral anticonvulsive therapy should be made on an individual case basis and will depend on factors such as:

- The identified or suspected cause: Transient? Progressive or non-progressive?
- The number and severity of seizures
- Response to initial parenteral treatment and the extent of parenteral treatment required
- Previous seizure history.

Oral anticonvulsive therapy is likely to be indicated in animals suspected of having an on-going seizure focus or those that have suffered severe or sustained seizure activity necessitating aggressive parenteral treatment. Although completely normal previously, animals that have suffered severe seizures secondary to intoxication may require short-term (months) tapered oral anticonvulsive therapy due to seizure-induced neuronal damage.

Head trauma may rarely be associated with seizures in the short term. In addition, animals occasionally develop seizures some time after the traumatic incident and it is presumed that the seizures are a result of a seizure focus resulting from the prior traumatic brain injury. On-going oral anticonvulsive therapy is likely to be indicated in these cases.

STATUS EPILEPTICUS

CLINICAL TIP

- Status epilepticus carries a very real risk of both permanent neuronal damage and multiorgan injury. Immediate and aggressive intervention is essential.

Although older texts describe a longer period of time, the current definition of status epilepticus is sustained generalized seizure activity for more than 5 minutes, or multiple consecutive seizures without return of consciousness in between. Status epilepticus can cause severe hyperthermia which can have marked and potentially life-threatening consequences (see Ch. 38), and may be associated with significant cardiovascular abnormalities (often tachycardia and hypertension early on, followed by bradycardia and hypotension). Hypoglycaemia and hypoxaemia may also occur. There is a significant risk of permanent neuronal damage due to sustained seizure activity and timely and aggressive intervention is warranted. Neurogenic pulmonary oedema may develop rapidly following status epilepticus.

Treatment

Management of status epilepticus typically starts with rectal diazepam administration (1 mg/kg; 2 mg/kg if receiving concurrent phenobarbital) as above to facilitate intravenous catheter placement, and flow-by oxygen supplementation is provided. Further diazepam administration (0.5 mg/kg i.v.) is then performed in an attempt to control the clinical signs. However, typically no more than three boluses are administered before the use of an additional drug is considered. In general, this involves heavily sedating or anaesthetizing the patient for a variable period of time in order to stop or minimize motor activity associated with seizuring.

If financial constraints do not exist, a constant rate infusion of propofol is used. The appropriate dose is administered (2 mg/kg aliquots slowly i.v. to effect), followed by a constant rate infusion starting at 6 mg/kg/hr and titrating upwards (or downwards) to effect. The use of a syringe driver here is preferred although a solution of propofol in normal saline can be made and administered via a fluid administration set using an infusion pump. These patients are recumbent and immobile, and although not ideal, it may therefore be possible to manage them adequately without the use of an infusion pump if one is not available. In cases in which high rates of propofol infusion prove necessary, additional agents should be considered in a propofol-sparing capacity. In particular, midazolam has been used either as intermittent boluses (0.1–0.5 mg/kg i.v.) or preferably as a constant rate infusion (0.1–0.8 mg/kg/hr). The dose of propofol generally starts to be tapered after 24 hours (e.g. reducing by 25% every 2–4 hours).

If financial or practical constraints preclude the use of a propofol infusion, pentobarbital boluses may be a viable alternative. However, to the author's knowledge, a sterile formulation of this agent for injectable use is no longer readily available and the risks associated with using nonsterile preparations available for euthanasia must clearly be borne in mind and discussed with the owner. The recommended dose is 5–20 mg/kg slowly i.v. to effect (e.g. 3 mg/kg aliquots q 90 s). The use of thiopentone and inhalational anaesthesia may also be considered.

Endotracheal intubation should be performed in all anaesthetized patients to protect the airway and prevent aspiration. Oxygen supplementation is not mandatory unless specific indications exist. Vital parameters should be monitored and recorded regularly, and fluid therapy administered to maintain hydration and electrolyte concentrations. In some cases general anaesthesia or heavy sedation is required for 48 hours or more.

Phenobarbital loading should be performed in all animals presenting in status epilepticus. The most aggressive intravenous protocols (e.g. 3 mg/kg slow i.v. q 30–60 min, up to total dose of 18–24 mg/kg in 24 hours) are typically reserved for those cases requiring anaesthesia. The delay in onset of action of phenobarbital means that it is generally not helpful in controlling signs very early on but its sedative effects are likely to facilitate propofol dose reduction. Blood for serum drug concentration measurement should be obtained prior to loading if possible in animals already on phenobarbital therapy. Following loading, patients are usually maintained on 3–5 mg/kg slow i.v. q 12 hr for 24–48 hours before changing to enteral therapy.

The approach to status epilepticus is summarized in Box 24.2.

BOX 24.2 Management of status epilepticus

- Administer rectal diazepam (1 mg/kg) using proprietary tube(s) or diluted injectable preparation
- Provide flow-by oxygen supplementation
- Place intravenous catheter and obtain blood for glucose and electrolyte measurement ± more extensive emergency database:
  - Administer glucose supplementation (0.25–0.5 g/kg diluted i.v.) if indicated; provide on-going glucose supplementation in such cases
- Administer up to three intravenous diazepam boluses (0.5 mg/kg i.v.)
- Administer propofol (2 mg/kg aliquots slowly i.v. to effect) if diazepam ineffective (pentobarbital, thiopentone or inhalational anaesthesia may also be considered)
- Perform endotracheal intubation and provide on-going oxygen supplementation if specifically indicated
- Perform major body system examination and check rectal temperature; provide active cooling measures if indicated
- Perform intravenous phenobarbital loading (3 mg/kg slow i.v. q 30–60 min, up to total dose of 18–24 mg/kg in 24 hours) – obtain blood for serum drug concentration measurement first in animals already on anticonvulsant therapy
- Provide intravenous fluid therapy for maintenance purposes and to correct volume deficits as required
- Perform close monitoring of vital parameters; be aware of possibility of neurogenic pulmonary oedema
- Provide standard nursing measures as for any recumbent animal
- Start to taper anaesthetic doses after 24 hours (e.g. reduce by 25% q 2–4 hr)
- Continue intravenous phenobarbital (3–5 mg/kg slow i.v. q 12 hr) for 24–48 hours before changing to enteral therapy

NURSING ASPECT

Standard nursing measures for recumbent patients should be implemented in animals anaesthetized or heavily sedated to control seizures. These measures include:

- Regular eye lubrication to prevent corneal drying and ulceration; and oral care (q 6 hr)
- Use of well-padded bedding to prevent pressure sores and ensuring bedding is dry, clean and comfortable
- Regular turning (q 4 hr) to prevent atelectasis (lung collapse)

NURSING ASPECT—cont'd

- Appropriate bladder management: express or catheterize if necessary and prevent urinary soiling
- Minimizing external stimuli (placing cotton wool balls/swabs in the ears; dim lighting and minimum passage of personnel)
- Deflate and reposition endotracheal tube regularly (q 4–6 hr) if present

25 Sudden loss of vision

Depending on the disorder in question, sudden loss of vision may occur unilaterally or bilaterally, and there may or may not be changes in the appearance of the eye(s). It is also noteworthy that some animals that present for apparent sudden loss of vision are in fact afflicted by a chronic slowly progressive disorder with which they had previously been coping. Often a change of environment brings their loss of vision to the owner's attention. Some causes of sudden blindness are shown in Table 25.1. In addition some causes of acute red eye (see Ch. 10) may also result in loss of vision.

Table 25.1 Causes of sudden loss of vision

Cause	Unilateral or bilateral blindness	Other comments
Retinal separation (detachment)	Usually unilateral initially, potentially becoming bilateral	Causes include systemic hypertension, trauma, neoplasia, immune-mediated disease, exudate caused by inflammatory disease, and congenital disorders; also idiopathic Vision may return with early treatment
Sudden acquired retinal degeneration syndrome (SARDS)	Bilateral	Cause unknown; permanent blindness Typically middle-aged to older dogs Often obese or recent weight gain History of polyuria/polydipsia common
Intracranial lesions	Often bilateral	Especially neoplasia Additional neurological signs may be present
Hypoxic brain injury	Bilateral	Central loss of vision Especially in cats following general anaesthesia
Toxicity	Bilateral	e.g. ivermectin (especially Collie breeds); fluoroquinolones in cats (retinal toxicity causing permanent blindness)
Optic neuritis	Often bilateral	Cause often unknown May be related to inflammatory central nervous system disease or systemic infection

26 Urticaria, angio-oedema and anaphylaxis

Urticaria, angio-oedema and anaphylaxis may occur as a result of a variety of different stimuli, predominantly immunological but also nonimmunological, that induce mast cell (and basophil) degranulation. The predominant immunological mechanism is a type I hypersensitivity (HS) reaction whereby antigen activates mast cells (and basophils) by binding to immunoglobulin E (IgE) molecules on surface receptors. Previous exposure to the antigen in question (sensitization) results in an exaggerated immune response and excessive production of IgE which is then available for binding to mast cells and mediating an abnormally intense response to repeat antigen exposure.

Type I HS is 'immediate' as a reaction occurs within seconds or minutes of antigen exposure. This may then be followed by an additional late phase reaction 6–12 hours later due to the release of mediators from activated eosinophils (and neutrophils). Nonimmunological mast cell activation does not require prior sensitization and occurs either directly or more commonly through complement activation.

Clinical signs result from the sudden and excessive release of inflammatory mediators from mast cells (and perhaps basophils) and subsequently eosinophils. The severity and location of the response depend on the number and location of the cells involved that in turn depend on the degree of sensitization of the animal (immunological), the amount of antigen involved and the route of exposure. Mast cell degranulation and mediator release can be localized or systemic in more severe cases.

LOCALIZED REACTIONS

Localized reactions are most common, with the site dependent on the route of antigen exposure. For example:

- Antigens affecting the skin cause localized dermatitis, urticaria (hives) and angioedema
- Inhaled/aerosolized antigens cause respiratory tract responses; may also contact the eyes causing conjunctivitis and lacrimation
- Ingested antigens cause diarrhoea (possibly haemorrhagic), abdominal pain.

URTICARIA AND ANGIO-OEDEMA

Urticaria refers to local superficial (dermis) lesions grossly visible as discrete erythematous wheals. Lesions usually develop within 30 minutes to a few hours and are variably pruritic. Lesions usually disappear within 24–48 hours (but may be more chronic). Differential diagnoses for urticaria include:

- Superficial folliculitis
- (Early) erythema multiforme
- Vasculitis
- Neoplasia.

In angio-oedema, subcutaneous tissues and deep blood vessels become affected by the inflammatory process, resulting in oedema and consequent diffuse swelling that is usually not pruritic. Angio-oedema typically affects the face (especially around the eyes, mouth and ears) although other areas, in particular the extremities, may be involved (Figure 26.1).

Angio-oedema of the laryngeal or pharyngeal mucosa may cause potentially severe upper respiratory tract obstruction. Differential diagnoses for angio-oedema include:

- Early juvenile cellulitis
- Early bacterial cellulitis
- Vasculitis
- Neoplasia.

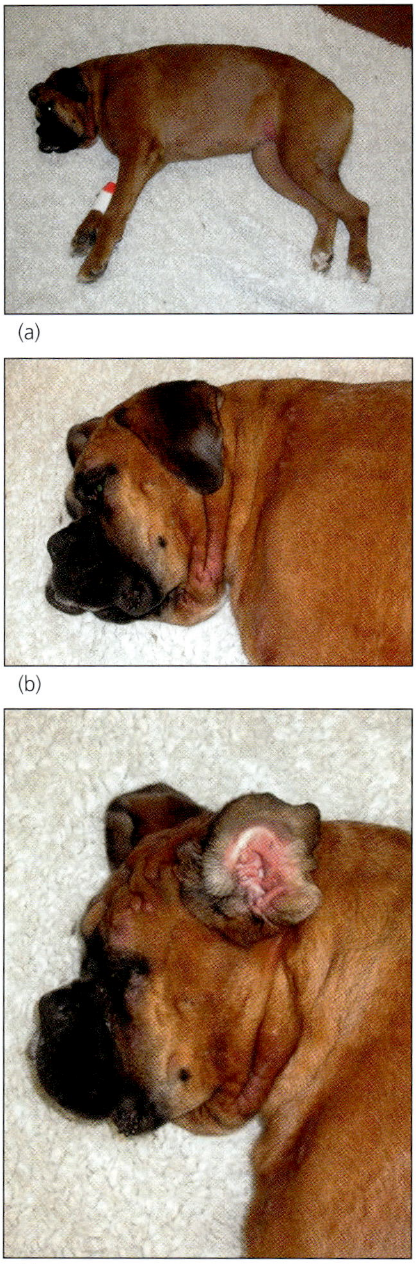

(a)

(b)

(c)

Figure 26.1 (a–c) Photographs of a Boxer dog showing cutaneous erythema, urticaria and angioedema especially affecting the head. (Photographs courtesy of Filippo de Bellis)

Treatment of urticaria and angioedema is described in the case example.

SYSTEMIC REACTIONS – ANAPHYLAXIS/ ANAPHYLACTIC SHOCK

A severe sudden systemic release of inflammatory mediators from activated mast cells (and perhaps basophils) is the underlying pathogenesis of acute anaphylaxis/anaphylactic shock. The rate of mediator release exceeds the animal's ability to compensate for their effects. The majority of mast cell mediators have vasoactive properties and systemic vascular effects are therefore most prominent.

Maldistributive shock occurs and in addition a marked increase in capillary permeability causes significant loss of fluid from the intravascular to the extravascular compartment, resulting in hypovolaemic shock (see Ch. 2). The cardiovascular picture during anaphylaxis (hypoperfusion that is refractory to appropriate fluid therapy) is also a hallmark of maldistributive shock secondary to systemic inflammatory response syndrome (SIRS) or sepsis (SIRS due to infection, most commonly bacterial). Thorough evaluation to exclude sepsis may be indicated in some cases prior to making a presumptive diagnosis of anaphylaxis.

Treatment of anaphylaxis

The aims of therapy in anaphylaxis are to correct systemic hypoperfusion and to attempt to address some of the underlying pathogenic mechanisms. If appropriate, suspected inciting causes must be discontinued and reexposure prevented. Aggressive individually tailored intravenous fluid therapy and adrenaline (epinephrine) are the mainstay of treatment, and regular monitoring of cardiovascular and other major systems is vital. Recommended doses of adrenaline (epinephrine) are:

- 0.01 mg/kg slow i.v. (or i.m., s.c. in less severe cases)
- If intravenous access cannot be obtained:
  - 0.01 mg/kg into tongue vein or parenchyma
  - 0.02 mg/kg via endotracheal tube (e.g. using a urinary catheter to administer at the level of the carina).

Adrenaline (epinephrine) should be administered immediately once the diagnosis is made and administration can be repeated after 20–30 min (or sooner if necessary). Appropriate fluid therapy and adrenaline (epinephrine) administration should bring about clinical improvement within minutes.

Corticosteroids may also be administered in the treatment of anaphylaxis (e.g. methylprednisolone sodium succinate 1–2 mg/kg i.v. over 15–20 min; dexamethasone 0.25–1 mg/kg i.v. bolus). However, they should not be used in place of adrenaline (epinephrine) as they are likely to be much less effective in the immediate life-threatening phase. Corticosteroids may be helpful, however, in controlling on-going mediator release following initial stabilization. Additional therapy may include the use of bronchodilators (e.g. terbutaline, aminophylline), furosemide and antihistamines.

CLINICAL TIP

- Urticaria, angioedema and anaphylaxis can be thought of as the same disease process with variations in severity and target organ(s). Dogs are uncommonly affected and cats rarely so.
- Appropriate treatment depends on the severity of the clinical signs and there is a spectrum from no intervention being required for mild self-limiting signs to the need for aggressive and life-saving intervention for anaphylactic shock.

Causes of urticaria, angioedema and anaphylaxis are listed in Box 26.1. There are a large number of potential causes (not all have been reported in dogs/cats) but in a significant proportion of cases the responsible antigen cannot be identified; fortunately this does not impact on short-term emergency management.

Case example 1

PRESENTING SIGNS AND CASE HISTORY

A 2-year-old male neutered Boxer dog presented for treatment of a suspected allergic reaction. The dog had been out in the garden with his owners and shortly after returning indoors, he was noted to have progressive skin changes. The dog's eyes had also puffed up en route to the practice and he appeared to be irritated by his skin. The owners reported a similar milder self-limiting episode the previous year but there was no other significant history.

BOX 26.1 Potential causes of urticaria, angioedema and anaphylaxis in dogs and cats

Venoms

- Hymenoptera stings (bees, wasps, ants)
- Snakes – including common adder
- Spiders, lizards

Drugs

- Antibiotics – penicillins, chloramphenicol, sulphonamides, cephalosporins, tetracycline
- Nonsteroidal antiinflammatory agents – aspirin, ibuprofen
- Anaesthetics/sedatives – acepromazine maleate, ketamine hydrochloride, barbiturates, local anaesthetics, diazepam
- Parasiticides (generally older or supermarket products)
- Others – opiates, aminophylline; asparaginase; neostigmine; amphotericin B

Hormones

- Insulin
- Exogenous adrenocorticotrophic hormone (ACTH)
- Vasopressin (antidiuretic hormone, ADH)
- Oestrus
- Oxytocin

Miscellaneous

- Food hypersensitivity
- Atopic dermatitis
- Blood products
- Plants
- Heparin
- Vaccines
- Vitamins – vitamin K, thiamine, folic acid
- Dextrans, gelatins
- Radiocontrast dyes
- Sunlight
- Excessive heat or cold
- Peanuts in dogs?

Major body system examination

On presentation the dog was alert and responsive but appeared mildly agitated. Cardiovascular examination was unremarkable but the dog was panting. Abdominal palpation was unremarkable and rectal temperature was mildly elevated at 39.3°C. Facial oedema was present along with diffuse cutaneous erythema and urticaria of the inguinal region, ventral abdominal and thoracic walls. The lesions were variably pruritic.

Assessment

Urticaria and angioedema were present but the dog's cardiovascular and respiratory systems were unremarkable and there was no evidence at presentation of anaphylactic shock.

Case management

Although the dog's respiration was normal at presentation, given his breed, there was some concern over the potential for him to develop upper respiratory tract obstruction. Bearing in mind the potential for a late phase hypersensitivity reaction 6–12 hr following the initial signs as well, it was decided to hospitalize the dog for treatment and observation. As the dog appeared agitated and pruritic, both chlorpheniramine (8 mg total dose i.m.) and dexamethasone (0.25 mg/kg i.m.) were administered parenterally.

The dog was discharged after 12 hr of hospitalization at which time urticaria and angioedema were still present but no longer progressing, and the dog appeared stable and comfortable. He was discharged on oral prednisolone (1 mg/kg q 24 hr for 48 hr) and chlorpheniramine (8 mg total dose p.o. q 12 hr for 48 hr). It was discussed with the owners that while avoidance and elimination of aetiological antigens are ideal, in this case – as in many others – it was not possible to identify specifically such an antigen.

27 Wounds and open fractures

A large variety of wounds may be seen in emergency patients, resulting from a range of different causes, and an extensive discussion is beyond the scope of this book. This chapter briefly presents some general considerations and the reader is referred to other texts for more extensive wound-specific management and surgical closure.

> **CLINICAL TIP**
>
> - A large proportion of patients presenting with wounds or open fractures have suffered significant multisystemic injury (see Ch. 28). It is essential to ensure that as far as possible the fundamental principles of emergency medicine are not sacrificed at the expense of focusing on the wound(s). Major body system examination, cardiorespiratory stabilization and adequate pain relief should be prioritized as always; wounds and fractures are rarely life-threatening.

Wound management centres on the following steps:

- Haemostasis is provided if required
- Further contamination should be minimized
- Non-viable tissues should be debrided
- Contaminating material should be removed
- Drainage should be ensured
- A viable vascular bed should be encouraged
- The wound should be closed appropriately.

Providing haemostasis

In most cases adequate haemostasis can be provided by direct pressure over the wound using sterile gauze swabs. Occasionally it is necessary to clamp a bleeding artery or arteriole until further intervention can be performed.

Minimizing further contamination

Traumatic wounds that receive adequate debridement and lavage within 6–8 hours of injury may be converted from contaminated to clean. However, a number of animals presenting with wounds require extensive major system stabilization before such wound management can be instituted, and stabilization should never be sacrificed over concerns regarding wound contamination.

Until such time that more thorough wound cleansing can be performed, it is important to adhere to certain guidelines:

- Aseptic technique should be employed when handling wounds as far as possible.
- As soon as possible, and typically after administration of analgesia, wounds should be protected using a temporary dressing; sterile swabs soaked in 0.05% chlorhexidine for example may be used as the primary layer. In some cases, cling film, or a similar type of wrap, can be used as a rapid short-term means of protecting a wound while initial patient evaluation and stabilization are performed; the temporary dressing is then applied. Preventing contamination with potentially resistant hospital bacteria is essential.
- Depending on the nature and aetiology of the wound, it may be appropriate to take a bacterial swab from the site and start broad-spectrum intravenous antibiosis immediately.

> **CLINICAL TIP**
>
> - Antibiotics are not required for either clean wounds or contaminated wounds that are debrided and lavaged appropriately within 6–8 hours of injury.
> - If antibiotics are indicated, a broad-spectrum agent that can be given intravenously should be chosen (e.g. amoxicillin/clavulanate, cephalosporin) and treatment reassessed based on subsequent culture results.

When the patient is sufficiently stable, appropriate sedation or general anaesthesia can be instituted for more thorough wound cleansing. The wound is protected with a sterile water-soluble lubricant (e.g. KY Jelly®, Johnson & Johnson) and a large area of hair surrounding the wound is clipped to prevent further contamination. The skin surrounding the wound is then cleaned with a surgical scrub solution.

Debriding nonviable tissue

Surgical debridement is performed to remove any tissue that is already obviously non-viable. In some cases, tissue with questionable viability may need to be left (e.g. if there is limited tissue availability) and further debridement performed subsequently if indicated.

Removing contaminated material

Depending on the nature and aetiology of the wound, marked contamination can occur with a variety of foreign material (e.g. dirt, leaves, hair). The 'solution to pollution is dilution' is a commonly employed phrase to emphasize the fact that copious wound lavage must be performed. Wounds are lavaged using warm 0.9% sodium chloride (normal, physiological saline). Recommendations regarding the ideal needle and syringe size for lavage vary depending on the reference consulted but the author typically uses a 21 gauge needle and a 20 ml syringe. Bacterial swabs are usually collected once debridement and lavage have been performed.

Ensuring drainage

It is essential to ensure that infected wounds have adequate drainage. In some cases, this involves leaving (a part of) the wound open; however, passive (or active) drains are desirable in many cases to reduce dead space and facilitate drainage. Penrose drains are used most commonly and work by capillary action (passive).

CLINICAL TIP

- The author would strongly recommend a liberal approach to the use of Penrose drains in wound management. These drains are cheap, easy to use and associated with few complications, and the benefits they offer in terms of wound management can be invaluable.

Encourage a viable vascular bed

Debridement and lavage are essential in reducing the risk of wound infection and encouraging healing. Most wounds are subsequently covered using sterile dressings to prevent further contamination and patient interference, and to provide a moist environment for repair. Wet-to-dry dressings should be used to provide ongoing debridement in the early stages if indicated.

Open fractures

All open fractures should be considered to be contaminated as a minimum and potentially infected (more than 8 hours since injury). The principles of wound management described above are entirely appropriate for open fractures and intravenous broad-spectrum antibiosis should be administered in all cases. Temporary fracture stabilization (e.g. splint, support bandage) may be required to provide analgesia and prevent further injury pending definitive repair.

CLINICAL TIP

- Animals with open fractures are liable to require more aggressive analgesia than those with soft tissue injuries alone, and this must not be overlooked while focusing on their wound(s). In addition, manipulation for wound management must be done with due concern not to exacerbate the orthopaedic injury further.

SECTION 3

SPECIFIC DISORDERS

28 The trauma patient

Trauma is one of the most common reasons for emergency presentation and can also be one of the most stressful to the patient, owner and veterinary personnel. A calm and rational approach is therefore paramount. Trauma is especially common in cats, amongst which motor vehicle accidents (road traffic accidents) are very common, and more so than dogs, severely injured cats can decompensate very easily without appropriate management. The majority of this chapter therefore focuses on cats although most of the principles and information provided are equally applicable to dogs.

The most common causes of trauma in companion animals are motor vehicle accidents, animal (especially dog) bite injuries, tail pull injuries and falls from a height (especially feline high-rise syndrome). Puppies and kittens are also relatively commonly trodden on and dogs may be kicked by horses. The most common injuries that occur following motor vehicle accidents are listed in Box 28.1. Cranial, thoracic and pelvic injuries are especially common in cats.

> **BOX 28.1 Common injuries following motor vehicle accidents**
>
> **Head**
> - Traumatic brain injury
> - Ocular injury
> - Skull fracture
> - Dental injury
>
> **Thorax**
> - Pulmonary contusions
> - Pneumothorax
> - Haemothorax
> - Rib fractures
> - Diaphragmatic rupture
>
> **Abdomen**
> - Abdominal wall rupture
> - Haemoabdomen
> - Uroabdomen
> - Bile peritonitis
> - Septic peritonitis from gastrointestinal rupture
>
> **Spine (vertebral column)/spinal cord**
> - Vertebral fracture
> - Vertebral luxation/subluxation
> - Intervertebral disc extrusion/herniation/prolapse
>
> **Pelvic fractures**
>
> **Limbs**
> - Long bone fracture
> - Joint luxation/subluxation
> - Tendon/ligament injury
> - Degloving injury
>
> **Wounds**

TRAUMATIC BRAIN INJURY

Theory refresher

Minimizing secondary brain injury

> **CLINICAL TIP**
> - The prime aim in the management of traumatic brain injury (TBI) is to limit secondary brain injury. This is done by ensuring that the brain receives an adequate supply of well-oxygenated arterial blood.

The prime aim in the management of traumatic brain injury (TBI) is to limit secondary brain injury that may occur as a result of various mechanisms including hypoxia, ischaemia due to hypoperfusion, raised intracranial pressure (ICP) or active haemorrhage. Earlier discussions of TBI tended to focus on the detrimental effects of raised ICP via impairment of cerebral blood flow and the potential for brainstem compression and herniation. However, secondary brain injury is significantly perpetuated by hypoxia and systemic hypoperfusion, and the priority is therefore to ensure that the brain receives an adequate supply of well-oxygenated arterial blood. Treatment for possible raised ICP is just one part of this therapy.

Ensuring adequate oxygenation and ventilation

Hypoxia must be avoided at all costs and pulse oximetry (and arterial blood gas analysis if available) should be used. A percentage saturation of haemoglobin with oxygen (SpO_2) on room air of more than 95% is satisfactory. Animals with low SpO_2 should be provided with oxygen supplementation immediately and a liberal 'if in doubt, supplement oxygen' approach is strongly encouraged. In addition, any processes that may interfere with adequate ventilation (e.g. pneumothorax, pain) must be addressed appropriately.

Ensuring adequate cerebral perfusion

Cerebral blood flow, and hence oxygen and nutrient delivery to the brain, is driven by the cerebral perfusion pressure (CPP) gradient between mean arterial pressure (MAP) and ICP:

$$CPP = MAP - ICP$$

Normal homeostatic mechanisms protecting cerebral blood flow may be lost in TBI and cerebral blood flow becomes largely dependent on systemic blood pressure. Maintenance of an adequate CPP is a cornerstone of modern brain injury therapy.

Mean arterial pressure The head trauma patient may well present with systemic hypotension (i.e. decreased MAP). Mean arterial pressure can be measured noninvasively using an oscillometric device and a reasonable target MAP is 80 mmHg. If only Doppler sphygmomanometry is available, then a systolic blood pressure of 100 mmHg is considered equivalent.

> **CLINICAL TIP**
>
> - Regardless of whether blood pressure monitoring is or is not available, it is essential to ensure that hypoperfusion identified on the basis of physical examination is corrected. Blood pressure monitoring is not a substitute for regular assessment of physical perfusion parameters.

Raised intracranial pressure ICP is the pressure exerted between the skull and the three intracranial compartments – brain parenchyma, blood and cerebrospinal fluid. Direct measurement of ICP is not practical in veterinary medicine at this time and the presence of elevated ICP is therefore inferred. The Cushing response is the most specific marker available – intracranial hypertension causes systemic hypertension and a consequent reflex bradycardia. These findings should prompt aggressive treatment for raised ICP. Other less specific findings that may suggest intracranial hypertension include otherwise unexplained deterioration of mental status, dilated nonresponsive pupils, loss of physiological nystagmus and decerebrate posturing.

Neurological examination

Once potentially life-threatening extracranial abnormalities have been addressed, a thorough baseline neurological examination should be performed.

1. Mentation: normal, depressed/obtunded, stuporous, comatose; hysterical.
2. Pupils: symmetry; size; pupillary light reflexes (PLR), direct and consensual
   (a) Normal size pupil with slow PLR (least severe)
   (b) Miotic pupil with intact PLR
   (c) Pinpoint pupil with no PLR
   (d) Mydriatic pupil with no PLR (most severe).
3. Other cranial nerves: especially menace responses, blink and gag reflexes and jaw tone.
4. Oculocephalic reflex: in a normal animal, moving the head from side to side and up and down elicits physiological nystagmus. At the end of each movement, the head should be stabilized and cessation of nystagmus noted. An abnormality of this reflex following head trauma is typically due to a lesion of the brainstem (Box 28.2).
5. Respiratory pattern: irregular respiratory patterns may be seen due to brain injury, including:

BOX 28.2 Findings consistent with brainstem injury

- Mentation: comatose
- Bilateral fixed (mid-position) dilated unresponsive pupils
- Absence of gag reflex
- Irregular respiratory patterns or apnoea
- Abnormal oculocephalic reflex

(a) Hyperventilation
(b) Cheyne–Stokes respiration
(c) Ataxic respiration (irregular rate, rhythm and excursion)
(d) Apnoea.

6. Motor function and posture: animals that are not comatose should maintain voluntary motor activity unless trauma has occurred to the brainstem, the spinal cord, or a peripheral nerve.
   (a) Hemiparesis/plegia: unilateral brainstem damage (also some spinal cord lesions)
   (b) Tetraparesis/plegia: more diffuse brainstem damage (also cervical spinal cord lesion)
   (c) Decerebrate rigidity: extreme extensor rigidity of all four limbs with no periods of relaxation; lateral recumbency and possible opisthotonos; marked changes in mentation and very grave prognosis
   (d) Decerebellate rigidity: extensor rigidity of all 4 limbs but with periods of relaxation and flexion of the pelvic limbs; mentation may be normal; better prognosis than decerebrate rigidity.
   (e) Schiff–Sherrington phenomenon: decerebrate and decerebellate rigidity must be distinguished from this phenomenon which may occur as a result of an acute severe lesion of the spinal cord between T2 and L3. Pelvic limb paralysis accompanied by extensor rigidity of the thoracic limbs is seen when the animal is in lateral recumbency.

Treatment

Treatment of TBI is summarized in Table 28.1 and illustrated further in Case example 1.

Prognosis

Some clinicians use a Modified Glasgow Coma Scale (The Small Animal Coma Scale) as a quantitative way of grading and monitoring brain injury and assisting with prognosis. Ultimately, signs of slow but steady improvement on repeat neurological evaluation may be the most practical guide.

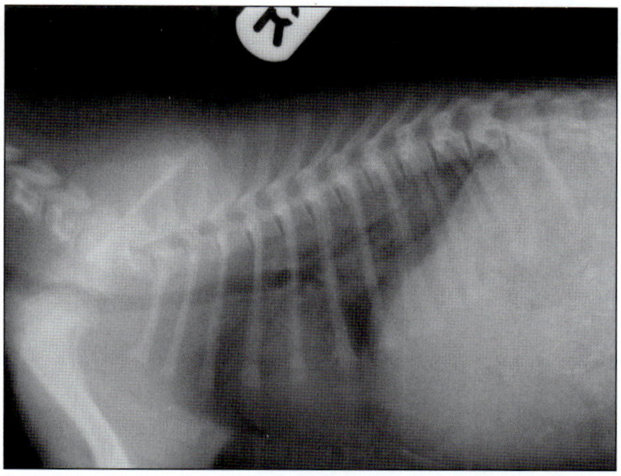

Figure 28.1 Thoracic radiograph of a puppy with head trauma showing caudodorsal lung changes consistent with neurogenic (noncardiogenic) oedema.

NURSING ASPECT

Patients with traumatic brain injury may be recumbent for prolonged periods and the value of adequate nursing in such cases should not be underestimated. The most important measures are as follows:

- TLC, gentle handling (independent of interventions)
- Minimize stress: be calm and quiet around the patient, provide a dimly lit quiet environment, use gentle restraint and minimize/group interventions
- Use well-padded bedding to prevent pressure sores and ensure bedding is dry, clean and comfortable
- Turn every 2–4 hours if recumbent to prevent atelectasis (lung collapse)
- Lubricate eyes every 4–6 hours to prevent corneal drying and ulceration
- Appropriate bladder management: express or catheterize if necessary and prevent urinary soiling
- Tempt to eat if appropriate
- Perform regular physiotherapy in patients that are likely to be recumbent for prolonged periods

Table 28.1 Treatment of traumatic brain injury

Treatment	Comments
Oxygen supplementation	Liberal approach encouraged Maintain SpO_2 above 95% Ideally intubate and ventilate if SpO_2 remains below 90% but there may be practical and financial considerations
Intravenous fluid therapy	Early fluid resuscitation to correct systemic hypoperfusion and ensure adequate cerebral blood flow Isotonic crystalloid typical first choice; may need synthetic colloid if inadequate response Hypertonic saline appropriate choice in some cases (see below) Avoid hypervolaemia as may increase intracranial pressure – but only be conservative once hypovolaemia corrected
Intracranial hypertension therapy	Promote venous drainage from the brain – keep head elevated 15–30° above horizontal; minimize jugular compression (e.g. avoid jugular venepuncture, do not restrain around the neck area) Medical therapy for cerebral oedema: • Mannitol: hyperosmolar; induces osmotic diuresis reducing cerebral oedema; other potential beneficial effects; contraindicated in hypovolaemic patients • Hypertonic saline (e.g. 7.5% sodium chloride): especially indicated in hypovolaemic patients with suspected raised ICP to both restore intravascular volume and reduce cerebral oedema; osmotically active; other potential beneficial effects
Minimize increases in cerebral metabolic rate	Antiseizure therapy if indicated Sedate if distressed (flailing, constant vocalization) – use opioids and anticonvulsant medications preferentially Treat hyperthermia secondary to brain injury and/or seizure activity
Analgesia	Rapid baseline neurological examination first Pure opioid May also contribute to sedation
Nutritional support	Important once patient is stable and improving – do not start too soon Avoid syringe feeding – provides inadequate calorific intake; potential for aspiration and interference with head injuries Oesophagostomy tube preferred once stable for anaesthesia

ICP, intracranial pressure; SpO_2, percentage saturation of haemoglobin with oxygen.

Case example 1

PRESENTING SIGNS AND CASE HISTORY

A 3-year-old male neutered domestic long hair cat presented shortly after a presumed motor vehicle accident. The cat had been healthy prior to going out that evening but had returned home some time later in respiratory distress. Notable deterioration had occurred in the time it had taken the owners to bring the cat to the clinic. No other significant preceding history was reported.

Major body system examination

On presentation the cat was stuporous. Heart rate was 160 beats per minute with no murmur or gallop sound heard and femoral pulses could not be palpated. Mucous membranes were pale pink with a prolonged capillary refill time and extremities were cold. The cat was tachypnoeic but lung sounds were appropriate for the rate and effort. Percentage saturation of haemoglobin with oxygen (SpO_2) on room air was 97%. Abdominal palpation was unremarkable but the cat was mildly hypothermic (rectal temperature 36.5°C). There were palpable skull fractures in the region of the left frontal bone and left-sided scleral and nasal haemorrhage was identified. Blood pressure could not be obtained initially by sphygmomanometry.

Assessment

The cat was assessed as moderately to severely hypovolaemic and the presence of hypothermia was not considered unusual in a cat with this presentation. Although the cat's mental status could in part be attributed to the hypovolaemia, it was felt to be too severely altered and, given the clear evidence of head injury, a component of TBI was therefore suspected. The cat's respiratory status seemed appropriate and neither significant intrathoracic injury nor a central effect on respiration was suspected. At this stage it was not possible to make a reliable assessment of the cat's pain status.

Emergency database

An intravenous catheter was placed in a cephalic vein and blood obtained via the catheter for an emergency database. This revealed low–normal manual packed cell volume (PCV) (32%, reference range 31–45%) with low serum total solids (TS) (50 g/l, reference range 61–80 g/l) suggestive of recent haemorrhage. The cat was moderately hyperglycaemic (15.0 mmol/l, reference range 4.2–6.6 mmol/l).

CLINICAL TIP

- Jugular vein occlusion for venepuncture should be avoided as far as possible in patients with raised intracranial pressure as impaired drainage from the brain may significantly exacerbate intracranial hypertension.

CLINICAL TIP

- Hyperglycaemia may be identified in dogs and cats following head trauma and is thought to result from a response involving the sympathetic nervous system and the adrenal medulla. The degree of hyperglycaemia often correlates with the severity of traumatic injury but a relationship with outcome has not been shown in dogs and cats.

Case management

CLINICAL TIP

- Treatment of extracranial potentially life-threatening abnormalities is the immediate

CLINICAL TIP—cont'd

priority in the management of patients with traumatic brain injury (TBI). In reality, treatment of such abnormalities often concurrently achieves the prime aim with respect to intracranial trauma management which is to limit secondary brain injury, i.e. as primary brain injury (including disruption of blood vessels and tearing/crushing of parenchyma) will already have occurred at the time of presentation.

Hypertonic saline was not available and a 20 ml/kg bolus of 0.9% sodium chloride (normal, physiological saline) was therefore administered intravenously over 15 minutes. No warming measures were implemented at this time and the cat was kept in sternal recumbency with his head elevated at a 30° angle to the table. A more thorough baseline neurological evaluation was performed at this time. Anisocoria was present with the right pupil larger than the left but a menace response could not be elicited in either eye. Bilateral pupillary light responses, both direct and consensual, were intact. Blink and gag reflexes were present and jaw tone was adequate. The cat's posture seemed appropriate. Oculocephalic reflex was not tested at this time.

A low dose (0.1 mg/kg slow i.v.) of methadone was administered during the initial fluid bolus. At the end of the bolus the cat's perfusion had improved but he remained mildly hypovolaemic. A further conservative bolus of 5 ml/kg was administered over 10 minutes, after which the cat was assessed as euvolaemic.

Despite the improved perfusion, the cat's mentation remained inappropriately reduced and it was therefore suspected that this was the result of raised intracranial pressure secondary to traumatic brain injury. Mannitol (0.5 g/kg i.v. bolus over 20 minutes) was therefore administered, following which a slow but notable clinical improvement was detected. The anisocoria resolved and the cat was able to raise his head voluntarily. Systolic blood pressure at this time was within normal limits (105 mmHg). No free peritoneal fluid was detected on abdominal ultrasound. Thoracic radiographs were not taken because it was felt that the index of suspicion for significant intrathoracic injury was too low to justify the additional stress involved for the cat.

CLINICAL TIP

Animals with traumatic brain injury must be monitored very closely, in particular for the following three developments.

- Seizure activity: seizure activity will increase cerebral metabolic rate, increasing cerebral oxygen demand and therefore the risk of hypoxic injury. It may also worsen cerebral oedema, thereby exacerbating raised intracranial pressure (ICP), and can cause hyperthermia. Antiseizure medication must therefore be administered at the first sign of seizure activity.
- Bradycardia: the onset of previously undetected bradycardia may signal an increase in ICP and should prompt immediate treatment.
- Respiratory distress: brain injury can give rise to neurogenic (non-cardiogenic) pulmonary oedema that usually develops within minutes to a few hours of the event. Thoracic radiographs typically show a caudodorsal distribution of lung field changes consistent with pulmonary oedema (interstitial to alveolar pattern) (Figure 28.1). Treatment involves oxygen supplementation and minimal stress; neurogenic pulmonary oedema is likely to be of mixed cause and a single low dose of furosemide may be rational. Clinical improvement is typically noted within 24–48 hours.

CLINICAL TIP

- Although the use of corticosteroids, in particular methylprednisolone succinate, for traumatic brain injury has been a longstanding practice in both human and veterinary medicine, it is not one based on clinical evidence.
- More recent clinical trials in humans have not shown positive effects on outcome and some have suggested possible increases in morbidity and/or mortality.
- Considering the potential adverse effects (e.g. gastrointestinal ulceration, increased risk of infection, hyperglycaemia) of these agents, current recommendations are that corticosteroids should not be used for traumatic brain injury.

The cat was maintained on intravenous fluid therapy and analgesia (buprenorphine 0.02 mg/kg i.v. q 6 hr), and monitored closely including repeat neurological examinations. He improved steadily with respect to his neurological status and, although not further investigated, the skull fractures were therefore not suspected to be surgical in nature.

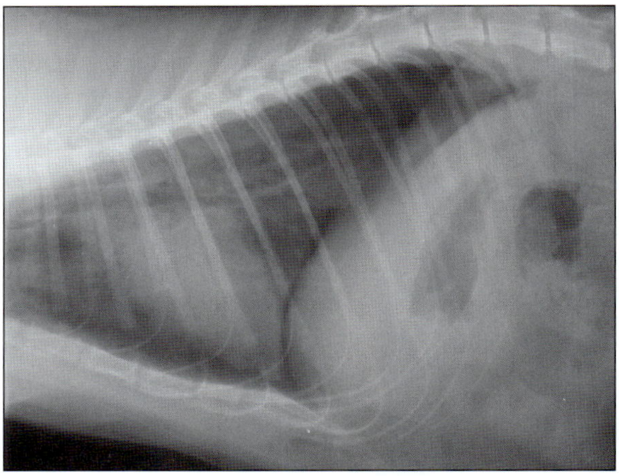

(a)

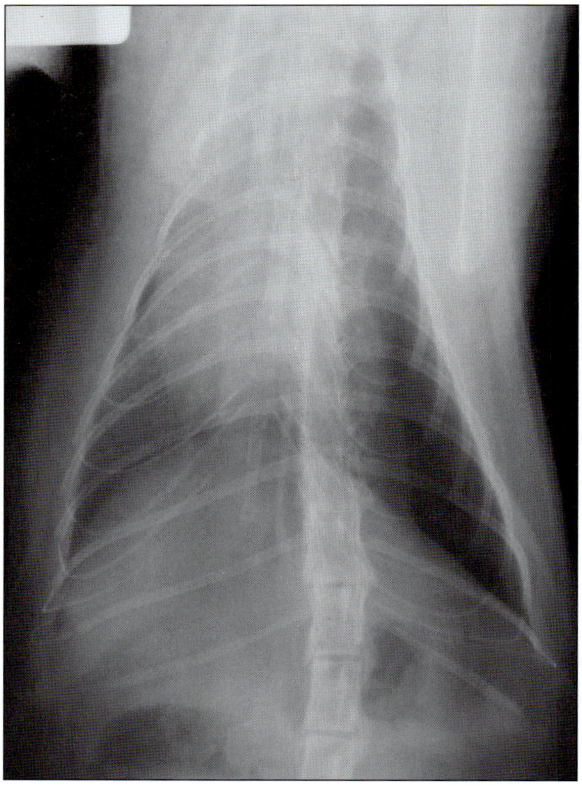

(b)

Figure 28.2 (a) Right lateral and (b) dorsoventral thoracic radiographs of a cat showing pneumothorax and pulmonary contusions following trauma.

However, the cat remained anorexic and an oesophagostomy tube was therefore placed under general anaesthesia 3 days after initial presentation. The cat made an uneventful recovery from this procedure and was subsequently discharged. His owner was asked to tempt him to eat but to feed him via the oesophagostomy tube regardless until he was eating satisfactorily on his own. Meloxicam oral suspension was dispensed, to be administered via the feeding tube initially.

CLINICAL TIP

- Diagnostic imaging of the head may be advisable in animals that do not show steady improvement, or that demonstrate acute deterioration. Although plain skull radiographs may reveal fractures, it can be difficult to obtain radiographs of interpretable quality and plain radiographs are unlikely to provide clinically useful information with respect to brain injury. Referral to a specialist centre for advanced imaging (computed tomography (CT) or magnetic resonance imaging (MRI)) should therefore be considered if affordable and once the patient has been stabilized.

THORACIC INJURY

Theory refresher

Thoracic injuries following blunt trauma include:

- Pneumothorax
- Pulmonary contusions
- Haemothorax
- Rib fractures and flail segment
- Diaphragmatic rupture.

In the author's experience, pneumothorax and pulmonary contusions are the most common.

Pneumothorax

Closed pneumothorax usually results from leakage of air secondary to a lesion within the lung parenchyma, although it may also occur for example due to damage to the airways or oesophagus (Figure 28.2). Open pneumothorax involves loss of integrity of the thoracic wall (e.g. following penetrating trauma) while a tension pneumothorax occurs if a one-way valve is formed at the site of air leakage such that air taken in during inspiration leaks into the pleural space but cannot be expelled (Figure 28.3). The result is a rapid and potentially life-threatening increase in intrapleural pressure with severe respiratory and cardiovascular compromise and immediate thoracocentesis is required. In the author's experience tension pneumothorax is rare.

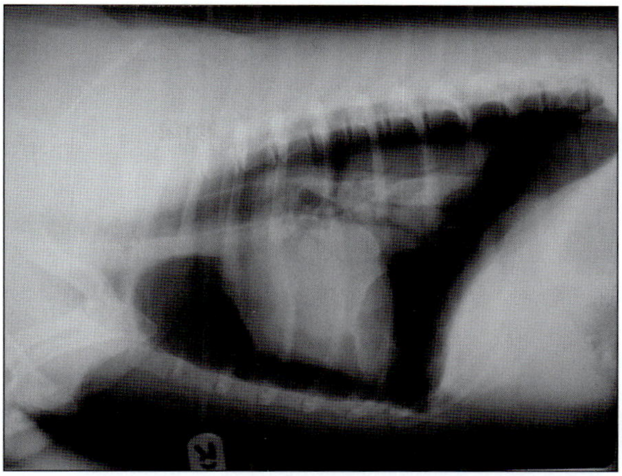

Figure 28.3 Right lateral thoracic radiograph of a dog showing traumatic tension pneumothorax. The dog underwent cardiopulmonary arrest just prior to arrival at the hospital and the owner did not want resuscitation to be attempted.

CLINICAL TIP

- Thoracocentesis is by no means required in all cases of traumatic closed pneumothorax and the air will be resorbed over days to weeks. The decision to perform thoracocentesis should be guided by whether the pneumothorax is thought to be compromising respiration in a clinically significant way.

Thoracocentesis is by no means required in all cases of traumatic closed pneumothorax and the air will be resorbed over days to weeks. The decision to perform thoracocentesis should be guided by whether the pneumothorax is thought to be compromising respiration in a clinically significant way. Clinical improvement following thoracocentesis is generally associated with aspiration of 20–30 ml/kg or more of air although improvement may be noted with removal of smaller volumes in animals with other concomitant thoracic injuries, most commonly pulmonary contusions. In the author's experience thoracocentesis does not usually need to be performed more than twice for traumatic pneumothorax and chest drain placement is infrequently indicated. The need for surgical intervention is rare.

As well as occurring as a result of trauma, pneumothorax may also be spontaneous following rupture of pulmonary lesions (e.g. bullae, tumours, subpleural blebs) or iatrogenic (e.g. following thoracocentesis or fine needle lung aspiration). Pneumothorax that occurs spontaneously is often more severe than following trauma, and chest drain placement and surgical intervention are more likely to be indicated.

Pulmonary contusions

Pulmonary contusions represent areas of alveolar and interstitial haemorrhage and oedema, and probably represent the most common thoracic injury in dogs and cats following trauma. Not all affected animals develop associated clinical signs and pulmonary contusions may occur with or without other thoracic injuries. Clinical signs may develop acutely or over several hours, and radiographic changes may lag behind clinical signs by up to 24 hours. Radiographic abnormalities (patchy or diffuse alveolar or interstitial lung changes) may persist for a variable period of time despite clinical improvement (Figure 28.4). There is no specific treatment for pulmonary contusions and management typically involves oxygen supplementation, cage rest, analgesia as indicated for concurrent injuries, minimal stress and time.

Intravenous fluid therapy does not have to be withheld but caution is advised. Hypovolaemia is common in patients with pulmonary contusions at time of presentation and the aim of fluid therapy should be to restore acceptable tissue perfusion while avoiding excessive fluid administration. It may be acceptable in some cases to leave the patient mildly hypovolaemic rather than risk worsening pulmonary contusions. Diuretics are not recommended in the treatment of pulmonary contusions and are contraindicated in hypovolaemia.

The incidence of bacterial pneumonia following pulmonary contusions is very low and the indiscriminate use of antibiotics in these cases is not recommended.

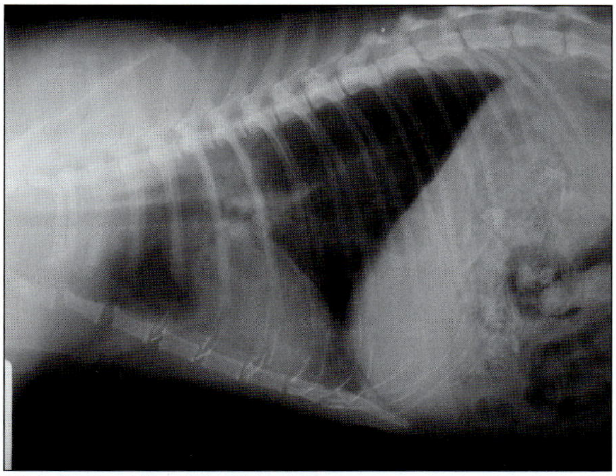

Figure 28.4 Right lateral thoracic radiograph of a cat showing pulmonary contusions.

CLINICAL TIP

- In the author's experience clinical signs associated with pulmonary contusions resolve in most cases (generally within 2–7 days) but their presence may necessitate that management of other non-life-threatening injuries (e.g. long bone fractures) be postponed until respiratory status has improved adequately.

Haemothorax

Haemothorax is accumulation of blood in the pleural space. It is not uncommon to detect a small volume of pleural effusion following blunt thoracic trauma that is presumed to be secondary to haemorrhage. However, in the author's experience, clinically significant haemothorax is relatively rare. The pleural space can accommodate a considerable volume of blood without causing clinically significant respiratory compromise and haemothorax should not be drained unless it is thought to be significantly contributing to dyspnoea; the blood will be resorbed over several days. This is especially important as anaemia secondary to haemorrhage is relatively common following trauma, particularly in cats.

If haemothorax is drained, it is sensible to remove as small a volume (e.g. 20 ml/kg) as possible that is expected to allow clinical improvement in respiratory status (i.e. so that the remainder may be resorbed). Surgical intervention for traumatic haemothorax is seldom required.

Aside from trauma, haemothorax may also occur as a result of severe coagulopathy, in particular due to anticoagulant rodenticide intoxication; other less common causes are neoplasia, pulmonary thromboembolism, lung lobe torsion and iatrogenic causes.

Rib fractures and flail segment

It is very unusual for rib fractures to occur in dogs and cats without at least one other significant thoracic injury. Rib fractures are often only diagnosed radiographically and they typically do not require specific intervention. Rib fractures are, however, reported to be very painful and a liberal approach to analgesia is therefore recommended in these cases. Ventilation may be compromised in painful animals, especially if rib fractures are present.

A flail segment may be created if two or more adjacent ribs are fractured both dorsally and ventrally, i.e. so that the segment is no longer stabilized by attachment to the sternum or spine. This flail segment then moves paradoxically in relation to the rest of the chest wall during respiration, i.e. the flail segment moves in on inspiration and out on expiration. Although large flail segments may cause hypoventilation, flail segments typically do not contribute significantly to dyspnoea and stabilization is not usually indicated. Their significance lies more in the fact that they are typically associated with other significant thoracic injuries, especially pulmonary contusions, and that they are often very painful. These factors are more likely to be responsible for any respiratory compromise identified.

Case example 2

PRESENTING SIGNS AND CASE HISTORY

A 3-year-old male neutered domestic short hair cat presented shortly after a presumed motor vehicle accident. The cat had been seen sitting in the front lawn by his owner 1 hour prior to dragging himself through the cat flap. The cat was vocalizing and had increased respiratory effort. His owner reported limited movement in the left pelvic limb and tail but no movement in the right pelvic limb. No other significant history was reported.

Major body system examination

The cat was initially briefly observed in his carrier. He was depressed with an obvious increase in respiratory effort and had bilaterally symmetrical mid-sized pupils. The front half was in sternal recumbency. The top of the transport carrier in this case could be removed and the rest of the initial assessment was therefore performed with the cat remaining in his carrier. Flow-by oxygen supplementation was commenced. Heart rate was 220 beats per minute with no murmur or gallop sound heard and the dorsal pedal pulse could just be palpated.

CLINICAL TIP

- In animals with suspected pelvic trauma, it is preferable to assess the arterial pulse at sites other than the femoral arteries (e.g. dorsal pedal artery, median artery). The potential to cause pain must be remembered when feeling for a femoral pulse in these cases.

Mucous membranes were pink with a normal capillary refill time. Respiratory rate was 42 breaths per minute with a marked increase in effort and lung sounds were dull dorsally. Lung sounds were possibly harsher cranioventrally than would be expected for the respiratory rate and effort but this was difficult to assess at this stage. The cat moved his left pelvic limb and tail during this initial examination but no deep pain perception or withdrawal reflex was elicited from the right pelvic limb. No further examination was performed at this time.

Assessment

Examination of the respiratory system in this case was highly suggestive of pneumothorax. The possible increase in harshness in the cranioventral lung field was potentially suggestive of pulmonary contusions that often accompany traumatic pneumothorax. As the dorsal pedal pulse could be palpated, the cat was not thought to be any more than mildly hypovolaemic and given the concern regarding pulmonary contusions, it was decided that intravenous fluid resuscitation was not a priority at this stage.

CLINICAL TIP

- It is often possible on the basis of observation and auscultation to make reliable judgements as to the most likely cause of dyspnoea in trauma patients and thoracic radiography is not recommended in distressed, painful or unstable patients. This is especially applicable to dyspnoeic cats as they may decompensate more easily than dogs.
- Where significant pleural space disease (pneumothorax, haemothorax) is suspected, thoracocentesis may be both diagnostic and therapeutic. This procedure is relatively simple and clinically significant complications are rare. It is recommended to perform thoracocentesis rather than subject unstable trauma patients to radiography initially. If radiography is performed, everything should be prepared before bringing the patient to the radiography room and minimal restraint should be used. If tolerated, oxygen supplementation should be provided by mask or flow-by. The intention here should be to produce an image that allows the anatomical area affected to be identified and not to

Continued

CLINICAL TIP—cont'd

produce the perfect thoracic radiograph. Even a rotated dorsoventral radiograph can provide more than enough information for the patient's initial management. A dyspnoeic animal should never be restrained in dorsal recumbency and it is typically best to minimize the amount of time spent in lateral recumbency.

Case management

Methadone (0.3 mg/kg i.m.) was administered and the cat was placed in an oxygen cage. While in the oxygen cage the cat was observed to urinate voluntarily, voiding a moderate amount of grossly haematuric urine. Preparation was made to perform thoracocentesis and this was then undertaken successfully (see p. 291). One hundred millilitres (approximately equivalent to 20 ml/kg) of air was aspirated from the right-hand side. Although the cat remained dyspnoeic, a significant improvement in respiratory status was observed and lung sounds were audible dorsally. It was therefore decided not to perform repeat thoracocentesis on the other side at this time. The previous suspicion of harsh lung sounds was confirmed, supporting the likelihood of pulmonary contusions.

As the cat remained compliant, further examination and interventions were performed at this time with flow-by oxygen supplementation provided throughout. Abdominal palpation was uncomfortable but no free fluid was detected ultrasonographically. The pelvis was painful on gentle palpation but there was good anal tone and perineal reflex.

An intravenous catheter was placed in a cephalic vein and blood obtained via the catheter for an emergency database that was unremarkable. The cat was returned to the oxygen cage and analgesia in the form of intermittent boluses of methadone (0.2 mg/kg i.v. q 4 hr) continued. It was envisaged that the cat would be anorexic but given the likelihood of pulmonary contusions, only maintenance intravenous isotonic crystalloid therapy (compound sodium lactate at 2 ml/kg/hr) was administered.

Forty-eight hours after initial presentation the cat's respiratory status had improved satisfactorily and he had been weaned off oxygen supplementation. General anaesthesia was performed and pelvic radiography confirmed multiple fractures with medial displacement of the caudal right hemipelvis, resulting in significant narrowing of the pelvic diameter. The fractures were therefore assessed as surgical in nature and the cat was referred for specialist repair and oesophagostomy tube placement.

TRAUMATIC DIAPHRAGMATIC RUPTURE

Theory refresher

Although listed here as a thoracic injury, acquired diaphragmatic rupture typically occurs as a result of blunt abdominal trauma. Circumferential and right-sided diaphragmatic tears are most common in dogs and cats and the liver is reportedly the most commonly herniated organ. In addition, the stomach, small intestine and spleen are often involved in left-sided hernias and the small intestine and pancreas in right-sided hernias.

Diagnosis

Radiography is commonly used in animals with suspected diaphragmatic rupture and consistent findings include complete or partial loss of the diaphragmatic line, mediastinal shift, obscuring of the cardiac silhouette, and cranial displacement of abdominal viscera and gas shadows (Figures 28.5 and 28.6). Orthogonal views are recommended but diagnosis may be difficult, for example if displaced viscera are obscured by pleural fluid or in the absence of visceral displacement. Positive contrast gastrography or peritoneography may be required in these cases.

CLINICAL TIP

- Timing of radiography must be carefully chosen and it is not a priority in unstable patients in which the additional stress may cause rapid decompensation.

If facilities and expertise allow, ultrasonography provides an alternative, reliable and less stressful means of diagnosing diaphragmatic rupture. This may be especially helpful earlier on in unstable patients or in those with significant pleural effusion obscuring radiographic detail.

Timing of surgical intervention

The timing of surgical intervention for diaphragmatic rupture has been the subject of some debate, with many

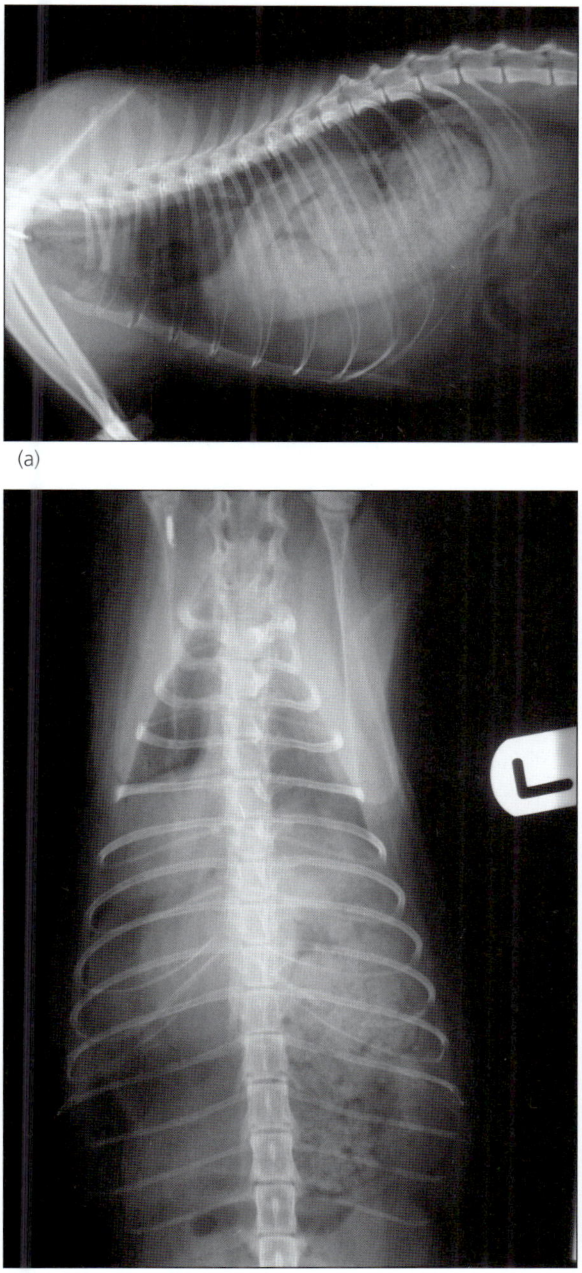

(a)

(b)

Figure 28.5 (a) Right lateral and (b) dorsoventral thoracic radiographs of a cat showing diaphragmatic rupture.

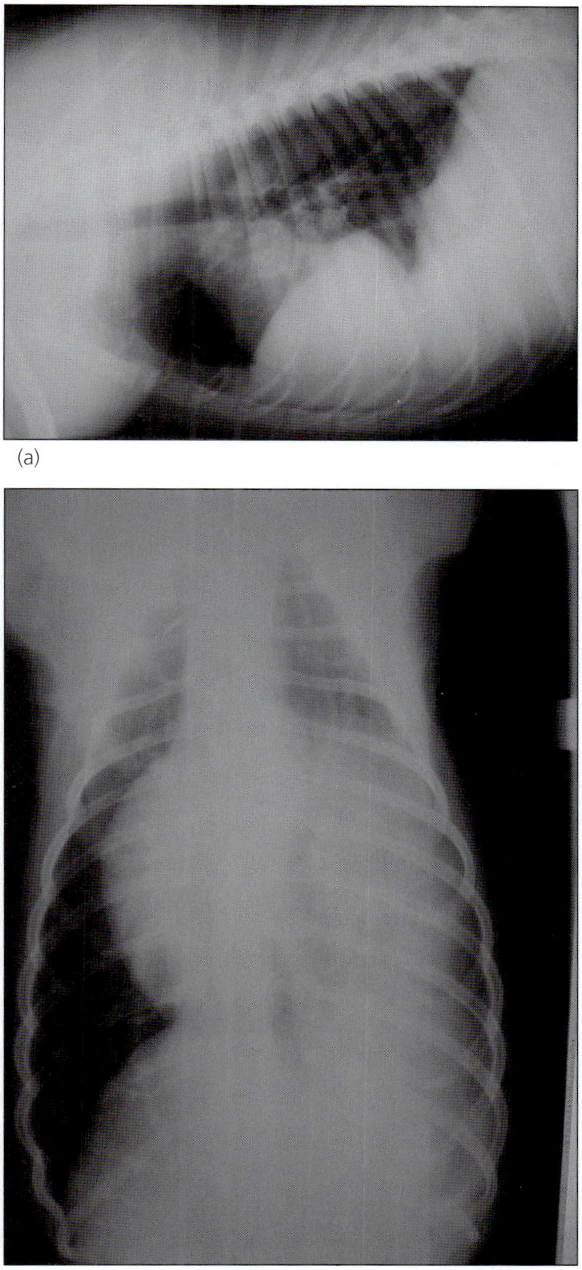

(a)

(b)

Figure 28.6 (a) Right lateral and (b) dorsoventral thoracic radiographs of a cross-bred dog showing diaphragmatic rupture.

authors recommending a delay of more than 24 hours following trauma to ensure adequate time for stabilization of other concurrent conditions (e.g. hypovolaemic shock) and injuries (e.g. pulmonary contusions), thereby reducing the risks associated with general anaesthesia and major surgery. However, current literature suggests that surgical intervention within 24 hours of admission in stable patients does not worsen the prognosis and therefore timing of surgical intervention should be made on an individual case basis.

CLINICAL TIP

- Diaphragmatic rupture repair is more likely to be associated with a successful outcome when performed as an elective procedure with adequate staffing and time for thorough planning and preparation.
- If a prolonged period of stabilization is provided, patients must be monitored very closely for any deterioration in clinical status that may for example occur as a result of gastric entrapment and distension or strangulation of displaced intestine. More emergent surgical intervention may then be required and needle decompression of the stomach is appropriate in a severely compromised patient while being prepared for surgery.

Case example 3

PRESENTING SIGNS AND CASE HISTORY

A 5-year-old female entire Yorkshire terrier presented a short time after a witnessed motor vehicle accident. The dog had remained conscious and ambulatory following the incident but she was noted to have some increased respiratory effort by her owner, prompting emergency presentation. No other significant history was reported.

Major body system examination

On presentation the dog was quiet and responsive although she had an unpredictable temperament, attempting to nip intermittently during examination. Cardiovascular examination revealed a heart rate of 212 beats per minute. Heart sounds could not be heard on the left side of the thorax but were readily audible in the right hemithorax. Peripheral pulses were hyperdynamic and ocular mucous membranes were pink; capillary refill time was not assessed. Respiratory rate was 48 breaths per minute with an increase in effort. Lung sounds were significantly decreased on the left side but were readily audible and diffusely harsh in the right hemithorax. No further examination was performed at this time.

CLINICAL TIP

Although respiratory dysfunction is a common presenting sign of traumatic diaphragmatic rupture, it may be minimal or even absent in a number of cases. The aetiology of respiratory compromise is usually multifactorial and may include:

- Loss of mechanical function of the diaphragm (most important muscle for inspiration)
- Pleural space-occupying material causing lung lobe compression and progressive atelectasis. This material predominantly constitutes abdominal organs but possibly also air (pneumothorax) and fluid (haemothorax, transudate)
- Concurrent thoracic injuries (e.g. pulmonary contusions, rib fractures)
- Other factors such as pain and hypovolaemia.

In some animals with diaphragmatic rupture acute respiratory decompensation may occur as a result of accumulation of a significant volume of abdominal viscera in the pleural space. In such cases, holding the animal upright to allow the abdominal contents to return to the peritoneal cavity is potentially life-saving.

Assessment

The findings on thoracic auscultation in this case were suggestive of possible diaphragmatic rupture with displacement of intra-abdominal contents predominantly into the left hemithorax. The harsh lung sounds audible on the right were likely due to pulmonary contusions. Cardiovascular examination may have suggested mild hypovolaemia; however, pain, anxiety and signalment were also thought to be contributing to the tachycardia. Given the concerns regarding pulmonary contusions, it was not felt that volume resuscitation was indicated at the outset.

Case management

Methadone (0.5 mg/kg i.m.) was administered. The fur over both cephalic veins was clipped and EMLA® cream 5% (AstraZeneca, see Ch. 5) applied topically. The sites were covered with an occlusive dressing and the dog was placed in an oxygen cage and monitored closely for 30 minutes. By the end of this time the dog's heart rate had reduced considerably and her temperament had also notably improved. Respiratory rate had reduced but there had been no notable change in effort.

An intravenous catheter was placed in one of the cephalic veins and blood obtained via the catheter for an emergency database that was unremarkable. Brief ultrasonography was suggestive of a loss of diaphragmatic integrity with displacement of at least the stomach into the left hemithorax. A small volume of pleural fluid was detected in the right hemithorax. A moderately sized urinary bladder was identified with no peritoneal fluid.

The dog was started on replacement isotonic crystalloid at 2 ml/kg/hr and returned to the oxygen cage. She was positioned on an incline and analgesia was continued in the form of intermittent boluses of methadone (0.2–0.3 mg/kg i.v. q 4 hr).

Thoracic radiography performed approximately 16 hours following presentation confirmed the presence of diaphragmatic rupture with probable displacement of the stomach into the left hemithorax. Midline exploratory coeliotomy and repair of the diaphragm was performed, with intermittent positive pressure ventilation (IPPV) provided as necessary, and the dog went on to make an uneventful recovery.

CLINICAL TIP

- A thoracostomy tube may be placed intraoperatively prior to closure of the diaphragmatic defect to allow residual air to be removed from the pleural cavity following repair. In order to avoid re-expansion pulmonary oedema, some authors recommend only aspirating a proportion of the residual air immediately postoperatively, i.e. as much as is necessary for satisfactory ventilation to occur, with the remainder being removed over the subsequent 8–12 hours. A thoracostomy tube will also allow monitoring for complications such as pneumothorax or haemothorax, as well as repeated administration of local anaesthesia.
- If a thoracostomy tube is not placed, it is important to remove residual air from the pleural cavity by other means to prevent respiratory compromise. This is ideally done through the diaphragm before the final suture is tightened but may be achieved via thoracocentesis during recovery.

PELVIC FRACTURES

CLINICAL TIP

- Considerable external force is required to fracture the pelvis and therefore animals with pelvic fractures are likely to have suffered other additional injuries. These injuries may be confined to the musculoskeletal system but they may also relate to the abdomen (e.g. urinary bladder rupture), thorax (e.g. pulmonary contusions, pneumothorax) or nervous system (e.g. lumbosacral plexus damage). Thus any animal with a suspected or confirmed pelvic fracture must be thoroughly evaluated for additional extrapelvic injuries.

As with all emergency patients, evaluation of an animal with a suspected pelvic fracture should begin with a major body system examination and initial stabilization should be provided as needed. Priority must be given to the identification and management of potentially life-threatening extrapelvic injuries. Radiographic evaluation of the pelvis must only be done once the patient has received adequate stabilization, including the provision of suitable analgesia.

CLINICAL TIP

- In animals with suspected pelvic trauma, it is preferable to assess the arterial pulse at sites other than the femoral arteries (e.g. dorsal pedal artery, median artery). The potential to cause pain must be remembered when feeling for a femoral pulse in these cases.

With respect to suspected lumbosacral or pelvic injury, it is important to find out whether the animal has been seen to walk and whether voluntary urination or defecation has occurred since the incident. Both pelvic limbs should be assessed for deep pain sensation and positive withdrawal reflex as a minimum. Anal tone and perineal reflex should be noted and the tail should be assessed for deep pain sensation and voluntary movement. Digital rectal examination performed at the appropriate time may provide information regarding both the degree of displacement of pelvic fractures and the width of the pelvic canal.

Pelvic fractures in cats most often involve the pelvic floor but sacroiliac luxation (potentially bilateral) and ilial body fractures are also common. A detailed discussion is beyond the scope of this book but not all pelvic fractures require surgical intervention. Conservative management may be appropriate in a proportion of cases and is more likely to be suitable for cats and small dogs than larger dogs. Surgical intervention is generally indicated in any animal in which there is, for example, significant narrowing of the pelvic canal, marked pain, neurological deficits or acetabular involvement.

Pelvic injury may be associated with damage to the lumbosacral plexus and/or the sciatic nerve. Sciatic nerve damage may manifest as severe pelvic limb paresis as well as loss of limb sensation to all but the medial aspect (supplied by the saphenous branch of the femoral nerve) including the medial digit. Lack of deep pain sensation in the other digits indicates severe sciatic nerve injury and a poor prognosis for recovery. Signs associated with damage to the pudendal, pelvic or caudal nerves may range from an inability to empty the bladder fully to complete loss of anal tone, voluntary urination, and perineal sensation (see Sacro-caudal and tail pull injuries).

SACRO-CAUDAL AND TAIL PULL INJURIES

The sacro-caudal region of the vertebral column contains the peripheral nerve roots of the cauda equina rather than the spinal cord. Injury to the sacral and caudal (coccygeal) nerve roots most commonly occurs as a result of sacro-caudal fractures or luxations/subluxations secondary to motor vehicle accidents and bite wounds (Figure 28.7a). Distraction and possible avulsion of the nerve roots may also occur as a result of a tail pull injury. Complete or partial, reversible or irreversible neurological dysfunction may occur depending on the extent of the injury to the nerve roots.

The sacral spinal cord segments (S1 to S3) and nerve roots contribute to the pelvic and pudendal nerves (Box 28.3). Neurons from the S1 segment also contribute to the sciatic nerve. The caudal spinal cord segments provide sensory and motor innervation to the tail via the caudal (coccygeal) nerves.

Sacrocaudal and tail pull injuries are identified most commonly in cats and clinical findings may include:

- Perineal urinary and/or faecal soiling
- Flaccid distended bladder that is usually easy to express manually due to reduced urethral sphincter tone; urinary incontinence may occur (loss of the detrusor reflex may result in overflow of a full bladder with dribbling of urine)
- Sacral nerve injury causes reduced or absent perineal reflex and anal sphincter tone (dilated anal sphincter) with possible constipation and faecal incontinence (Figure 28.7b); perineal sensation may also be reduced or absent
- Pain on palpation of the tail head
- Reduced or absent tail sensation, motor function or tone

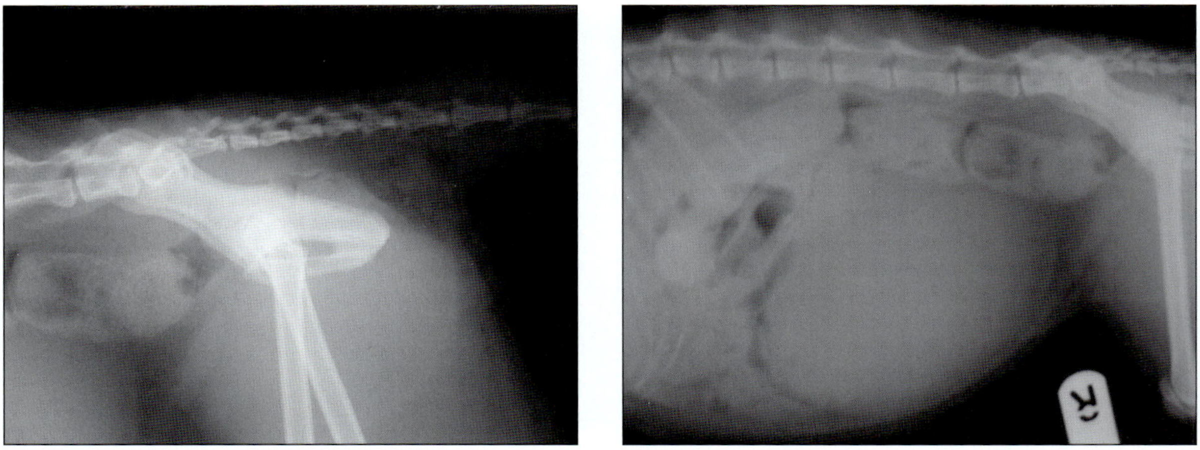

(a) (b)

Figure 28.7 Right lateral radiographs showing (a) sacro-caudal subluxation and (b) large distended bladder and faecal retention in a cat.

BOX 28.3 *Functions of the pelvic and pudendal nerves*

Pelvic nerve

- Transmits sensory information from and parasympathetic motor innervation to the detrusor muscle of the bladder
- Transmits sensory information from and parasympathetic motor innervation to smooth muscle of the descending colon

Pudendal nerve

- Transmits sensory information from the external urethral sphincter, anal sphincter and perineal area
- Provides motor innervation to the external urethral sphincter and the striated muscle of the anal sphincter

- Concomitant injuries depending on the aetiology
- Pelvic limb weakness, lameness or ataxia – may be due to sciatic nerve involvement and/or pelvic or pelvic limb fractures.

Prognosis

The prognosis for cats in which only the tail is affected is very good, including possible return of tail function. Thereafter the prognosis is generally associated with the severity of neurological injury and the most severely affected animals (dilated anus with no anal tone; absent tail sensation and motor function) may not recover. Recovery, in particular with respect to tail sensation and motor function, can take weeks to months to occur. As a guideline, most cats that do not recover urinary control after 4 weeks are likely to remain incontinent. A discussion of appropriate management for animals with prolonged recovery is beyond the scope of this book.

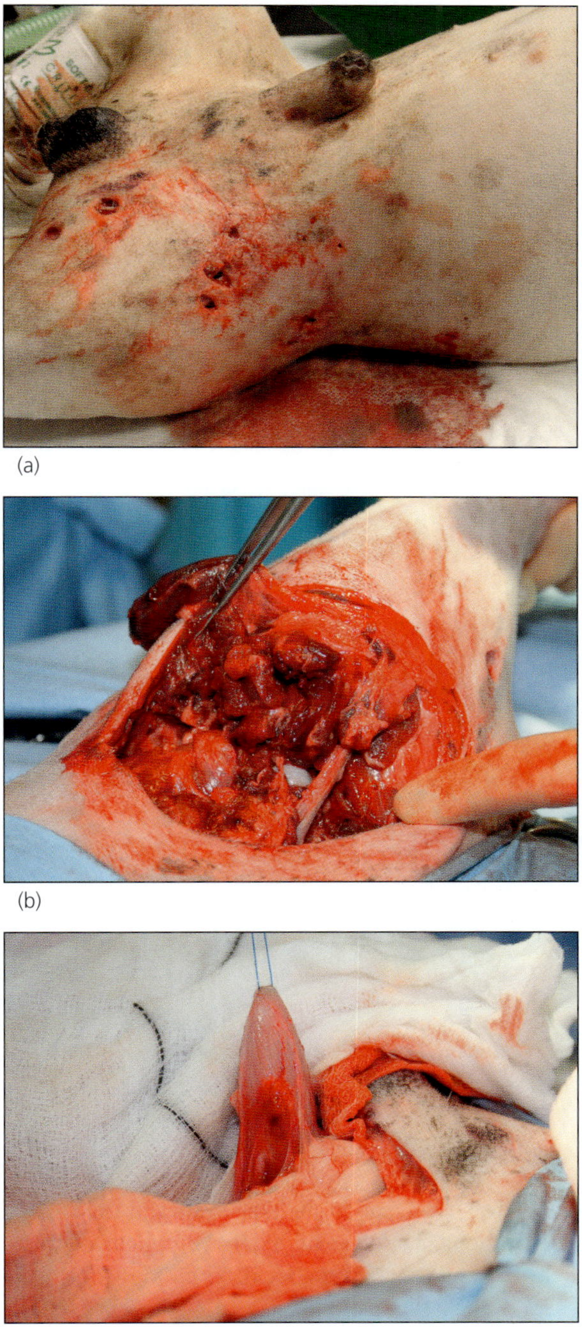

(a) (b) (c)

Figure 28.8 (a) A West Highland White terrier that had suffered dog bite wounds to the caudal abdominal, left inguinal and proximal left pelvic limb areas. (b) Traumatic limb amputation and (c) a puncture wound in the urinary bladder are evident. (Photographs courtesy of Zoe Halfacree)

BITE WOUNDS

Theory refresher

Although skin lacerations or puncture wounds may be the most visible result of a bite injury, these lesions should be considered as only the 'tip of the iceberg'. Crushing, shearing, tearing and avulsion may occur during biting and may cause extensive and deep tissue trauma (Figures 28.8–28.11) that may not be readily appreciable from the outside. It is therefore recommended that all but the

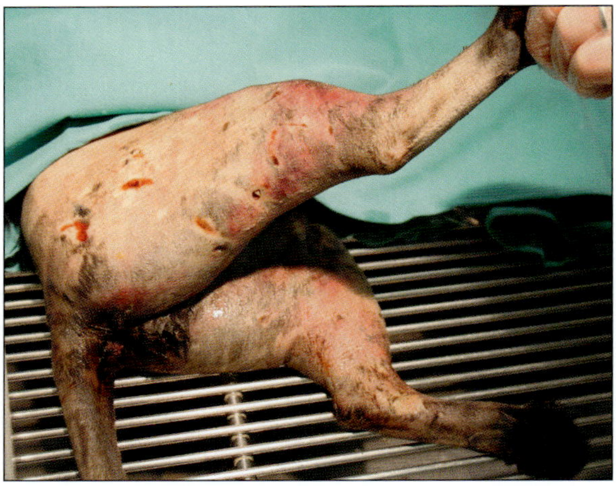

Figure 28.9 Severe perineal and bilateral pelvic limb swelling and bruising in a cat with dog bite wounds. (Photograph courtesy of Zoe Halfacree)

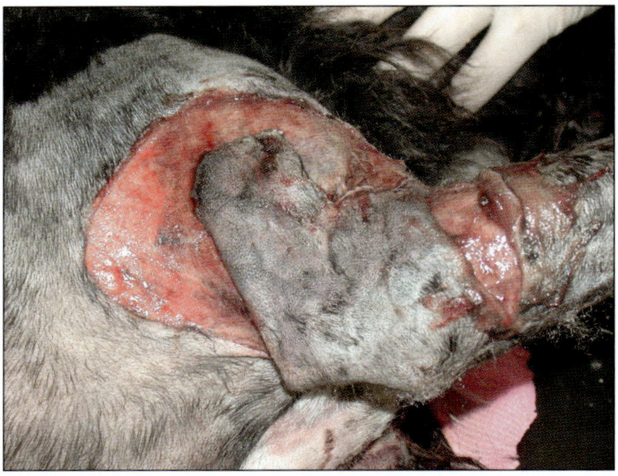

Figure 28.11 Extensive trauma to the thoracic limb of a dog following a dog attack. (Photograph courtesy of Stephen Baines)

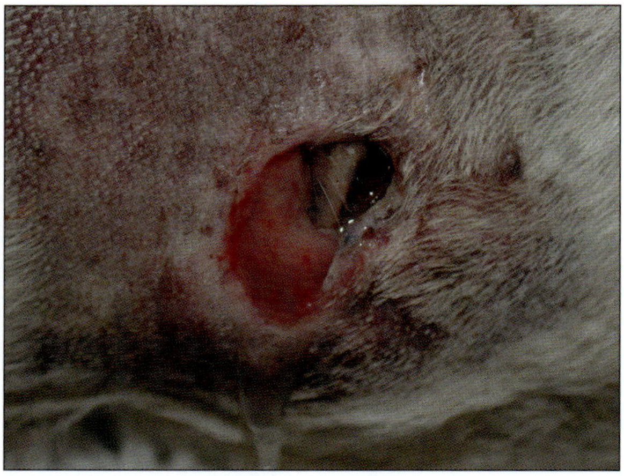

Figure 28.10 Deep penetrating dog bite wound to the flank of a dog. (Photograph courtesy of Stephen Baines)

mildest of bite wounds are explored – but only at the appropriate time following extensive patient stabilization. Diagnostic imaging should be performed as indicated by the location of the wounds and positive contrast sinography may be useful in determining whether wounds have penetrated into body cavities.

Bite wounds, whether open or closed, are invariably contaminated with bacteria. Bacteria may be inoculated deeply into traumatized tissue, with dead space and serum accumulation creating a highly suitable environment for severe infection to develop. All but the most superficial bite wounds should therefore be lavaged thoroughly and adequate drainage ensured. Primary closure of bite wounds without adequate drainage may result in disastrous consequences with respect to wound dehiscence, tissue devitalization and the development of sepsis (Figure 28.12).

Systemic antibiosis may not be required in mild low-risk bite injuries but should be provided parenterally (typically intravenously) and then orally in other cases. A broad-spectrum bactericidal antibiotic with activity against the most commonly cultured bacteria (*Staphylococcus* species, *Escherichia coli*, *Enterococcus* species) should be chosen. Amoxicillin/clavulanate is a good first choice. It must be remembered that antibiotics are not a substitute for appropriate lavage, debridement and drainage. Wound culture is recommended to guide further antimicrobial choice in bite wounds that become infected despite antibiosis.

Systemic inflammatory response syndrome (SIRS), sepsis and death may result from multiple or severe bite wounds, especially when not managed appropriately in a timely fashion.

Case example 4

PRESENTING SIGNS AND CASE HISTORY

A 1-year-old male neutered domestic short hair cat presented shortly after a presumed dog attack. The owners had been awoken by the cat's howling from outside the house and had gone out

PRESENTING SIGNS AND CASE HISTORY—cont'd

to find the cat cowering under a car with a Staffordshire bull terrier dog nearby. The owners had chased the dog away and then retrieved the cat from under the car. No other significant preceding history was reported.

Major body system examination

On presentation the cat was distressed but responsive. Heart rate was 240 beats per minute and no murmur or gallop sound could be heard. Femoral pulses were hyperdynamic, mucous membranes were pink, and capillary refill time was approximately 1.5 seconds. The cat was tachypnoeic (respiratory rate 60 breaths per minute with shallow pattern) but lung auscultation was appropriate for the rate and effort. Abdominal palpation was unremarkable and the bladder was palpable and small. The cat was mildly hypothermic (rectal temperature 37.0°C).

Multiple puncture wounds were identified caudally over the dorsal pelvis and right thigh. There was severe bruising and swelling associated with these areas. Voluntary movement and pain sensation were present in both pelvic limbs and in the tail, and there was good anal tone.

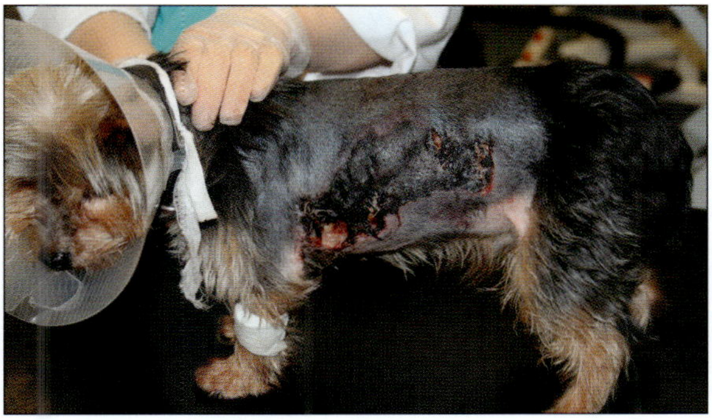

(a)

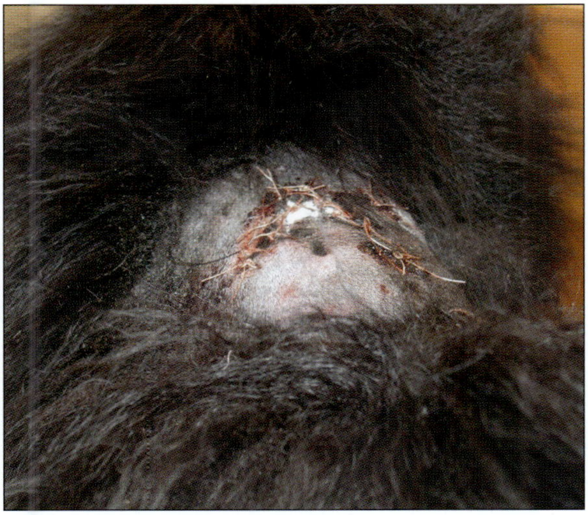

(b)

Figure 28.12 Tissue devitalization and wound dehiscence in two dogs in which dog bite wounds had been closed primarily without ensuring adequate drainage. (Photograph (a) courtesy of Zoe Halfacree; Photograph (b) courtesy of Chiara Valtolina)

Assessment

The tachycardia in this case was thought to be due to a combination of mild hypovolaemia, pain and anxiety. The cat's respiratory status was thought to reflect these abnormalities as opposed to a primary respiratory disorder and trauma appeared to be restricted to the caudal part of the body.

Emergency database

An intravenous catheter was placed in a cephalic vein and blood obtained via the catheter for an emergency database. This was consistent with haemoconcentration (packed cell volume 48%, reference range 31–45%) but total solids were potentially inappropriately low (65 g/l, reference range 61–80 g/l). The cat was also moderately hyperglycaemic (13.8 mmol/l, reference range 4.2–6.6 mmol/l).

Case management

A 10 ml/kg bolus of an isotonic replacement crystalloid solution was administered over 15 minutes and analgesia provided in the form of methadone (0.4 mg/kg i.v.). The cat was also started on intravenous amoxicillin/clavulanate (20 mg/kg i.v. q 8 hr) and a brief abdominal ultrasound was performed that revealed no detectable peritoneal fluid. Cardiovascular status improved after a single bolus and the cat was subsequently maintained on the same intravenous fluid at 4 ml/kg/hr.

The cat responded well to stabilization and approximately 4 hours following initial presentation underwent general anaesthesia. Systolic blood pressure obtained via Doppler sphygmomanometry prior to induction was normal (130 mmHg). Thoracic and abdominal radiography was performed and found to be unremarkable. In particular there was no evidence of pneumoperitoneum or pneumoretroperitoneum that was of concern given the location of the puncture wounds. The cat's pelvis was manipulated thoroughly and no significant abnormalities were detected.

All of the puncture wounds were lavaged with copious amounts of sterile normal saline. The wounds were variously explored, debrided and closed as appropriate, with a Penrose drain being placed strategically to maximize drainage. The cat recovered well from general anaesthesia and was initially maintained on buprenorphine (0.02 mg/kg i.v. q 8 hr) and amoxicillin/clavulanate as above. Meloxicam (0.3 mg/kg s.c.) was administered once the cat was fully recovered and he was subsequently discharged on oral amoxicillin/clavulanate and meloxicam.

CLINICAL TIP

- Severe bite wounds may require urgent referral to a specialist centre where suitable management can be implemented. This is particularly the case where a full thickness injury into the thoracic or abdominal cavity is considered a possibility.
- If a significant delay in referral is anticipated, and following initial stabilization, brief general anaesthesia for rapid initial management (lavage, debridement, drain placement) may be prudent, with more definitive surgery being performed if indicated once the patient has been admitted to the specialist centre.
- The possibility of visceral trauma despite the lack of a skin lesion should be borne in mind and may occur for example in a 'big dog/little dog' scenario.

FELINE HIGH-RISE SYNDROME

Feline high-rise syndrome refers to trauma sustained by a cat falling from a height, typically a balcony or window of a building in an urban area. This syndrome occurs most commonly in younger cats. An extensive list of traumatic injuries has been reported in cats falling from a height but the most frequently identified include limb fractures (most cats have only a single fracture), thoracic injuries (especially pneumothorax and pulmonary contusions), nonfracture-related contusions and facial injuries. A relationship between the height fallen and the distribution of injuries has been suggested but clearly each case needs to be evaluated on an individual basis.

29 The acute abdomen

Differential diagnoses of acute abdomen are discussed in Chapter 8 and some of the most common disorders are discussed in greater detail here using case examples.

SEPTIC (BACTERIAL) PERITONITIS

Theory refresher

Free peritoneal fluid and gas

Abdominal palpation is an insensitive means of detecting free peritoneal fluid. Ultrasonography is extremely useful in this respect even in relatively inexperienced hands. Small amounts of free peritoneal fluid are most readily detected at the apex of the urinary bladder and between liver lobes. If ultrasonography is not available, loss of serosal detail may be identified radiographically.

Abdominal radiography is useful for identifying free peritoneal gas (often most readily seen between the liver and diaphragm) as well as diagnosing intestinal foreign body material and obstruction. Radiography will be less useful in this respect if a large volume of free peritoneal fluid is present due to increased loss of contrast.

In animals without a history of recent (last 3–4 weeks) laparotomy or open system abdominocentesis, free peritoneal gas suggests rupture of a hollow viscus and is an indication for emergency surgical exploration. This also applies to animals that have suffered penetrating injuries as free peritoneal gas implies full thickness penetration into the abdomen.

Cytology of peritoneal fluid

Depending on the severity of peritoneal contamination, direct smears of peritoneal effusion may be less rewarding than smears made after centrifugation with respect to identifying bacteria. However, centrifugation may alter cell morphology, preventing accurate assessment. The author therefore routinely examines direct smears first and then smears made following centrifugation if appropriate – typically if no bacteria are identified on direct smears but there is a high index of suspicion for bacterial peritonitis or neutrophils appear degenerate. The exception to this approach is for samples obtained via diagnostic peritoneal lavage which are likely to contain only scant cellular and other material and must be centrifuged prior to cytological analysis.

The identification of even one intracellular (phagocytosed) bacterium is considered diagnostic for septic peritonitis which is a surgical emergency. Extracellular bacteria are suggestive of this condition but the possibility of contamination cannot be excluded and in such cases other considerations must be taken into account in making a diagnosis.

Case example 1 – surgical gastrointestinal wound dehiscence

PRESENTING SIGNS AND CASE HISTORY

A 1-year-old male entire Staffordshire bull terrier presented as an emergency 3 days after gastrotomy and enterotomy for removal of a linear foreign body. The dog had initially recovered well from surgery and had been discharged from the primary care clinic after 48 hours. However, he had become progressively more depressed and lethargic in the 12 hours prior to emergency presentation.

CLINICAL TIP

- Clinical signs associated with dehiscence of a surgical gastrointestinal wound are most likely to be seen 3–5 days following surgery. This period reflects the inflammatory phase of visceral wound healing.

Continued

CLINICAL TIP—cont'd

- The inflammatory phase is followed by the proliferative phase, during which there is a rapid increase in wound strength and dehiscence becomes much less likely.

Major body system examination

On presentation the dog was ambulatory but depressed. Cardiovascular examination was unremarkable with no evidence of hypovolaemia. Respiratory examination was unremarkable and rectal temperature was within normal limits. The dog's abdomen was rigid and diffusely painful on palpation but a fluid thrill was not detected. Digital examination per rectum was unremarkable.

Emergency database

An intravenous catheter was placed in a cephalic vein and blood collected via the catheter for an emergency database. This was unremarkable except for the presence of a subjective neutrophilia with mild to moderate toxic change (see Ch. 3).

Case management

Morphine (0.3 mg/kg slow i.v.) was administered for analgesia. An abdominal ultrasound was performed using a focused assessment with sonography for trauma (FAST) protocol. This involved scanning the dog in lateral recumbency and obtaining both transverse and longitudinal views at each of four sites – just caudal to the xiphoid process (last sternebra), on the midline over the urinary bladder, and at the right and left flank regions. Despite this thorough evaluation, no peritoneal fluid could be identified. However, given the dog's history and clinical signs, there was a very high index of suspicion for bacterial peritonitis secondary to surgical gastrointestinal wound dehiscence and a diagnostic peritoneal lavage (DPL) was therefore performed (see p. 294).

The peritoneal fluid subsequently obtained was centrifuged and smears made from the sediment. Cytology demonstrated degenerate neutrophils with occasional intracellular rod-shaped bacteria and a diagnosis of bacterial peritonitis was therefore confirmed. A peritoneal fluid glucose concentration of less than 2.8 mmol/l is reported to have high specificity for bacterial peritonitis and was found to be 2.0 mmol/l in this case.

Intravenous antibiosis using amoxicillin/clavulanic acid (20 mg/kg) was commenced and an exploratory laparotomy performed. This revealed dehiscence with leakage from the enterotomy incision that was debrided and repaired. Antibiosis was continued postoperatively, first intravenously and then *per os*, and culture of the fluid obtained from the abdomen following DPL revealed a scant growth of *Escherichia coli* that was sensitive to amoxicillin/clavulanic acid. The dog made an uneventful recovery from the surgery and was discharged after 5 days to complete a 2-week course of antibiotics.

CLINICAL TIP

- Broad-spectrum bactericidal intravenous antibiosis with activity against both Gram negative and Gram positive, aerobic and anaerobic bacteria should be used if the gastrointestinal tract is thought to be the source of bacterial peritonitis. Amoxicillin/clavulanic acid or a second generation cephalosporin are reasonable single agent choices initially. Metronidazole may be added to increase anaerobic coverage.

Case example 2 – uterine rupture

PRESENTING SIGNS AND CASE HISTORY

An 11-year-old female entire cross-bred dog presented with a 3-day history of intermittent vomiting and progressive lethargy and inappetence. She had also been panting excessively on the day of presentation. Her last season had finished apparently uneventfully 3 weeks earlier and no vulval discharge had been noted by her owners prior to presentation.

Major body system examination

On presentation the dog was obtunded. Cardiovascular examination revealed a heart rate of 200 beats per minute with very weak femoral pulses and absent dorsal pedal pulses. Mucous membranes were hyperaemic with a rapid capillary refill time. Respiratory examination revealed tachypnoea with appropriate lung auscultation. The abdomen was tense and painful on palpation but a more thorough examination could not be performed due to the dog's recumbency. Marked pyrexia (rectal temperature 40.4°C) was identified. The vulva was swollen but no discharge was detected. A brown-tinged serous mammary discharge was present but the mammary glands were not enlarged or obviously inflamed.

Assessment

The dog was assessed as being in moderate to severe mal-distributive shock that was most likely secondary to acute abdomen. Given the dog's signalment and history, there was a high index of suspicion for pyometra. The cardiovascular picture in this case was highly suggestive of sepsis as the cause of the mal-distributive shock that raised the index of suspicion for septic peritonitis secondary to uterine rupture following closed-cervix pyometra.

CLINICAL TIP

- Closed-cervix pyometra is more commonly associated with pyrexia and is expected to cause more severe systemic compromise than open-cervix pyometra (see p. 150). Closed-cervix pyometra requires more rapid intervention. Medical therapy is less advisable for bitches with closed-cervix pyometra due to a greater risk of potentially fatal complications.

Emergency database

An intravenous catheter was placed in a cephalic vein and blood collected via the catheter for an emergency database. This revealed marked haemoconcentration (manual packed cell volume (PCV) 72%, reference range 37–55%; plasma total solids (TS) 95 g/l, reference range 49–71 g/l) and a subjective degenerate neutrophilic left shift.

Case management

Aggressive intravenous fluid resuscitation with an isotonic crystalloid solution was commenced and morphine (0.3 mg/kg slow i.v.) administered. Abdominal ultrasound revealed the presence of enlarged uterine horns distended with hypoechoic fluid consistent with pyometra and peritoneal fluid was detected (Figure 29.1).

Abdominocentesis (see p. 293) was performed and a sample of the fluid retrieved. Cytology demonstrated large numbers of degenerate neutrophils with intracellular bacteria as well as a considerable number of extracellular bacteria (Figure 29.2). A diagnosis of bacterial peritonitis secondary to uterine rupture was made. Regrettably, due to financial constraints, the dog was euthanased.

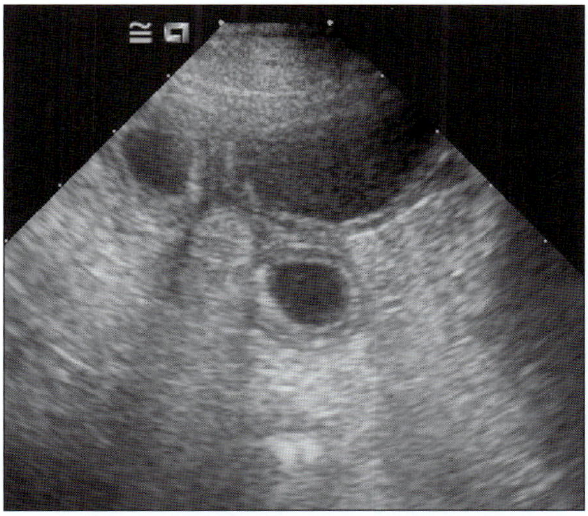

Figure 29.1 Ultrasound image of pyometra showing enlarged uterine horns distended with hypoechoic fluid; the urinary bladder is also visible.

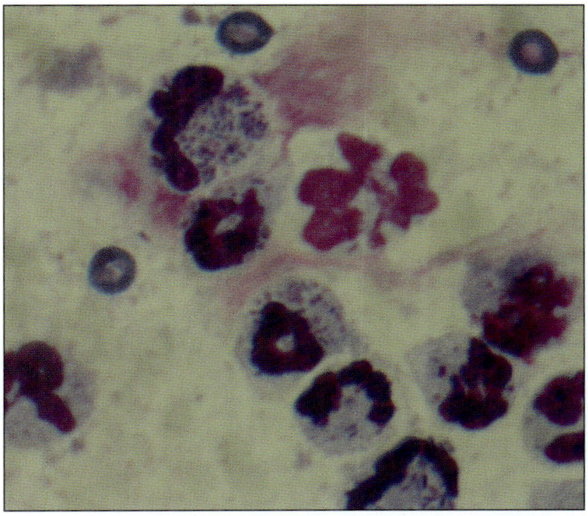

Figure 29.2 Septic peritoneal fluid secondary to uterine rupture; several degenerate neutrophils with intracellular bacteria are visible.

HAEMOABDOMEN

Causes of haemoabdomen are listed in Box 29.1.

Theory refresher

Canine haemangiosarcoma

Canine haemangiosarcoma is most commonly diagnosed in German shepherd dogs followed by golden retrievers.

BOX 29.1 Causes of haemoabdomen

Non-traumatic

- Rupture of intra-abdominal neoplasm (especially splenic; also hepatic, adrenal and others)
- Coagulopathy (e.g. anticoagulant rodenticide intoxication; *Angiostrongylus vasorum* infection)
- Splenic torsion
- Splenic infarction
- Splenic haematoma rupture
- Liver disease (including neoplasia, necrosis, amyloidosis, rupture), especially in cats
- Liver lobe torsion
- Gastric dilatation/volvulus syndrome (GDV)

Traumatic (usually causes rupture of intra-abdominal viscera, especially liver, spleen)

- Blunt trauma, especially motor vehicle accident
- Penetrating trauma

Other large breed dogs, such as Labrador retrievers and Boxers, are also over represented. The spleen is the most common site of origin but right atrial, pericardial and hepatic canine haemangiosarcoma are also reported relatively frequently. Any site in the body that contains vascular endothelium can theoretically be affected.

Haemangiosarcoma is presumed to have metastasized at the time of diagnosis in the vast majority of cases, regardless of whether or not metastases are detected by currently available imaging modalities. The prognosis is very poor, with survival times in the region of 2–4 months reported for splenic haemangiosarcoma following splenectomy alone; survival may in some cases be improved modestly by additional chemotherapy and immunotherapy.

In dogs presenting with haemoabdomen presumed to be secondary to rupture of a splenic lesion, splenectomy will be palliative and remove the risk of recurrent haemorrhage in the short term. It should be remembered that the nature (benign or malignant) of hepatic nodules that may be identified in such cases cannot be determined based on ultrasonographic appearance and surgical intervention therefore remains a rational choice. Palliative surgery is unlikely to be an option in primary hepatic haemangiosarcoma.

Abdominal counterpressure bandage

The purpose of an abdominal bandage is to apply external pressure that will increase intra-abdominal pressure and thereby tamponade bleeding. Realistically, intra-abdominal pressure is only likely to be increased sufficiently to exceed venous pressure and reduce venous haemorrhage. Therefore, excessively tight bandages do not offer any significant advantage and are likely to be associated with greater complications.

Traditionally a soft material has been used as the primary layer of an abdominal pressure bandage with an elastic material applied on top. In the author's experience, however, these bandages are more likely to slip and the author prefers to use an elastic adhesive primary layer despite the inherent difficulties in subsequent removal. The bandage should be placed starting caudally, approximately at the level of the pubis, and moving in a cranial direction up to the xiphoid, stopping before the caudal rib margin.

The bandage should be removed once the patient has remained stable for a reasonable period. Removal should commence at the cranial end (i.e. in the opposite direction to how the bandage was placed) and should be staggered by cutting a small section every 30–60 minutes over a period of several hours. The patient should be monitored closely for signs of deterioration during removal of counterpressure.

Abdominal bandages should not be used in animals with respiratory compromise or those suffering from diaphragmatic rupture.

Case example 3

PRESENTING SIGNS AND CASE HISTORY

A 10-year-old male neutered German shepherd dog presented with a 7-day history of intermittent lethargy and exercise intolerance. The dog had been found collapsed and tachypnoeic with a distended abdomen on the day of presentation.

Major body system examination

On presentation the dog was obtunded. Cardiovascular examination revealed a heart rate of 180 beats per minute with no murmur detected; femoral and dorsal pedal pulses were absent. Mucous membranes were very pale with a prolonged capillary refill time. Respiratory examination revealed tachypnoea with appropriate lung auscultation and both marked distension and recumbency precluded reliable abdominal palpation.

Assessment

The dog was assessed as being in severe hypovolaemic shock that was most likely due to acute abdomen. Given the dog's signalment and history, there was a high index of suspicion for haemoabdomen secondary to rupture of an intra-abdominal haemangiosarcoma lesion. The fact that some colour remained in the mucous membranes despite the severity of hypovolaemia suggested that severe anaemia was not present.

Emergency database

An intravenous catheter was placed in a cephalic vein and blood collected via the catheter for an emergency database. This revealed mild anaemia (PCV 31%, reference range 37–55%) with a more significant decrease in TS (40 g/l, reference range 49–71 g/l), findings that were compatible with acute haemorrhage. Peripheral blood smear examination showed the anaemia to be regenerative (moderate polychromasia, moderate anisocytosis). As a regenerative response often takes a minimum of 3 days to be detectable clinically in dogs, this suggested one or more prior episodes of haemorrhage in the days preceding presentation. Platelet count was considered adequate and a neutrophilia with left shift suspected.

Case management

Aggressive intravenous fluid resuscitation with an isotonic crystalloid solution was commenced (60 ml/kg bolus via pressure infusor). Abdominal ultrasonography revealed the presence of a large volume of echogenic peritoneal fluid. Abdominocentesis (see p. 293) was performed and the non-clotting haemorrhagic fluid was found to have a PCV of 30%; cytology of the fluid revealed red blood cells, occasional erythrophagocytosis, no platelets and no evidence of sepsis. An abdominal counterpressure bandage was applied and fluid therapy discontinued as soon as the dog was assessed as being adequately perfused. The dog remained stable subsequently and the abdominal bandage was removed gradually over several hours.

The following day the dog was referred for further management. Abdominal ultrasonography revealed a cavitary splenic lesion and although the liver was hyperechoic, no focal lesions were identified. Thoracic radiography was performed under general anaesthesia and found to be unremarkable. Complete splenectomy and a liver biopsy were then carried out, from which the dog made an uneventful recovery. Histopathology confirmed the suspicion of splenic haemangiosarcoma although no neoplastic cells were identified in the sample of liver submitted.

CLINICAL TIP

- In the author's experience, free peritoneal fluid is readily detected and sampled in most animals presenting with clinically significant haemoabdomen and DPL is typically not required. However, if this technique is used, the subsequent dilution must be kept in mind when interpreting the results of fluid analysis. A packed cell volume of DPL fluid of 2–5% or more is reportedly suggestive of significant haemorrhage.

UROABDOMEN

Causes

Trauma is the most common cause of uroabdomen:
- Especially blunt abdominal/pelvic trauma – urine leakage usually from the bladder
- Also iatrogenic – especially urethral rupture during urethral catheter placement.

Neoplasia and prolonged urinary tract obstruction are less common causes.

CLINICAL TIP

- The presence of a palpable bladder does not rule out leakage of urine from the bladder and definitely does not rule out uroabdomen due to rupture elsewhere in the urinary tract. In addition, the ability to urinate also does not exclude uroabdomen.
- Leakage of urine from the kidneys or proximal ureters will result in uroretroperitoneum potentially without uroabdomen.

Diagnosis

Animals with uroabdomen typically have severe azotaemia, and variable hyperkalaemia may be present. Blood urea nitrogen (BUN), creatinine and potassium concentrations in the peritoneal fluid are typically higher than plasma concentrations measured at the same time. Creatinine and potassium in peritoneal effusion equilibrate more slowly with the intravascular space and are therefore considered more reliable than BUN for detecting uroabdomen. Blood and peritoneal fluid samples should be collected within a few minutes of one another and an intravenous fluid bolus should not be administered in the interim if the peritoneal fluid is collected first (dilution of plasma BUN, creatinine and potassium by the bolus may create concentration gradients consistent with uroabdomen and lead to misdiagnosis).

Positive contrast radiography of the urinary system (intravenous urography, retrograde urethrocystography) is helpful in determining the site of urinary tract rupture.

> **CLINICAL TIP**
>
> - Aside from the bladder, surgical repair or management of urinary tract rupture in other sites is often best done in the hands of a specialist surgeon. As such it may be appropriate to refer animals with uroabdomen following initial stabilization without performing general anaesthesia for contrast radiography.

BILE PERITONITIS

Causes

Bile peritonitis occurs due to leakage from or rupture of the gallbladder and/or biliary tract. This may result from:

- Blunt or penetrating abdominal trauma; also iatrogenic
- Inflammation with or without infection (e.g. necrotizing cholecystitis)
- Obstruction (e.g. cholelithiasis, neoplasia).

Diagnosis

Clinical jaundice and hyperbilirubinaemia may be identified in animals with bile peritonitis, depending on the cause, along with varying degrees of cardiovascular compromise. Marked elevations in liver enzymes may also be seen.

Peritoneal fluid may be greenish in appearance and clusters of golden refractile pigment are identified. The bilirubin concentration of the peritoneal fluid is considerably higher than the plasma bilirubin concentration.

> **CLINICAL TIP**
>
> - Bile peritonitis is a surgical emergency but the author cannot stress strongly enough the importance of referral of these cases to a specialist surgeon. Biliary tract surgery is highly challenging with the potential for disastrous consequences in inexperienced hands.

GASTRIC DILATATION/ VOLVULUS SYNDROME (GDV)

Theory refresher

Risk factors

A large number of risk factors have been suggested for acute gastric dilatation/volvulus syndrome (GDV). Some are supported by sound clinical evidence; others are more controversial or anecdotal. The cause of this condition, however, remains unknown and is likely to be multifactorial. Suggested risk factors are listed in Box 29.2.

Pathophysiology

The pathophysiology of GDV is multifactorial and involves the cardiovascular and gastrointestinal systems

> ***BOX 29.2 Suggested risk factors for gastric dilatation/volvulus syndrome (GDV)***
>
> - Large/giant breed
> - Purebred
> - Narrow and deep chest
> - Feeding of single daily meal
> - Large amount of food consumed per meal
> - Exercise after eating
> - Eating quickly, especially if accompanied by aerophagia
> - Increasing age
> - Fearful/agitated demeanour
> - Hereditary factors
> - Increased length/laxity of hepatogastric ligaments
> - Reduced gastric motility
> - Delayed gastric emptying
> - Increased gastrin levels
> - Abnormal oesophageal motility
>
> *Small breed dogs and cats can be affected but this is rare.*

in particular. Respiratory compromise may also be severe. Significant pathophysiological mechanisms are as follows.

- An increase in intraabdominal pressure that compresses the caudal vena cava, portal vein and splanchnic vasculature. This causes a decrease in venous return to the heart, reducing cardiac output and potentially arterial blood pressure. As dilatation progresses, an increasing amount of blood is sequestered in the abdominal vasculature.
- Myocardial function is further compromised by dysrhythmias and reduced contractility that occur due to the effects of reactive oxygen species produced in the abdomen as well as ischaemia and acidosis.
- Perfusion of the gastric wall is compromised as a result of both compression of capillaries due to raised intraluminal pressure and a reduced blood supply due to systemic hypoperfusion. This results in ischaemia, necrosis and potentially perforation. Intraluminal haemorrhage occurs due to mucosal necrosis.
- The short gastric arteries branch off the splenic artery and supply the greater curvature of the stomach. They may be avulsed when the stomach rotates during acute GDV, resulting in potentially severe haemorrhage and further reducing perfusion to the stomach wall.
- Gastric and intestinal motility is severely diminished and significant volumes of fluid may be sequestered in the gastrointestinal tract.
- The distended stomach presses on the diaphragm, reducing intrathoracic volume and impairing movement of the diaphragm during inspiration. This results in hypoventilation due to reduced tidal volume and a compensatory increase in respiratory rate occurs.

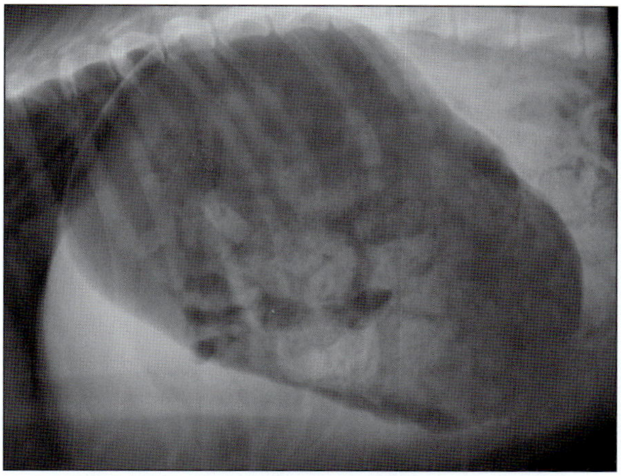

Figure 29.3 Right lateral abdominal radiograph showing gastric dilatation without volvulus.

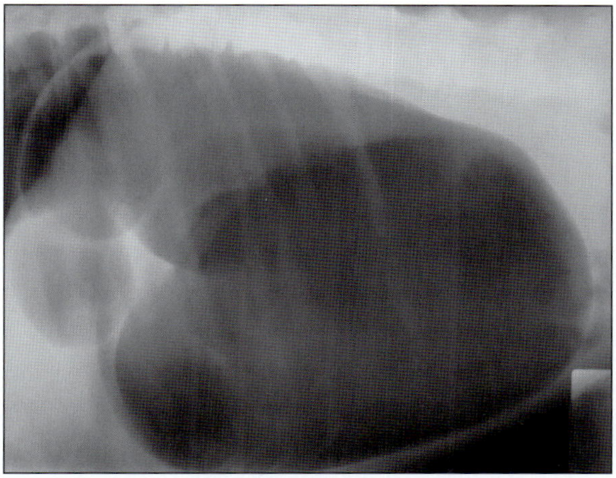

Figure 29.4 Right lateral abdominal radiograph showing gastric dilatation with volvulus with the Popeye arm (double bubble, reverse C) configuration.

Radiography

Acute GDV can usually be diagnosed on the basis of history, signalment and physical examination; radiography is generally not required. However, radiography may allow differentiation of gastric dilatation alone from gastric dilatation with volvulus. Radiography should not be performed until after fluid therapy and analgesia have been commenced and only if the patient is compliant as is usually the case. Radiography may be performed during the initial fluid resuscitation but should not delay gastric decompression. A single radiograph with the patient in right lateral recumbency is all that is typically required. Examples of radiographic findings are shown in Figures 29.3–29.6.

Thoracic radiography may be indicated in dogs suspected of having cardiac disease or inappropriate respiratory compromise (e.g. due to aspiration), or to rule out co-existing disease (e.g. neoplasm) in older animals.

Intra-operative considerations

Patients require close monitoring of vital signs during anaesthesia, and blood pressure and electrocardiogram monitoring is recommended. Cardiovascular depression can be minimized by careful dosing of induction and maintenance agents to effect. A crystalloid rate of 10–40 ml/kg/hr is advisable and colloids may be required. If orogastric intubation is performed during surgery, the

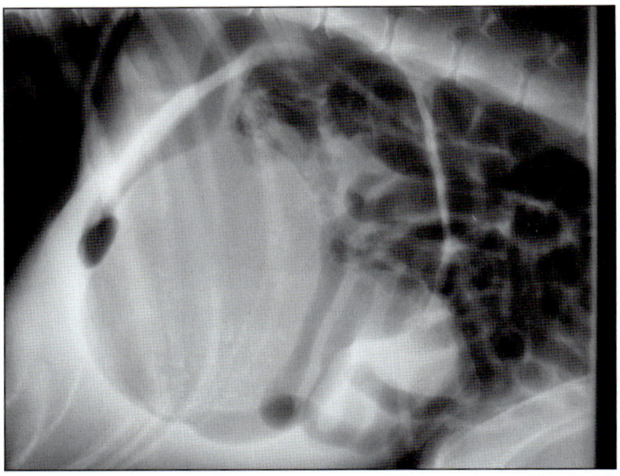

Figure 29.5 Right lateral abdominal radiograph showing gastric dilatation with volvulus; compartmentalization by a soft tissue fold is present. Gas-filled intestines are often identified as in this example.

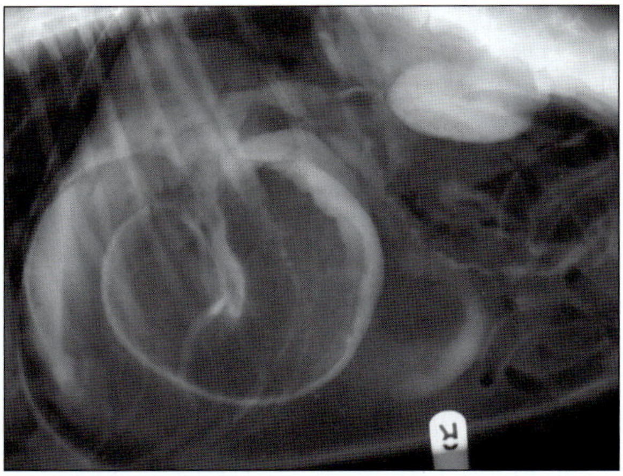

Figure 29.6 Right lateral abdominal radiograph showing gastric dilatation with volvulus and perforation of the stomach wall. Free air is visible within the abdominal cavity.

risk of aspiration of oesophageal reflux means that use of a cuffed endotracheal tube is mandatory, and great care must be taken at extubation.

Postoperative considerations

Fluid therapy is continued postoperatively and adjusted on the basis of regular assessment. Serum potassium levels should be monitored and supplemented as necessary, in particular if lidocaine administration is required. Analgesia must be continued using a dynamic approach and the usual postoperative considerations such as wound management, appropriate bedding and bladder management should not be forgotten. The time at which food and water are provided will depend to an extent on the nature of the surgical intervention in each case.

Electrocardiogram abnormality has been reported to occur in approximately 40% of dogs with acute gastric dilatation/volvulus. Ventricular premature complexes (VPCs) and ventricular tachycardia (VT) are the most common, both pre- and postoperatively (see Figures 12.4 and 12.5). In general, ventricular dysrhythmias arising secondary to another condition such as acute GDV only warrant antidysrhythmic therapy if they are considered to be compromising the patient's perfusion based on physical examination and blood pressure measurement if available. In addition, VT should be treated if it occurs at rates greater than 180 beats per minute or if R-on-T phenomenon is identified (see Ch. 12).

Is surgery always necessary?

The aims of surgical intervention in dogs with acute GDV are:

- To decompress, empty and lavage the stomach if this has not already been achieved
- To derotate the stomach if necessary
- To evaluate the viability of the stomach and perform a gastrectomy if indicated
- To perform gastropexy to prevent volvulus in the future
- To evaluate the viability of the spleen and perform a splenectomy if indicated
- To lavage the abdomen to remove haemorrhage and possibly gastrointestinal contents.

In animals in which gastric volvulus persists despite decompression or in which the presence of volvulus cannot be excluded, surgical intervention is mandatory but should only be performed when the patient is haemodynamically stable.

As described above, there are compelling reasons for surgical intervention in patients presenting with gastric dilatation alone. There are cases, however, in which owners may not be willing to provide consent, for example due to financial constraints or because of the age of the pet. Such cases can be successfully managed conservatively but the owner must be advised of the risks associated with this approach, particularly a lack of information regarding the viability of the stomach and spleen, and the possibility of recurrence both overnight and subsequently.

Case example 4

PRESENTING SIGNS AND CASE HISTORY

A 10-year-old male neutered weimaraner presented with a 2-hour history of nonproductive retching and drooling that began shortly after eating his evening meal. He had become progressively more lethargic and the owner had noticed abdominal distension.

Major body system examination

On presentation the dog was ambulatory but depressed and drooling. Cardiovascular examination revealed a heart rate of 160 beats per minute with absent dorsal pedal pulses and weak femoral pulses. Mucous membranes were pink with a capillary refill time of approximately 2 seconds. The dog was panting but lung sounds were appropriate when this was temporarily stopped. Abdominal palpation revealed tympany cranially and was uncomfortable. Rectal temperature was within normal limits.

Assessment

The dog was assessed as being in moderate hypovolaemic shock. The signalment, history and physical examination findings were highly suggestive of gastric dilatation with possible volvulus.

Emergency database

A large bore (16 gauge) intravenous catheter was placed into each cephalic vein and blood collected via one of the catheters for an emergency database. This was largely unremarkable except for hyperlactataemia (4.0 mmol/l, reference range 0.6–2.5 mmol/l).

CLINICAL TIP

- Intravenous catheters should be placed in the cephalic veins (or a single jugular catheter). Administration of resuscitative fluids via saphenous catheters will be much less effective due to obstruction of the caudal vena cava.

Case management

Aggressive intravenous fluid therapy was commenced with 1 l of Hartmann's solution being administered as a bolus via each cephalic catheter using pressure infusors (see Figure 4.1). Electrocardiography demonstrated sinus tachycardia with occasional ventricular premature complexes (see Figure 12.4). As radiography facilities were readily accessible, a right lateral abdominal radiograph was taken during initial fluid resuscitation that confirmed the presence of gastric dilatation with volvulus.

The dog's cardiovascular status improved noticeably and fluid therapy was continued but less aggressively. Sedation was administered using methadone (0.2 mg/kg i.v.) and diazepam (0.5 mg/kg i.v.) and orogastric decompression performed using a stomach tube (see p. 294). This resulted in a noticeable reduction in abdominal distension and further improvement in cardiovascular status.

CLINICAL TIP

In the majority of cases fluid resuscitation can be achieved through the use of an isotonic crystalloid alone (e.g. Hartmann's solution). In some cases, the additional use of small volume resuscitation fluids (colloids, hypertonic saline) may be applicable if available. Examples are:

- Cases that fail to respond adequately to crystalloid therapy alone
- Extremely large dogs where administration of large volumes of crystalloid may take too long
- Animals in which only limited intravenous access has been established.

CLINICAL TIP

- Opioid analgesia should be provided early on in dogs with acute GDV. As morphine has a greater emetic effect, another pure agonist such as pethidine or methadone is recommended initially.
- Nonsteroidal antiinflammatory agents should not be used in any animal with hypovolaemia. Furthermore, the inevitable compromise to the gastrointestinal mucosa during acute GDV warrants judicious and delayed use of these agents.

The combination of methadone and diazepam already administered acted as premedication to reduce the dose of cardiovascular depressant drugs subsequently required for general anaesthesia. Exploratory laparotomy was performed that confirmed 180° clockwise volvulus of the stomach. This was reduced manually after further decompression and emptying of the stomach contents. Both the gastric wall and spleen appeared to be viable. An incisional gastropexy was performed between the pyloric antrum and the right abdominal wall. The abdomen was lavaged thoroughly prior to closure. Intravenous broad-spectrum antibiosis (amoxicillin/clavulanic acid 20 mg/kg i.v) was commenced preoperatively and repeated during surgery; however, it was stopped thereafter based on the relatively benign findings at laparotomy.

CLINICAL TIP

- Although anticlockwise rotation has been reported, the stomach usually twists clockwise. A 180° rotation – such that the pylorus comes to lie craniodorsally to the body of the stomach on the left of the abdomen – is most common, but 90°, 270° and 360° rotations may also occur. The spleen usually rotates with the stomach (attached by gastrosplenic ligaments) to a position right of midline.

The dog was monitored closely following surgery, in particular for clinically significant cardiac dysrhythmia, but made an uneventful recovery. Water was introduced as soon as the dog was fully recovered from general anaesthesia and food was offered 12 hours postoperatively.

SMALL INTESTINAL FOREIGN BODY

Case example 5

PRESENTING SIGNS AND CASE HISTORY

A 2-year-old female neutered cross-bred dog presented with a 24-hour history of vomiting, depression and anorexia. The dog was still drinking and no other signs were reported. The dog was known to be a notorious scavenger although the owner was unaware of a specific episode of dietary indiscretion prior to the onset of signs. The dog had had an enterotomy 1 year previously for removal of a linear foreign body.

Major body system examination

On presentation the dog was ambulatory but depressed. Heart rate was 140 beats per minute but the dog was assessed as euvolaemic and not obviously clinically dehydrated. Respiratory examination revealed tachypnoea but auscultation was unremarkable. Abdominal palpation revealed moderate discomfort but this could not be localized. The dog was mildly pyrexic (rectal temperature 39.3°C).

Emergency database

An intravenous catheter was placed in a cephalic vein and blood collected for an emergency database that was suggestive of dehydration (high-normal PCV and TS) but was otherwise unremarkable.

Case management

Methadone (0.2 mg/kg i.v.) was administered and plain abdominal radiography performed. This revealed focal areas of gaseous small intestinal dilatation consistent with possible mechanical obstruction (Figure 29.7).

The options of contrast radiography or referral for ultrasonography were discussed; however, given the dog's history of scavenging and the highly suggestive plain radiographs, it was decided to perform an exploratory laparotomy. A cloth intestinal foreign body was subsequently removed via enterotomy. The dog recovered uneventfully from surgery.

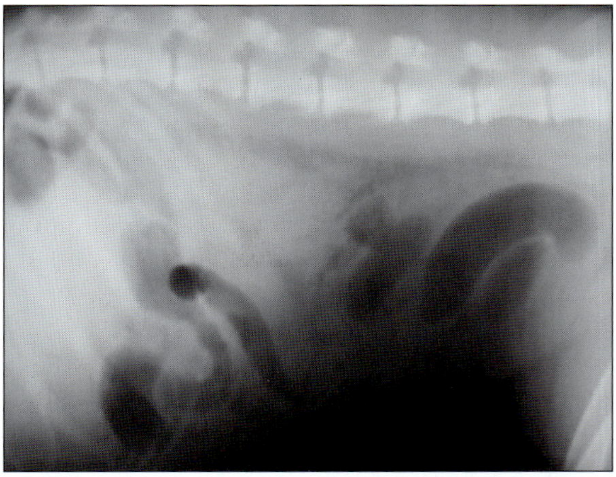

Figure 29.7 Right lateral abdominal radiograph showing focal areas of gaseous small intestinal dilatation consistent with obstruction.

CLINICAL TIP

- Linear foreign bodies (e.g. string, thread) may be identified trapped around the base of the tongue; this finding is more common in cats. Linear foreign bodies may also become fixed at the pylorus. Pleated or plicated small intestine bunched in the cranial to mid-ventral abdomen may be identified radiographically. Sacculation and small intraluminal gas bubbles may be present. Surgical removal is likely to be the safest option in most animals.

INTUSSUSCEPTION

Theory refresher

Intussusception may involve any part of the gastrointestinal tract but a significant proportion of published cases in dogs and cats are enterocolic and in particular ileocolic. Affected animals are often young, especially less than 1 year of age, and a variety of intestinal disorders (e.g. gastroenteritis/enteritis, parasitic infestation, mass lesions, foreign bodies) may potentially predispose to intussusception. Acute enteritis or gastroenteritis has been shown to be the most likely predisposing factor in young dogs. However, the majority of cases in dogs and cats are thought to be idiopathic.

Survey abdominal radiographic findings may be suspicious for intussusception and positive contrast studies are often diagnostic. However, in experienced hands abdominal ultrasonography is the preferred method of diagnosis. A target-like mass consisting of multiple hyperechoic and hypoechoic concentric rings in transverse section (Figure 29.8), or the appearance of multiple hyperechoic and hypoechoic parallel lines in longitudinal section, is considered virtually diagnostic of an intussusception.

Case example 6

PRESENTING SIGNS AND CASE HISTORY

A 13-year-old female neutered domestic short hair cat presented with a 2-day history of anorexia, progressive depression and a small amount of diarrhoea. No vomiting had been noted but the cat had retched once and had been drinking more

PRESENTING SIGNS AND CASE HISTORY—cont'd

than normal over the last 48 hours. The cat's diet had been changed 2 weeks prior to the onset of signs. A small intestinal intussusception had been manually reduced 1 year previously.

Major body system examination

On presentation the cat was quiet but alert and responsive. Cardiovascular examination revealed a grade IV/VI holosystolic heart murmur but was otherwise unremarkable. Respiratory examination was unremarkable. Abdominal palpation revealed a nonpainful sausage-shaped mass approximately 5 cm long in the ventral abdomen suggestive of an intussusception. Rectal temperature was within normal limits.

Case management

An intravenous catheter was placed into a cephalic vein and blood collected for an emergency database that was unremarkable except for mild hypokalaemia. Abdominal ultrasonography revealed a small intestinal intussusception (see Figure 29.8) and exploratory laparotomy was performed.

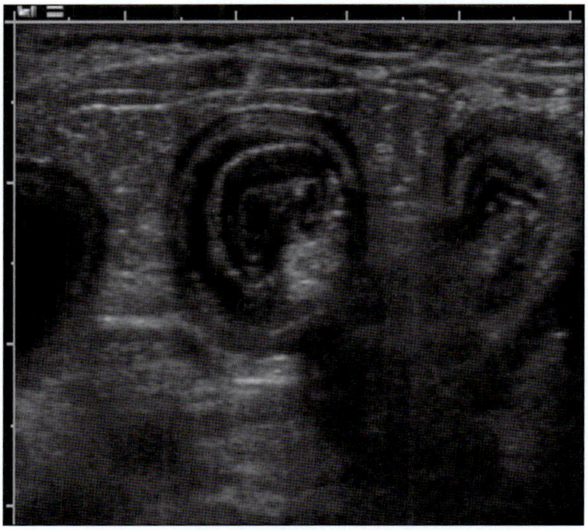

Figure 29.8 Target-like ultrasonographic appearance of intussusception in transverse section. (Photograph courtesy of Andrew Parry)

The intussusception was manually reduced and enteroplication performed in an attempt to reduce the likelihood of recurrence. Multiple full thickness small intestinal biopsies and several mesenteric lymph node biopsies were taken and the abdomen thoroughly lavaged prior to closure. The cat made an uneventful recovery from surgery. Histopathology revealed moderate lymphoplasmacytic–eosinophilic enteritis and the lymph nodes were hyperplastic with moderate eosinophilic infiltration.

The heart murmur in this case warranted caution with intravenous fluid therapy and the cat was therefore kept on Hartmann's solution at a conservative 3 ml/kg/hr while under general anaesthesia. Vital parameters, including systolic blood pressure, were monitored closely throughout and the cat remained normotensive.

SEVERE ACUTE PANCREATITIS

Theory refresher

Diagnosis

Detection of elevated serum amylase and lipase activities show relatively poor sensitivity and specificity for diagnosing acute pancreatitis. Hyper-amylasaemia may also for example be seen in pancreatic neoplasia, intestinal disorders and in association with renal insufficiency/ azotaemia. Hyper-lipasaemia may also for example be seen in pancreatic neoplasia, liver disease (especially neoplasia) and in association with renal insufficiency/ azotaemia. Consideration must be given to the severity of elevation during interpretation. It is noteworthy that hypovolaemia and/or dehydration that may be a feature of some of the differential diagnoses of acute pancreatitis (e.g. intestinal obstruction, haemorrhagic gastroenteritis) can cause elevations in serum amylase and lipase activities that may prompt misdiagnosis of pancreatitis. Measurement of canine pancreatic lipase (cPLI) is now the preferred diagnostic test.

Abdominal radiography has relatively poor sensitivity and specificity for acute pancreatitis but should help to exclude some of the differential diagnoses (e.g. intestinal obstruction). Signs consistent with acute pancreatitis in dogs include loss of serosal detail and increased density in the right cranial abdomen, displacement of the descending duodenum to the right with widening of the angle between the proximal duodenum and the pylorus, and caudal displacement of the transverse colon. Ultrasonographic changes are usually present in severe acute pancreatitis but this modality requires considerable expertise.

Analgesia in acute pancreatitis

Opioids are the mainstay of analgesia in pancreatitis. Some authors have argued that pethidine is the most appropriate initial choice but this would appear to be based on theoretical considerations adopted from human literature and is unlikely to be of clinical significance in dogs and cats. Pethidine cannot be administered intravenously and has a short duration of action, making it a poor choice for on-going analgesia in pancreatitis. The author therefore prefers to use morphine, given as intravenous boluses titrated to effect initially and then as a constant rate infusion. Following adequate improvement, analgesia is then stepped down to intermittent boluses of buprenorphine. Again, suggested contraindications of using this agent in pancreatitis are more likely to be of theoretical concern rather than of clinical significance.

Nonsteroidal anti-inflammatory agents are generally not used and should definitely not be administered to animals with acute pancreatitis that are cardiovascularly unstable, dehydrated or azotaemic.

Feline pancreatitis

Most cats with severe acute pancreatitis present with vague signs of lethargy, anorexia and dehydration, with vomiting and abdominal pain featuring less commonly than in dogs. Testing of serum feline pancreatic lipase immunoreactivity (fPLI) is available, and concurrent inflammatory bowel disease (IBD) and/or cholangitis–cholangiohepatitis are reported relatively frequently in cats (this is the so-called 'triad disease' of cats); hence icterus is relatively common in cats with pancreatitis. Serum amylase and lipase activities are of little diagnostic value in feline pancreatitis.

Treatment of feline and canine acute pancreatitis is similar. However, these cats are especially vulnerable to developing potentially fatal hepatic lipidosis. Nutritional support must therefore be emphasized and early feeding tube placement is recommended. Given the inherent difficulties in reliably detecting abdominal pain in animals in general and especially in cats, analgesia is indicated in all cases. Buprenorphine may be a suitable first line agent in this species although its onset of action is likely to be slower than that of the pure opioids. Low plasma ionized calcium concentration may be associated with a worse outcome in cats with acute pancreatitis.

Case example 7

PRESENTING SIGNS AND CASE HISTORY

A 9-year-old female neutered Cocker Spaniel presented with a 1-day history of anorexia, restlessness, vomiting and intermittently adopting the praying position. No diarrhoea had been noted. The dog had been seen to scavenge from the rubbish bin several days prior to the onset of signs.

CLINICAL TIP

- Dogs affected by acute pancreatitis are generally middle-aged or older. Canine breeds most commonly implicated include the Miniature Schnauzer, the Cocker Spaniel and the Yorkshire terrier, and affected dogs are often overweight.

CLINICAL TIP

- The praying position describes the upright posture adopted by some dogs with abdominal pain whereby the thoracic limbs are extended with the sternum on the ground and the pelvic limbs upright.
- The proportion of dogs with abdominal pain that are reported or witnessed to adopt the praying position is low. However, it is a relatively specific sign of significant abdominal discomfort and should not be discarded lightly when present.

Major body system examination

On presentation the dog was depressed and recumbent. Cardiovascular examination revealed a heart rate of 160 beats per minute and absent pedal pulses with weak femoral pulses. Mucous membranes were markedly hyperaemic with a very rapid capillary refill time. Respiratory rate was 80 breaths per minute with a shallow pattern and abdominal palpation was painful cranially. An abdominal fluid thrill could not be detected. The dog was moderately pyrexic (rectal temperature 39.7°C) and had a body condition score of 7/9 (heavy fat cover over ribs, lumbar area and tail base; absent waist).

Assessment

The dog was assessed as being in mal-distributive shock. Given the history and the other physical examination findings of tachypnoea and pyrexia, the dog was likely to be suffering from systemic inflammatory response syndrome (SIRS) and potentially sepsis (i.e. SIRS secondary to confirmed or highly suspected infection). A primary intra-abdominal process was suspected and there was a high index of suspicion of severe acute pancreatitis given the dog's signalment.

Emergency database

An intravenous catheter was placed in a cephalic vein and blood collected for an emergency database that showed mildly lipaemic plasma, hyperlactataemia, and a subjective neutrophilia with left shift. The dog was found to be normocalcaemic. Blood was also submitted in a serum gel tube for measurement of cPLI concentration.

CLINICAL TIP

- Lipaemia is a relatively frequent finding in dogs with acute pancreatitis and may artefactually increase refractometric total solids measurement.

Case management

A 40 ml/kg bolus of Hartmann's solution was administered to which there was a noticeable but relatively short-lived positive response. Two 5 ml/kg boluses of a synthetic colloid (6% hydroxyethyl starch, Voluven®) were then administered, following which the dog remained stable. The dog was subsequently maintained on a combination of Hartmann's solution (4 ml/kg/hr) and hydroxyethyl starch (2 ml/kg/hr).

CLINICAL TIP

- Animals with a severe inflammatory focus, such as septic peritonitis or severe acute pancreatitis, are likely to have vasculitis. Decreased plasma total solids due to panhypoproteinaemia may be identified and is thought to reflect exudation of protein into the peritoneum.

Continued

CLINICAL TIP—cont'd

- Colloidal fluid therapy may be required in such cases for effective and sustained correction of hypovolaemia as crystalloid solutions are likely to be less effective (due to increased vascular leakage and reduced intravascular oncotic pressure).

Morphine (0.3 mg/kg slow i.v.) was administered for analgesia. The dog was reassessed after a short period and although improved, still showed signs of abdominal discomfort. A further dose of morphine (0.1 mg/kg slow i.v.) was administered and the dog was started on a constant rate infusion of morphine (0.1 mg/kg/hr).

Abdominal ultrasonography revealed a significantly enlarged pancreas with a small amount of localized peritoneal effusion. There was hyperechogenicity of the peripancreatic mesentery. This provided further evidence for the suspected diagnosis of acute pancreatitis although an inciting cause was not identified, as is often the case.

The dog was managed intensively with fluid therapy, analgesia and anti-emetic treatment, and in keeping with more recent recommendations, first water and then food (low fat) was offered as soon as vomiting had resolved for 12 hours. The dog was eventually discharged after satisfactory improvement 5 days later. The sample submitted on the day of presentation showed an elevation in serum cPLI concentration (650 μg/l, reference range 0–200 μg/l), confirming inflammatory pancreatic disease.

CANINE PARVOVIRAL GASTROENTERITIS

Theory refresher

Canine parvovirus infection is seen most commonly in dogs under 6 months old but may occur in older animals. Existing passive maternal immunity may impair an effective response to vaccination in very young animals and clinical signs may therefore occur in vaccinated animals. The enteritis and leucopenia syndrome is the most common clinical manifestation and diarrhoea usually follows initial clinical signs by 12–48 hours.

Antimicrobial therapy

It is generally argued that any dog with blood in its faeces is at increased risk of translocation of intestinal bacteria into the bloodstream and therefore requires antibiotic therapy. However, the true clinical significance of this remains to be clearly elucidated. The author only uses antimicrobial therapy in neutropenic dogs and those with pyrexia or evidence of sepsis. A broad-spectrum bactericidal antibiotic is used and given intravenously early on while vomiting and delayed gastric emptying are likely.

Case example 8

PRESENTING SIGNS AND CASE HISTORY

A 9-week-old male neutered cross-bred dog presented with a 36-hour history of vomiting and progressive lethargy and inappetence. Haemorrhagic watery diarrhoea had also been noted on the morning of presentation. The puppy had been acquired from a rescue centre 1 week previously and had received the first dose of his primary vaccination course 2 weeks prior to being rehomed.

Major body system examination

On presentation the puppy was recumbent and depressed. Cardiovascular examination revealed a heart rate of 200 beats per minute and hyperdynamic peripheral pulses. Mucous membranes were mildly hyperaemic with a brisk capillary refill time. Respiratory examination was unremarkable. Abdominal palpation was not obviously uncomfortable but fluid filled intestinal loops were detected. Mild pyrexia was identified (rectal temperature 39.3°C) and moderate dehydration (estimated 8%) was suspected. Body weight was 4.0 kg at presentation.

Case management

Local anaesthetic cream (EMLA® cream 5%, AstraZeneca) was applied to the skin over both cephalic veins in the consultation room and the sites lightly dressed. While waiting for the topical anaesthesia to take effect, a rectal swab was tested for faecal canine parvovirus-2 antigen using an ELISA test kit (SNAP® Parvo Test, Idexx Laboratories) and found to be strongly positive. Barrier nursing and isolation measures were immediately instituted.

An intravenous catheter was placed in a cephalic vein and blood collected for an emergency database.

Manual PCV was 43% and plasma TS 65 g/l. Although these values fall within commonly cited reference ranges for adult dogs, both PCV and TS (considered approximately equivalent to total protein) would be expected to be lower than adult reference ranges in a puppy of this age. These values were therefore considered consistent with dehydration. The rest of the emergency database, including peripheral blood smear examination and blood glucose concentration, was unremarkable.

The puppy was assessed as mildly hypovolaemic on presentation and a bolus (20 ml/kg) of Hartmann's solution was given initially, after which euvolaemia was restored. Thereafter the puppy was kept on Hartmann's solution at 13 ml/kg/hr with appropriate potassium supplementation, but perfusion parameters were monitored regularly. This rate was calculated based on the following assumptions:

- An estimated 8% dehydration
- A maintenance isotonic crystalloid rate of 4 ml/kg/hr given the puppy's age
- Replacement of existing deficit to be achieved over 24 hours
- On-going losses equating to one and a half extra maintenance requirements over this period.

The puppy was also started on anti-emetic therapy (maropitant 1 mg/kg s.c. q 24 hr) and analgesia (buprenorphine (0.02 mg/kg q 6 hr)) and monitored regularly for possible hypoglycaemia. A nasogastric feeding tube was placed and used to aspirate stomach contents intermittently (q 6 hr).

Over the next 24 hours the vomiting persisted but improved significantly; however, the diarrhoea worsened considerably. An emergency database was repeated that showed a marked decrease in TS to 35 g/l and panleucopenia. The Hartmann's solution was reduced to 8 ml/kg/hr and a synthetic colloid (6% hydroxyethyl starch, Voluven®) infusion commenced at 1 ml/kg/hr. Broad-spectrum antibiosis was commenced using amoxicillin/clavulanic acid (20 mg/kg i.v. q 8 hr). A constant rate infusion of a complete liquid diet was commenced at a rate that would meet a third of the puppy's resting energy requirement (RER) over the initial 24 hours.

The puppy was monitored closely, including regular weighing and gentle abdominal palpation in case of intussusception, and supported intensively as required. Therapy was weaned as appropriate and the puppy was eventually discharged 1 week following presentation, by which time normal faeces had been observed.

CANINE IDIOPATHIC HAEMORRHAGIC GASTROENTERITIS (HGE)

Case example 9

PRESENTING SIGNS AND CASE HISTORY

A 6-year-old male neutered Border Collie presented with a 2-day history of vomiting and diarrhoea. The diarrhoea had become progressively more haemorrhagic and the dog was increasingly inappetent and lethargic. No significant preceding history was reported.

Major body system examination

On presentation the dog was ambulatory but depressed. Cardiovascular examination revealed a heart rate of 160 beats per minute with absent dorsal pedal pulses and weak femoral pulses. Intermittent pulse deficits were identified. Mucous membranes were pale with a prolonged capillary refill time and the dog's extremities were cold. Respiratory examination was unremarkable. The dog's abdomen was tense and painful on palpation but a fluid thrill could not be detected. Mild hypothermia was identified (rectal temperature 37.0°C) and severe dehydration suspected.

Assessment

The dog was assessed as being in moderate to severe hypovolaemic shock that may in part have been due to severe dehydration.

Emergency database

An intravenous catheter was placed in a cephalic vein and blood collected for an emergency database that showed marked haemoconcentration (manual PCV 74%, reference range 37–55%) with normal TS (60 g/l, reference range 49–71 g/l). The emergency database also revealed:

- Moderate hyponatraemia (134.1 mmol/l, reference range 140.0–153.0 mmol/l): as the dog was hypovolaemic on presentation, this was considered secondary to sodium loss in excess of water loss.
- Normokalaemia (4.0 mmol/l, reference range 3.6–4.6 mmol/l); sodium to potassium ratio 33.5:1
- Mild to moderate azotaemia (urea 17.8 mmol/l, reference range 3.0–10.0 mmol/l; creatinine 319 μmol/l, reference range 50–140 μmol/l): this was considered

most likely to be prerenal in origin although urine specific gravity could not be determined prior to commencing intravenous fluid therapy.

- Hyperlactataemia (4.6 mmol/l, reference range 0.6–2.5 mmol/l).
- Unremarkable peripheral blood smear examination.

Electrocardiography revealed sinus rhythm with intermittent uniform ventricular premature complexes (VPCs) (see Figure 12.4).

CLINICAL TIP

- In the author's experience, it is quite common for dogs diagnosed presumptively with HGE to present with a severely elevated PCV (65% or more). In addition, ventricular premature complexes and ventricular tachycardia are occasionally identified, although in the author's experience it is relatively rare for antidysrhythmic therapy to be indicated in these cases.
- The diarrhoea in these cases may contain fresh blood as well as sloughed intestinal mucosa (raspberry jam appearance).

Case management

Aggressive fluid resuscitation was performed starting with a 60 ml/kg bolus of 0.9% sodium chloride solution (normal, physiological saline). This produced some improvement but the dog remained mildly hypovolaemic and a further 20 ml/kg bolus was administered, after which euvolaemia was restored. Thereafter fluid therapy was administered at a rate calculated (8 ml/kg/hr) to treat the dog's dehydration, and perfusion and hydration parameters were monitored regularly. Fluid therapy was adjusted as indicated and colloidal support was not required.

Abdominal radiography showed mild focal gaseous dilation of the small intestine and no peritoneal fluid was detected ultrasonographically. Faecal analysis (cytology, microbiology and testing for parvoviral antigen) was unremarkable although a sample was not submitted for clostridial enterotoxin. Although the electrolyte abnormalities in this case were not consistent with classic hypoadrenocorticism, an adrenocorticotrophin (ACTH) stimulation test was performed to rule out atypical hypoadrenocorticism (see Ch. 34) and found to be unremarkable. A presumptive diagnosis of canine idiopathic HGE was made based on typical clinical presentation and progression, and exclusion of other differential diagnoses.

The dog was discharged 4 days after initial presentation following satisfactory improvement.

CANINE OPEN-CERVIX PYOMETRA

Pyometra typically affects mature bitches but may occur in bitches of any age. Most present within 12 weeks of the end of the previous oestrus but the condition may occur at any stage of the oestrus cycle as well as during pregnancy. No association has been shown between pseudopregnancy and pyometra but an increased incidence is reported in nulliparous bitches.

CLINICAL TIP

- Pyometra should be considered as a differential diagnosis in any sick intact bitch.

Diagnosis

Common clinical signs include polyuria/polydipsia and a malodorous mucopurulent vaginal discharge. An enlarged viscus may be palpable in the caudal abdomen and the cervix is found to be open on vaginal examination. Neutrophilia is a common finding and cytology of vaginal discharge reveals large numbers of degenerate neutrophils with intracellular bacteria.

CLINICAL TIP

- Many dogs with pyometra have a mild to moderate, normocytic normochromic anaemia (PCV 30–35%, reference range 37–55%). However, evaluation at time of presentation may be complicated by concurrent dehydration.

Abdominal radiography reveals convoluted loops of tubular fluid opacity in the caudal abdomen with dorsal displacement of the descending colon (Figure 29.9), and ultrasonography shows enlarged uterine horns distended with hypoechoic fluid (Figure 29.10).

Treatment

Ovarohysterectomy remains the recommended treatment for pyometra in bitches without significant reproductive value or when the owner has no particular desire

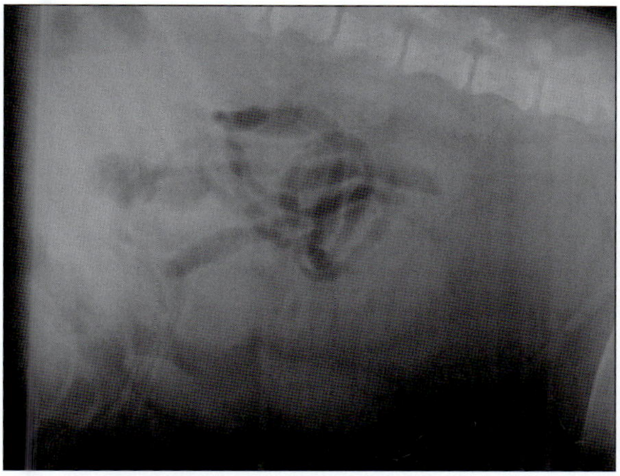

Figure 29.9 Right lateral abdominal radiograph in a dog with pyometra. Convoluted loops of tubular fluid opacity are visible in the caudal abdomen.

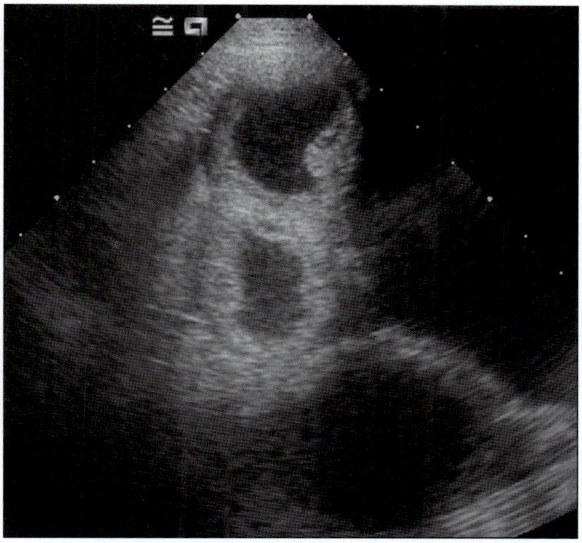

Figure 29.10 Ultrasonographic appearance of pyometra. Enlarged uterine horns distended with hypoechoic fluid are visible in proximity to the urinary bladder.

to breed from the bitch. However, good success rates have been reported with medical therapy when used in dogs with open-cervix pyometra. Protocols implemented include the use of prostaglandin, prolactin inhibition and/or progesterone receptor antagonists. Medical therapy is not recommended for bitches with closed-cervix pyometra due to a greater risk of potentially fatal complications.

Broad-spectrum antimicrobial therapy should be administered to all cases, regardless of whether surgical or medical therapy is used. The bacteria most commonly isolated from the uterus in pyometra include *Escherichia coli*, *Staphylococcus aureus*, and *Streptococcus*, *Pseudomonas* and *Proteus* species. Amoxicillin/clavulanic acid, a cephalosporin or potentiated sulphonamide are good empirical choices. Longer courses will be needed in dogs receiving medical therapy.

Toxicological emergencies

Suspected or witnessed poisoning is a common reason for presentation of small animals to emergency clinics, with dogs being much more commonly affected than cats. This chapter presents a general approach to the poisoned patient before going on to describe some of the more commonly implicated poisons in greater detail using a number of case examples.

APPROACH TO THE POISONED PATIENT

Telephone communication

Initial telephone communication is perhaps no more important than in the intoxicated patient. The important questions to ask are summarized in Box 30.1.

NURSING ASPECT

Nurses are frequently the first members of staff with whom owners ringing about suspected or witnessed poisoning will communicate. It is therefore imperative that all nurses are well rehearsed in the questions that are important to ask (Box 30.1) and advice should be sought from the veterinary surgeon if there is any concern.

On the basis of the information obtained, a recommendation should be made as to whether the animal needs to be presented to the practice or may be managed conservatively at home. In some cases, the animal will be exhibiting marked clinical signs and questioning should be kept to a minimum with immediate transport to the practice being the only appropriate recommendation. In other cases, it is necessary to obtain further information before a recommendation can be made.

BOX 30.1 Important questions to ask owners ringing with respect to intoxication

- Was exposure witnessed or is it suspected? If suspected, based on what evidence?
- What poisons are involved? Can the owner provide more specific details – quantity, concentration, etc.?
- Where appropriate, does the owner have access to the container?
  - The owner should be asked to bring this with them if the animal is presented to the practice
- What is the animal's signalment and estimated body weight?
- How long ago did exposure occur?
- By what route did exposure occur?
- Is the animal showing clinical signs? If so, what are they, when did they start and what is their progression?
- Is the owner sure that this is the only animal to be affected?
- Does the animal have any preexisting medical conditions? Is the animal currently taking any medications?

Further information

The purpose of seeking additional information about the poison in question is to ascertain if possible the severity of exposure that has or may have occurred (see Box 30.2).

A number of sources of information are available with respect to veterinary toxicology that includes:

- The Veterinary Poisons Information Service (VPIS) in the United Kingdom (practice registration required)
- The ASPCA Animal Poison Control Center in North America

BOX 30.2 Important additional information about specific poisons

- Has potentially toxic exposure occurred?
- Has lethal exposure occurred?
- What are the expected clinical signs?
- Would the animal be expected to have developed clinical signs by now?
- If signs are present, are they reported to be early or late signs of intoxication? Is their progression typical?

BOX 30.3 Useful information for calculating dosage of toxin exposure

- 1 standard teaspoon = ~5 ml; 1 standard tablespoon = ~15 ml
- 1 fluid ounce (oz) = 29.6 ml; 1 ml = 0.034 oz
- 1 lb = 0.454 kg; 1 kg = 2.2 lb
- 1% solution = 10 mg/ml = 1 g/100 ml
- 1 part per million (ppm) = 1 mg/kg for solid substances, 1 mg/l for liquid substances
- w/w: an abbreviation for 'by weight'; used to describe the concentration of a substance in a mixture or solution. In strict terms, 8% w/w means that the mass of the substance in question is 8% of the total mass of the solution or mixture. The metric symbol g/g has the same meaning as w/w.

- Books on veterinary toxicology (see Further Reading)
- The internet: only reliable up-to-date sources should be used (e.g. http://www.vin.com, http://www.ivis.org). The internet is also useful for determining ingredients and concentrations in cases where for example only a proprietary product name is available.

Some information that may be useful when calculating exposure dosages is presented in Box 30.3.

Home management

If the decision is made for the animal to be monitored at home, the owner must be thoroughly briefed both on what signs to observe the animal for and the typical time frame for their onset and progression. In general, if there is any doubt as to the animal's condition, veterinary examination should be recommended. Owners should be advised on appropriate measures to implement during transportation (e.g. keeping unconscious animals warm or keeping seizuring animals cool and protected from injury).

BOX 30.4 Contraindications to induction of emesis

- Significantly altered mentation due to increased risk of aspiration of vomitus; in particular in depressed animals in whom there may be dysfunction of the gag reflex
- Respiratory distress and pre-existing conditions (e.g. laryngeal paralysis) that may predispose the animal to aspiration
- Animals that are already vomiting
- Ingestion of a caustic or corrosive agent (e.g. acids or alkalis) – emesis will potentially expose the oropharyngeal and oesophageal mucosa to further injury. Consumption of milk or water should be encouraged if not contraindicated

Inducing emesis at home

In some cases in which poison ingestion has occurred within a suitable period of time, it may be appropriate for the owner to induce emesis at home, for example if financial concerns or practical constraints preclude presentation to the practice. In addition, if a considerable delay is anticipated prior to presentation, and the owner has ready access to an appropriate emetic, inducing emesis prior to departure from home may be advisable to minimize further absorption of the poison in transit. The owner must be questioned carefully to ensure that contraindications to inducing emesis do not exist; these are summarized in Box 30.4.

Agents that may be used to induce emesis at home are shown in Table 30.1.

CLINICAL TIP

- It is very important to make sure that soda crystals (washing soda) are used for emesis, as owners have inadvertently administered caustic soda (sodium hydroxide) instead. This is very harmful following ingestion, causing severe injury to the oropharyngeal and oesophageal mucosa with potentially fatal consequences (Figure 30.1).

Table 30.1 Agents for inducing emesis at home

Agent	Dose	Comments
Soda crystals (washing soda)	1 crystal	Place on tongue at back of mouth Emesis usually within 10 minutes Can be repeated NB. Not caustic soda (sodium hydroxide)
Syrup of ipecacuanha (7%)	D: 1–2 ml/kg p.o. C: 3.3 ml/kg p.o.	Emesis usually within 30 minutes Can be repeated once Bitter taste therefore poor compliance
Hydrogen peroxide (3%)	D, C: 1–3 ml/kg	Emesis usually within 10 minutes Can be repeated once Care to avoid aspiration
Table salt (sodium chloride)	Not recommended	Unreliable May induce or exacerbate hypernatraemia with potentially severe consequences Ad lib access to water imperative if used

C, cats; D, dogs.

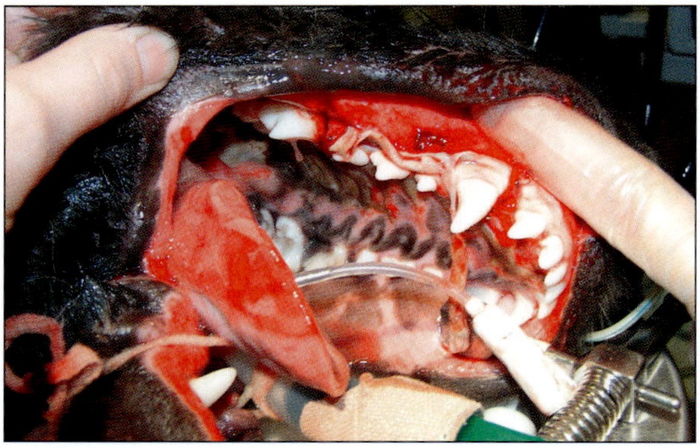

Figure 30.1 Severe oral cavity injury in a dog inadvertently given caustic soda by her owners for emesis. Severe mucosal injury extended all the way down the oesophagus. (Photograph courtesy of Tammy Ford)

General Clinical Approach

See Box 30.5.

History

CLINICAL TIP

- In a patient presents with severe clinical signs (e.g. seizures, severe muscle tremors) history-taking should not be prioritized over initial stabilization, especially as specific antidotes are not available for the majority of poisons to which dogs and cats are exposed. Ultimately treatment is directed at the patient and not the poison.

BOX 30.5 General approach to the poisoned patient

- Perform major body system examination and institute immediate life-saving measures as necessary
- Perform emergency database
- Obtain thorough history at first reasonable opportunity
- Minimize further systemic absorption of poison
- Administer antidote if available
- Promote elimination of any poison already absorbed
- Perform further clinical evaluation as appropriate
- Provide symptomatic, supportive and nursing care as appropriate
- Ensure close monitoring and regularly repeat clinical evaluation as appropriate

All the information in Boxes 30.1 and 30.2 should be obtained at the appropriate time. In some emergency patients, clinical signs and progression are compatible with possible intoxication without an immediately suggestive history. In such cases, the owner must be carefully and thoroughly questioned to establish whether a potential source of poison exists that the owner has not considered.

Initial management of ingested poisons

As for all emergency patients, a major body system (cardiovascular, respiratory, neurological) examination (see Ch. 1), including measurement of rectal temperature, should be performed and immediate measures taken to correct potentially life-threatening problems. Intravenous fluid therapy (see Ch. 4) may be required to correct hypovolaemia and/or dehydration. Fluid therapy is also indicated in the management of poisons that are nephrotoxic (e.g. nonsteroidal antiinflammatory agents) and those that are largely dependent on renal excretion. Oxygen supplementation is indicated in patients with respiratory compromise, for example from aspiration following vomiting, and in the context of certain poisons such as carbon monoxide.

Emergency database

An emergency database (see Ch. 3) for the intoxicated patient should consist of the following if possible:

- Manual packed cell volume (PCV) and serum total solids (TS)
- Blood glucose, electrolyte, urea and creatinine concentrations
- Peripheral blood smear examination
- Electrocardiogram (ECG)
- Noninvasive blood pressure (NIBP).

Additional tests that may be indicated at the appropriate time in certain cases include acid–base analysis, urinalysis (e.g. oxalate crystals in ethylene glycol poisoning) and calcium measurement (e.g. hypocalcaemia may occur in ethylene glycol poisoning). Abdominal radiographs taken at the appropriate time may reveal ingestion of items containing heavy metals or certain enteric-coated or sustained-release drug formulations. Routine haematology and biochemistry profiles may become indicated as case management progresses and may also identify pre-existing conditions that may have implications with respect to management of individual patients.

Treatment of seizures and muscle tremors

A variety of poisons include neurotoxicity amongst their mechanisms of action – examples include metaldehyde, pyrethroids, strychnine, caffeine, theobromine, organophosphates and tremorogenic mycotoxins. Seizures and/or muscle tremors are common signs of poisoning requiring symptomatic treatment (see Ch. 24).

In patients intoxicated with tremorogenic poisons (e.g. metaldehyde, permethrin), it can be difficult to differentiate severe muscle tremors from seizure activity. However, if the poison in question is known to be one associated with severe tremors or sufficient clinical suspicion exists, the use of methocarbamol may be indicated and may avoid the need for anaesthesia. This is a centrally acting muscle relaxant related to guaiphenesin whose precise mechanism of action remains unclear. The manufacturer's recommended dose in dogs and cats is 44–220 mg/kg i.v. with a typical upper limit of 330 mg/kg in a 24 hour period. However, to the author's knowledge, an injectable preparation of this agent is not currently available in the United Kingdom. In the absence of methocarbamol, the management of patients with tremors is the same as for those with seizures.

CLINICAL TIP

- The aim of treatment is to achieve adequate control of tremors; complete abolition of tremors is neither likely nor necessary and may require excessive drug administration.

Hyperthermia is a potentially serious development in patients suffering from seizures or muscle tremors. Hypothermia may also occur following bathing or sedation. Close monitoring of rectal temperature for either development and appropriate intervention (see Chs 16 and 17) is therefore required.

Gastrointestinal decontamination (GID)

Toxin exposure is usually via ingestion and gastrointestinal decontamination (GID) is frequently indicated. This consists of emptying of the stomach followed by administration of an adsorbent to minimize absorption of any poison remaining in the gastrointestinal tract.

Gastric emptying In the absence of contraindications (see Box 30.4), induction of emesis is the most expeditious means to empty the stomach; feeding a small meal

Table 30.2 Drugs used to induce emesis

Drug	Dose	Comments
Apomorphine	D: 0.04–0.1 mg/kg s.c., i.m., ocular	Drug of choice, emesis usually in 5–15 min Centrally acting Sedation, respiratory depression, ataxia, protracted vomiting possible (rare) Naloxone reverses sedative but not emetic effects Ocular route: apply to conjunctival sac; lavage thoroughly following emesis to minimize drug absorption; highly dependent on compliance
	C: 0.01–0.02 mg/kg s.c., i.m.	Use lowest possible dose Not recommended by some due to possible significant sedation Naloxone reverses sedative but not emetic effects
Medetomidine	C: 20 μg/kg i.m., i.v.	Alpha$_2$-adrenergic agonist Use atipamezole (50 μg/kg i.m.) to reverse effects once emesis has occurred Use very cautiously due to potential cardiorespiratory depression
Xylazine	C: 0.4–0.5 mg/kg i.m., s.c.	Alpha$_2$-adrenergic agonist Atipamezole may reverse effects Use very cautiously due to potential cardiorespiratory depression

C, cats; CNS, central nervous system; D, dogs; i.m., intramuscular; i.v., intravenous; s.c., subcutaneous.

first may increase the effectiveness of this approach. The author has performed gastric emptying up to 4–6 hours following ingestion with some good results. Drugs used to induce emesis are summarized in Table 30.2.

Activated charcoal Activated charcoal acts as an adsorbent binding to toxins and allowing their passage through the gastrointestinal tract while preventing or minimizing further systemic absorption. It is typically administered once gastric emptying has been performed and should be given as soon as possible. If an emetic has been employed for gastric emptying, enough time must be allowed for the emetic effects to subside before activated charcoal is administered. In some cases activated charcoal is administered initially via stomach tube at the end of gastric lavage. The recommended dose in dogs and cats is 1–5 g/kg to be repeated as necessary (typically every 4–6 hours) until black faeces are detected. Doses up to 8 g/kg have been used. Activated charcoal is often successfully administered in food to dogs. However, compliance is likely to be much poorer in cats. Various proprietary preparations are available with accompanying dosing guidelines, including powdered formulations (e.g. BCK Granules®, Fort Dodge) that can be added to food or made into a slurry and administered by mouth, and suspensions (e.g. Charcodote®, Pliva Pharma Ltd).

Different substances are bound to different degrees by activated charcoal. However, unless contraindicated, the use of activated charcoal in almost all cases of oral poisoning is probably reasonable and may also help following topical poisoning (see below). Activated charcoal should not be used following ingestion of caustic or corrosive substances, in patients that are vomiting or seizuring, or where there is any possibility of gastrointestinal perforation. Vomiting and constipation following administration of multiple doses are the main complications reported.

Gastric and colorectal lavage In patients in which induction of emesis is contraindicated or unsuccessful, gastric lavage may be appropriate for gastric emptying (see p. 296). However, it is contraindicated following ingestion of caustic or corrosive substances and where the risks of general anaesthesia are considered unacceptable.

In some cases (e.g. metaldehyde poisoning), following gastric lavage, the author will perform additional lavage via a stomach tube inserted as proximally as possible per rectum. Colorectal lavage is continued until clear fluid is returned and activated charcoal suspension is then instilled. The anus may be plugged with a swab for example for a short period of time to minimize leakage of the activated charcoal.

Topical poisoning

Washing the patient is recommended to minimize irritation of and absorption via the skin; this should also minimize absorption through ingestion following grooming. Washing is usually done using mild soap or detergent, followed by copious rinsing with water and then drying the animal as thoroughly as possible. Powdered toxins may be vacuumed off before washing. All individuals involved in handling the animal should take care to wear gloves and preferably an apron so as to avoid self-contamination. In some cases it may be appropriate for the owner to wash the animal at home. However, in compromised or noncompliant animals, veterinary care is recommended.

Clipping the coat of long-haired patients may help to maximize decontamination. Chemical restraint may be preferable during washing to allow protection of the eyes and in some cases general anaesthesia with endotracheal intubation is safest to minimize the risk of aspiration. Vital parameters including rectal temperature should be monitored closely throughout.

Oily substances may be more successfully removed using commercial hand-cleaning degreaser formulations (e.g. Swarfega Hand Cleaner® products) but it is important to ensure that such preparations are thoroughly washed off the animal subsequently.

The use of activated charcoal is generally recommended following topical poisoning. This is to minimize gastrointestinal absorption that may occur following ingestion from grooming. In addition, some poisons undergo enterohepatic circulation following absorption from the skin and thereby become available in the gastrointestinal tract.

In cases in which the skin has come into contact with an acidic or caustic substance, the affected area should be lavaged very thoroughly ('the solution to pollution is dilution') using normal saline or indeed warm water. The same is true in cases of ocular contamination and in both cases the animal should be given appropriate analgesia and chemically restrained to allow comprehensive lavage to be performed. Damaged skin is highly susceptible to mechanical injury and gentle lavage is therefore mandatory.

Diuresis

Diuresis is most indicated in the treatment of poisoning by agents for which renal excretion of either the primary intoxicant or its metabolites is a significant feature (e.g. phenobarbital, salicylates). Standard intravenous isotonic crystalloid therapy is employed to promote renal excretion with or without additional diuretic administration. Isotonic crystalloid therapy is administered at a rate of 1–4 ml/kg/hr above calculated fluid requirements and the patient must be monitored closely to ensure that adequate urine production occurs. In cases of aggressive diuresis, close monitoring of hydration status and electrolyte concentrations is indicated.

Antidotes

In a significant proportion of canine and feline patients a diagnosis of poisoning is made presumptively with the poison in question remaining unknown. Furthermore, specific antidotes or antagonists do not exist for the majority of potentially poisonous substances to which dogs and cats may be exposed. That said, the majority of clinical cases reported are due to a relatively small number of poisons for which, in some cases, specific treatments are available. These will be alluded to in the discussion of specific poisons that follows.

SPECIFIC POISONS

Pyrethrins and pyrethroids

Theory refresher

Pyrethrins are naturally occurring insecticidal esters of chrysanthemic acid and pyrethric acid extracted from the *Chrysanthemum cinerariaefolium* plant; pyrethroids (e.g. permethrin) are synthetic pyrethrins. Many topical and household insecticidal preparations containing these compounds are marketed for the control of flea and lice infestations amongst others in dogs and cats. These preparations are widely available from a variety of outlets.

CLINICAL TIP

- Synthetic pyrethroid insecticides are now most commonly used in small animal patients as topical spot-on formulations and the accidental or misguided inappropriate use of canine products on cats is the most commonly encountered cause of poisoning. In addition, cats may directly contact or lick the product once applied to a dog in the same household.

Toxic dose

The toxic dose for permethrin in cats is unknown. Dermal application of 100 mg/kg permethrin may prove life-threatening if untreated.

Mechanism of toxicity

Pyrethrins and pyrethroids alter the kinetics of neuronal sodium channels causing repeated nerve firing. In addition, some of these compounds may also inhibit gamma aminobutyric acid (GABA) receptors, resulting in hyperexcitability of nervous tissue. Glucuronidation is one pathway involved in the metabolism of some of these compounds and glucuronyl transferase deficiency may be part of the explanation for the apparent sensitivity of cats to pyrethroids.

Oral exposure

Oral exposure should be treated by gastrointestinal decontamination if appropriate, including activated charcoal if patient compliance allows. Pyrethrins and pyrethroids are highly fat soluble and low fat foods should therefore be fed in the short term to reduce further absorption.

Case example 1

PRESENTING SIGNS AND CASE HISTORY

A 1-year-old female neutered domestic short hair cat (2.5 kg) presented 3 hours after topical application of a spot-on preparation containing 744 mg permethrin per millilitre. The preparation used was registered for use in dogs only but the owner had thought it would be safe to administer half of the pipette to the cat. The cat had developed clinical signs within 1 hour of administration and at the time of presentation was showing severe muscle tremors.

CLINICAL TIP

- Clinical signs usually develop within a few hours of exposure. Minor and usually self-limiting signs include hyperaesthesia, hypersalivation, ataxia, mydriasis, paw flicking and ear twitching. These signs may be accompanied by other nonspecific signs such as lethargy or transient vomiting and diarrhoea.
- Severe neurotoxicity resulting from excessive exposure may result in marked depression, ataxia, potentially violent muscle tremors, seizures and death. Protracted gastrointestinal signs may also occur.

Case management

Diazepam (5 mg) was administered per rectum to facilitate intravenous catheter placement and blood was obtained via the catheter for an emergency database to be performed; this was found to be unremarkable. Major body system examination was unremarkable except for the muscle tremors that were less severe but still marked.

Intravenous fluid therapy was commenced and anaesthesia was induced using propofol and maintained using isoflurane. The cat was washed thoroughly in a mild detergent and dried before being recovered with an Elizabethan collar in place. Muscle tremors were apparent in recovery but of lesser severity and a single intravenous bolus of midazolam (0.2 mg/kg) was administered.

Tremors resolved fully over the next 24 hours, during which time vital parameters, in particular temperature, were monitored closely and appropriate supportive and nursing measures instituted.

Permethrin dosage in this case was approximately 150 mg/kg.

CLINICAL TIP

- The prognosis for full recovery is reasonable despite severe poisoning in animals receiving early and appropriately aggressive intervention; neurotoxicity is fully reversible. In severe cases clinical signs may take 72 hours or more to resolve.

Metaldehyde

Theory refresher

Metaldehyde is a cyclic tetramer of acetaldehyde that is commonly used as a pesticide against slugs and snails (molluscicide). Commercial pellet preparations usually contain 1.5–8% metaldehyde w/w (see Box 30.3) in a cereal base. The pellets are often blue or green in colour and the cereals and other additives make slug/snail baits palatable to dogs. Cats as usual are more discerning and metaldehyde poisoning has only been reported in a few cases. Liquid preparations containing higher concentrations of metaldehyde are also available, as are granular and powdered preparations. Metaldehyde baits sometimes contain additional herbicides and pesticides, most commonly carbamate insecticides.

Toxic dose

A fatal oral dosage of metaldehyde in dogs of 60 mg/kg body weight has been reported although some authors quote much higher values. Clinical signs may be expected to occur at a range of typically much lower dosages. A lethal dose of 207 mg/kg has been reported in cats.

Toxicokinetics

Metaldehyde may be absorbed intact from the gastrointestinal tract but its subsequent distribution, metabolism and excretion remain to be fully clarified. Acid hydrolysis occurs in the stomach producing acetaldehyde which is then absorbed rapidly and converted to carbon dioxide (probably eliminated via the lungs) or excreted in urine. The half-life of metaldehyde in people is estimated at approximately 27 hours but is unknown in dogs.

Mechanism of toxicity

The precise mechanism of toxicity of metaldehyde remains to be elucidated but it is known to cross the blood–brain barrier readily and impairment of GABA activity is currently thought to be most implicated. As GABA is an inhibitory neurotransmitter, a decrease in its activity may be responsible for the increased neurological activity seen in metaldehyde poisoning. A decrease in the concentration of other neurotransmitters in the central nervous system (CNS), such as serotonin (5-HT) and noradrenaline (norepinephrine), may also be involved.

Case example 2

PRESENTING SIGNS AND CASE HISTORY

A previously healthy 2-year-old male neutered black Labrador retriever (30 kg) presented recumbent with marked twitching, muscle tremors, mydriasis and hyperthermia. The dog had been out unattended in the garden earlier that afternoon and would have had access to the shed in which the owner kept slug pellets. One hour after returning inside the dog was found to be twitching and salivating and the owner had rung the hospital for advice.

Given the dog's signalment and history, there was a high index of suspicion for poisoning and the owner was advised to come straight down to

PRESENTING SIGNS AND CASE HISTORY—cont'd

the hospital (a 15-minute car journey). The owner was advised not to travel alone and to ensure that the dog was kept cool and protected from injury during the journey. Meanwhile another member of the family went to investigate the shed where indeed it was found that the slug bait container had been disrupted. Details from the container were communicated directly to the practice while the dog was *en route*. Preparations had been made in the interim to manage the dog for a suspected diagnosis of metaldehyde poisoning.

CLINICAL TIP

- Clinical signs due to metaldehyde poisoning often occur quickly (e.g. within 1 hour of ingestion) but may take up to several hours to appear. The typical presentation involves CNS signs including twitching, tremors, muscle spasms and hyperaesthesia, with opisthotonos and seizures (including status epilepticus) being seen in severe cases.
- Hyperthermia is frequently identified in metaldehyde poisoning and is presumed to occur due to the marked neuromuscular activity (hence it is sometimes referred to as the 'shake and bake syndrome'). Hyperthermia may contribute significantly to the pathophysiology and clinical presentation.

Case management

After checking the dog's temperature, diazepam (1 mg/kg) was administered per rectum and an intravenous catheter subsequently placed. A further intravenous bolus of diazepam (0.5 mg/kg) was administered and a major body system examination performed. Anaesthesia was then induced using propofol and maintained using isoflurane following endotracheal intubation. Thorough gastric lavage was performed and revealed blue-green coloured material. Activated charcoal was then administered into the stomach. Colorectal lavage was also done and an activated charcoal enema administered.

CLINICAL TIP

- Treatment of metaldehyde poisoning should always be instituted as early as possible and should be aggressive. A conservative approach in a dog with severe neurological signs may result in preventable irreversible brain injury and potentially respiratory failure.
- Induction of emesis is only appropriate in asymptomatic animals, and dogs showing neuromuscular signs should be fully anaesthetized and subjected to thorough gastric and colorectal lavage.

The dog was maintained on a propofol infusion for the next 12 hours, during which phenobarbital loading was performed (3 mg/kg i.v. q 1 hr for six doses); thereafter the dog was gradually weaned off propofol (over 4 hours). External stimulation was kept to a minimum (e.g. cotton wool balls/swabs in the ears, dim lighting, minimal noise and passage of personnel). The dog remained markedly depressed for the following 24 hours but gradually became ambulatory and although ataxic initially went on to make a full recovery over the following 3 days. Fluid therapy and appropriate nursing measures were instituted throughout. Phenobarbital (3 mg/kg i.v. then p.o. q 12 hr) therapy was discontinued at discharge.

The slug bait container contained 1 kg of blue pellets with a metaldehyde composition of 4% w/w. Assuming the dog had ingested all 1 kg of bait, this was equal to 40 mg (i.e. 4% × 1000 mg) of metaldehyde and a maximum dosage of only 1.3 mg/kg.

CLINICAL TIP

- Clinical signs may persist for 24 hours or more but the prognosis for full recovery is good and survival rates are very high for animals that receive prompt and aggressive management and survive the initial 24-hours period following intoxication.
- Dogs recovering from severe metaldehyde intoxication may very occasionally have temporary blindness and liver failure is a serious but very infrequently reported delayed (2–3 days) development.

Ethylene glycol

Although ethylene glycol (EG) is a common cause of poisoning in companion animals in North America, its incidence is significantly lower in the United Kingdom. EG is a sweet-tasting liquid used primarily as an antifreeze, screen wash and windshield de-icing agent. Antifreeze ingestion is the most common source of EG poisoning, with many common preparations containing as much as 95% EG. Companion animal exposure is generally the result of environmental contamination from improper disposal or insecure storage, and poisoning is most likely to occur in late autumn and early spring when antifreeze usage increases.

Toxic dose

The minimum lethal dose of undiluted EG is reported to be 4.4–6.6 ml/kg in dogs and 1.5 ml/kg in cats.

Toxicokinetics

EG is rapidly absorbed from the gastrointestinal tract and distributed systemically. Its plasma half-life is approximately 3 hours and a variable proportion is excreted unchanged in urine. The remainder is metabolized predominantly in the liver. The first step in this metabolism is oxidation of EG to glycoaldehyde by alcohol dehydrogenase (ADH), a conversion that can be saturated. Glycoaldehdye is then converted to glycolic acid, glyoxylic acid and finally to oxalic acid. EG metabolic pathways may vary between species.

Calcium binds to oxalic acid, resulting in the formation of calcium oxalate crystals that are deposited widely but especially in the renal tubules, and calcium oxalate crystalluria is a common finding.

Mechanism of toxicity

CLINICAL TIP

- The effects of EG prior to metabolism are generally relatively minor. However, the metabolites of EG are highly toxic. Acute renal failure is the most severe consequence of EG poisoning in companion animals. Most of the metabolites of EG are thought to be toxic to the renal tubular epithelium and calcium oxalate deposition may cause further damage.

Metabolism of EG generates free oxygen radicals that are potentially cytotoxic to a variety of tissues. In addition, the organic acid metabolites produced interfere with normal cellular processes. Central nervous system (CNS) dysfunction is thought to be predominantly due to the effects of glycoaldehyde along with calcium oxalate deposition in nervous tissue. Both hypocalcaemia secondary to binding of calcium to oxalic acid and metabolic acidosis may contribute further to CNS signs. Metabolic acidosis may be severe and is due to the accumulation of acid metabolites, most notably glycolic acid.

Clinical signs

Clinical signs of EG poisoning are dose-dependent and in companion animals occur in two phases. The first is predominantly associated with EG itself prior to metabolism. Signs develop within an hour of ingestion and may persist for 12 hours. They include CNS depression, somnolence, ataxia, impairment of conscious proprioception, nausea, vomiting, and osmotic diuresis with consequent polyuria/polydipsia. In severe cases seizures, coma and death may occur. In dogs these signs may seemingly resolve with apparent recovery although they may occur earlier and be more persistent in cats.

The second phase of clinical signs is associated with the highly toxic metabolites of EG and is predominantly related to acute renal failure. Signs usually develop within 24–72 hours of ingestion in dogs, often earlier in cats, and may include reduced mentation from depression through to coma, seizures, anorexia, vomiting, and oliguria with low urine specific gravity or isosthenuria. Anuria may develop 3–4 days post-ingestion.

An intermediate phase between the two phases already described consists of cardiopulmonary manifestations (tachycardia, tachypnoea, pulmonary oedema) but this is recognized much less commonly in dogs and cats than in people.

Laboratory tests

Biochemistry, acid–base analysis Early changes are mainly due to accumulation of acid EG metabolites with normochloraemic metabolic acidosis, reduced plasma bicarbonate (HCO_3^-) and increased anion gap. If plasma HCO_3^- measurement is not available, reduced concentration may be reflected as a decrease in total carbon dioxide (total CO_2). These changes may be detectable 1–3 hours following ingestion and a high anion gap may persist for 12–48 hours. Total hypocalcaemia may occur due to chelation by oxalic acid, hyperglycaemia is also reported, and prerenal azotaemia may be detected with appropriately severe dehydration.

Later biochemical abnormalities reflect renal injury and reduced glomerular filtration rate with renal azotaemia and hyperphosphataemia. These changes are usually detectable 24–72 hours post-ingestion in dogs and earlier in cats.

Urinalysis

Osmotic diuresis and polydipsia (due to increased serum osmolality) result in reduced urine specific gravity, typically within 3 hours of EG ingestion. Dogs are usually isosthenuric (urine specific gravity 1.007–1.015) but urine specific gravity may be higher than this and often is in cats. Urine specific gravity remains low as renal insufficiency and impaired ability to concentrate urine develop in the later stages. Glucosuria with concurrent normoglycaemia may be detected in dogs as a result of proximal renal tubular damage.

Calcium oxalate crystals may be identified in urine 3–6 hours after EG ingestion. Calcium oxalate monohydrate crystals (clear six-sided prisms or dumbbell-shaped (Figure 30.2) crystals) are more common than the dihydrate form (envelopes or Maltese cross-shaped). Aciduria, haematuria, renal epithelial cells and casts are other common urinalysis findings.

Serum ethylene glycol concentration

Serum EG concentrations peak 1–6 hours post-ingestion and EG is usually no longer detectable in serum (or urine)

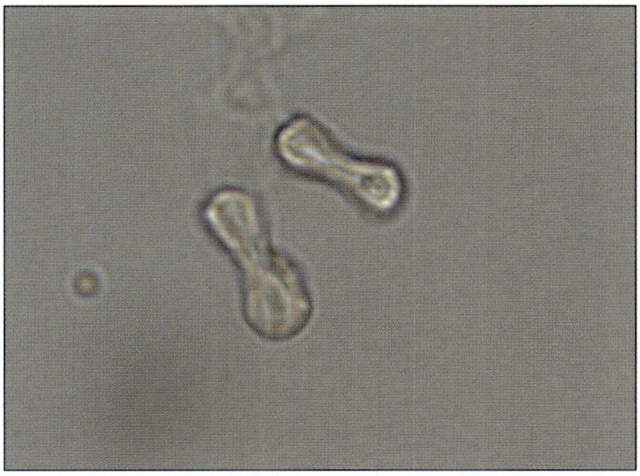

Figure 30.2 Dumbbell-shaped calcium oxalate monohydrate crystals in urine. (Photograph courtesy of Kate English)

by 48–72 hours post-ingestion. A commercial test kit (Ethylene Glycol Test Kit®, PRN Pharmacal Inc., Florida; http://www.prnpharmacal.com/egtkit/index.php) is available for estimating serum EG concentrations based on an enzymatic assay; it is both accurate enough for clinical use and relatively inexpensive. Results are available within 30 minutes. These kits have a minimum detectable level of 50 mg/dl of EG in the blood and it is noteworthy that cats may develop clinically significant poisoning despite serum EG levels lower than this threshold.

CLINICAL TIP

- The EG test kit may generate a false-positive result if propylene glycol or glycerol is present in the patient's blood. Propylene glycol is a constituent of some activated charcoal suspensions, diazepam formulations and semi-moist diets. Blood for this test should be drawn before administration of any preparations that may contain propylene glycol or glycerol.
- False-positive results may also occur following metaldehyde ingestion but do not occur in the presence of ethanol.

Serum osmolality

EG is an osmotically active substance and ingestion results in an increase in serum osmolality and osmole gap (equivalent to the measured serum osmolality minus the calculated osmolality). Measurement of serum osmolality is useful for identifying early EG poisoning. However, access to measured serum osmolality is likely to be very limited in general emergency practice.

Wood's lamp

A number of modern antifreeze preparations contain sodium fluorescein to aid in detection of radiator leaks. This dye is excreted in urine following ingestion; excretion usually only occurs for up to 6 hours post-ingestion (but it can be longer). Urine as well as the mouth, paws and vomitus can therefore be examined with a Wood's lamp for fluorescence due to the presence of this dye. However, it is noteworthy that a negative result does not exclude the possibility of EG ingestion as not all antifreeze preparations contain sodium fluorescein.

Treatment

Treatment of suspected EG poisoning should be instituted as early as possible because it is metabolized rapidly into highly toxic metabolites. Treatment consists of the following components:

- GID to minimize EG absorption
- Preventing metabolism of absorbed EG to more toxic metabolites
- Promoting urinary excretion of EG and its metabolites with intravenous fluid therapy
- Correction of fluid, acid–base and electrolyte abnormalities
- Supportive nursing care.

Gastrointestinal decontamination

EG is absorbed very rapidly from the gastrointestinal tract and GID may therefore only be of benefit very early post-ingestion (1–2 hr). Activated charcoal decreases ethanol absorption and should not therefore be administered if oral ethanol is being used as an antidote.

Preventing ethylene glycol metabolism

The prevention of EG oxidation by ADH is the most important component of therapy and may be achieved in one of two ways: inhibition of the enzyme or provision of a competitive substrate. Treatment should be administered in all animals presenting within 36 hours of EG ingestion.

Fomepizole ADH may be inhibited by the administration of fomepizole (4-methylpyrazole, 4-MP). This agent is a synthetic competitive ADH inhibitor and has become the treatment of choice in EG poisoning (Box 30.6). Minimal side effects have been reported

BOX 30.6 Guidelines for fomepizole administration

Dogs

- 20 mg/kg body weight i.v. for first dose, followed by 15 mg/kg i.v at 12 and 24 hr, and 5 mg/kg i.v. at 36 hr
- Continue with 5 mg/kg i.v. q 12 hr if recovery has not occurred by 36 hr

Cats

- 125 mg/kg body weight i.v. for first dose, followed by 31.25 mg/kg i.v. at 12, 24 and 36 hr
- Continue with 31.25 mg/kg i.v. q 12 hr if recovery has not occurred by 36 hr

following the use of this agent in companion animals and in particular it lacks the CNS depressive effects of ethanol (see below).

Ethanol Ethanol may be used in the treatment of EG poisoning as it has a higher affinity for ADH than EG and therefore acts as a preferential competitive substrate (Box 30.7). Injectable ethanol should be diluted in saline prior to administration. If a pure preparation for injection is not available, ethanol may be administered orally using an alcoholic beverage.

Perhaps the biggest disadvantage of the therapeutic use of ethanol is the associated CNS depression that may necessitate intensive and supportive care, especially with intermittent bolus administration and in cats. If oral ethanol is being used, direct administration via orogastric intubation may prove necessary in animals that are too sedated to swallow reliably.

BOX 30.7 Guidelines for therapeutic ethanol administration

Ethanol as intravenous injection

Dogs

- 5.5 ml of 20% ethanol/kg body weight i.v. q 4 hr for five doses then q 6 hr for four doses; or
- Give the same total dose over the same period as a constant rate infusion

Cats

- 5.0 ml of 20% ethanol/kg body weight i.v. q 6 hr for five doses then q 8 hr for four doses; or
- Give the same total dose over the same period as a constant rate infusion

Ethanol as an alcoholic beverage

Dogs

- 4.4–6.6 ml/kg of 40% ethanol alcoholic beverage p.o. q 4 hr for five doses then q 6 hr for four doses

Cats

- 4.4 ml/kg of 40% ethanol alcoholic beverage p.o. q 6 hr for five doses then q 8 hr for four doses

CLINICAL TIP

- Other ethanol-containing preparations such as surgical spirit or methylated spirits should be avoided as they contain methanol.
- Ethanol should not be administered to animals presenting in renal failure as ingested EG will already have been metabolized by that stage.

Other treatment considerations

Appropriate supportive therapy consists of intravenous fluid therapy to correct hypovolaemia and dehydration and to promote diuresis. Potassium and calcium supplementation should be provided as deemed necessary on the basis of regular monitoring. Patients presenting with oliguric renal failure should be treated with intravenous fluid therapy and diuretic agents to establish diuresis if possible (see Ch. 36). If adequate diuresis cannot be established, then referral for haemodialysis or peritoneal dialysis should be considered if available and affordable.

Renal tubular damage caused by EG may be reversible but can take weeks to months and urine concentrating ability may never return in some cases. Most dogs and cats surviving the acute renal failure phase of EG poisoning will eventually regain normal renal function.

NURSING ASPECT

Patients suffering from EG poisoning may be severely depressed and recumbent, both from the poisoning and from treatment if ethanol is used. Standard nursing measures for recumbent patients should be implemented, including provision of clean, dry, well-padded bedding, regular turning and bladder management. Regular eye lubrication and oral care may be needed and patients must be monitored closely for hypothermia.

Prognosis

Prognosis depends on the dosage of EG ingested, rate of absorption and, most importantly, the time to institution of specific therapy. The prognosis for dogs treated with fomepizole within 5 hours of ingestion is good, and most will recover if treatment is administered within 8 hours of ingestion. The prognosis is reasonable for cats receiving therapy within 3 hours of ingestion.

However, a grave prognosis for survival is heralded by the onset of oliguric renal failure in both species and unfortunately most animals present at this late stage.

Grapes/raisins

Theory refresher

Grape/raisin poisoning in dogs has been recognized since the late 1990s. No confirmed cases have been reported in cats at the time of writing but susceptibility is suspected. A similar syndrome has not been reported in people.

CLINICAL TIP

- The same poisoning syndrome may occur following consumption of all types of fresh grapes and commercially available raisins, including those manufactured organically. The potential for toxicity should be considered in all cases regardless of the dosage consumed.

Toxic dose, toxicokinetics, mechanism of toxicity

Grape/raisin ingestion may be associated with renal toxicity but the toxin or toxins involved have yet to be identified and the mechanism of toxicity is unknown. There does not appear to be a correlation between the quantity of grapes/raisins consumed and the subsequent renal pathology and clinical progression; an idiosyncratic reaction is suspected.

Case example 3

PRESENTING SIGNS AND CASE HISTORY

A previously healthy 3-year-old male entire Labrador retriever (30 kg) presented with a several hour history of acute onset severe vomiting. After extensive questioning the owners revealed that the dog had eaten 350 g of raisins the day before.

CLINICAL TIP

- Vomiting is reported in almost all cases, usually within 24 hr of ingestion, and grapes or raisins may be identified in the vomitus. Vomiting may be related to dietary indiscretion or the

CLINICAL TIP—cont'd

development of azotaemia, but a specific effect of grapes or raisins is also suspected due to the frequency with which this sign is reported. Subsequently anorexia, lethargy, diarrhoea and abdominal pain have been reported.

Major body system examination

Physical examination revealed the dog to be very depressed and moderately dehydrated but was otherwise unremarkable.

Emergency database

An intravenous catheter was placed in a cephalic vein and blood obtained via the catheter for an emergency database. This revealed severe azotaemia (blood urea nitrogen 45 mmol/l, reference range 3–9.10 mmol/l; creatinine 1250 μmol/l, reference range 98–163 μmol/l) and moderate hyperkalaemia (6.0 mmol/l, reference range 4.1–5.3 mmol/l). Dehydration was confirmed (manual packed cell volume 55%, reference range 37–55%; plasma total solids 75 g/l, reference range 49–71 g/l). The severity of azotaemia was consistent with a primary renal or postrenal cause but some prerenal contribution due to dehydration was also likely.

Case management

A soft indwelling Foley urethral catheter was placed with ease, thereby excluding urethral obstruction, and an emergency abdominal ultrasound revealed no free peritoneal fluid, thus excluding uroperitoneum; both kidneys had grossly normal architecture. Urinalysis on a sample collected via the urethral catheter revealed a specific gravity of 1.020 and mild proteinuria, glucosuria and haematuria. The azotaemia was diagnosed as renal in origin (with the caveat that the ureters had not been imaged to exclude completely a postrenal cause or component). A presumptive diagnosis of acute renal failure due to raisin poisoning was therefore made.

The dog was not felt to be hypovolaemic but moderate dehydration (7%) was suspected, and he was started on 0.9% sodium chloride (normal, physiological saline) at 10 ml/kg/hr to provide rehydration and maintenance requirements over approximately 8 hours. The bladder was emptied via the urethral catheter at the outset. After 10 hours of fluid therapy, urine output was calculated and the dog was found to have produced only

0.5 ml/kg/hr of urine. A diagnosis of oliguric acute renal failure was therefore made. The decision was made at this point to refer the dog.

Despite aggressive diuretic therapy at the referral centre, using furosemide and mannitol, oliguria persisted and the dog became overhydrated, showing chemosis, diffuse subcutaneous oedema and mild peritoneal and pleural effusion. Peritoneal dialysis was considered appropriate in this case (young previously healthy dog with potentially curable disease) and was performed successfully. Four months following discharge from the referral hospital mild persistent azotaemia was present (blood urea nitrogen 13 mmol/l, creatinine 190 μmol/l) but the dog was clinically well. Appropriate dietary management and on-going monitoring were recommended.

CLINICAL TIP

- Acute renal failure does not develop in all dogs following grape/raisin ingestion. Nevertheless, as grape/raisin poisoning is suspected to be due to an idiosyncratic nondose-related reaction, treatment should be instituted in all cases following ingestion as early as possible. Gastrointestinal decontamination including induction of emesis if the animal is not already vomiting and administration of activated charcoal is performed and intravenous fluid therapy provided for a minimum of 48 hours.
- Although a beneficial effect of fluid therapy on outcome in grape/raisin poisoning has yet to be convincingly demonstrated, both the potential benefits of this therapy and the gravity of this poisoning syndrome make it a recommended treatment in all cases.
- Serum chemistry and urine output should be monitored for 72 hours.

CLINICAL TIP

- Outcome is not correlated with the dosage of grapes or raisins ingested. The prognosis for survival following the onset of oliguric and, in particular, anuric acute renal failure is poor but some dogs may recover, especially if dialysis is available.
- Clinical signs are expected to resolve fully in recovering dogs while blood renal parameters

CLINICAL TIP—cont'd

may or may not normalize. Normalization of renal parameters, interpreted as resolution of renal dysfunction, may take several weeks or months.

Lilies

Domestic cats are the only animals thus far reported to be susceptible to lily nephrotoxicity. Earliest reports involved Easter lily (*Lilium longiflorum*) but it is now suspected that all species of the *Lilium* genera, including Tiger lily, as well as day lilies (*Hemerocallis* genera) may be potentially nephrotoxic to cats. All parts of the plants, including the flowers, are associated with poisoning and exposure is usually via access to household plants.

Toxic dose, toxicokinetics, mechanism of toxicity

Even very small amounts of plant ingest may be poisonous to cats and rapid absorption from the gastrointestinal tract is suspected as some cats still develop renal insufficiency despite early gastrointestinal decontamination. The toxin or toxins involved have yet to be identified and the metabolism is unknown. The precise mechanism of toxicity is unknown but renal tubular epithelial necrosis and subsequent acute renal failure are known to occur.

Pancreatitis and pancreatic degeneration have also been reported in cats with lily poisoning, as have seizures of unconfirmed pathogenesis.

Clinical signs

Clinical signs may develop in as little as 5–10 minutes following ingestion. Within 1–3 hours vomiting, salivation, depression, lethargy and anorexia may be apparent. Polyuria and consequent dehydration occur 12–30 hours following ingestion and this is followed by anuria.

Anuria typically occurs 24–48 hr following ingestion and death may occur within 7 days of exposure. Renomegaly and abdominal pain may be detected in some cats.

Laboratory tests

Depending on the time elapsed since ingestion, clinicopathological findings are likely to reflect acute renal failure with azotaemia, hyperphosphataemia and possible hyperkalaemia. These abnormalities are usually evident within 24–72 hours of ingestion. Urinalysis may reveal isosthenuria, tubular casts (Figure 30.3), proteinuria and glucosuria.

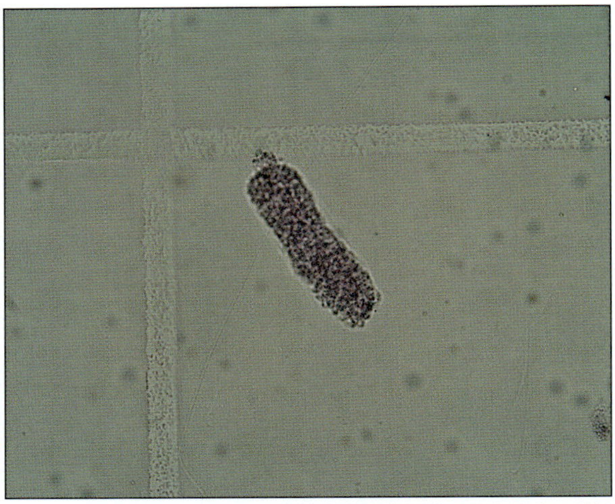

Figure 30.3 Tubular cast in urine (×200). (Photograph courtesy of Kate English)

Treatment

Depending on the time elapsed since ingestion, routine GID may be indicated to minimize absorption. Fluid diuresis should be implemented for 24–72 hours, with regular monitoring of serum biochemistry and urinalysis. Diuretic therapy (furosemide, mannitol) may be beneficial in cats with oliguric renal failure but is unlikely to induce urine production in anuric cats for which referral for dialysis may be the only treatment option if available and affordable. Mannitol should not be used in anuric animals.

Prognosis

Prognosis depends in large part on the time between ingestion and presentation for treatment. Early presentation with GID and fluid diuresis carries a good prognosis for clinical recovery although some chronic renal dysfunction may persist. The prognosis is grave with standard medical therapy following the onset of anuria. The prognosis for anuric animals receiving dialysis may be favourable but remains to be elucidated.

Nonsteroidal antiinflammatory agents

Nonsteroidal antiinflammatory agents (NSAIAs) are widely used in human and veterinary medicine as both prescription-only and over-the-counter (OTC) preparations. A large heterogeneous variety of agents exists but they share certain therapeutic antiinflammatory, antipyretic and analgesic effects as well as undesirable adverse effects. The following discussion presents general information about NSAIA intoxication.

Toxic dose

The pharmacokinetics of NSAIAs show differences between species and doses used in people should not be extrapolated to dogs and cats.

Toxicokinetics, mechanism of toxicity

NSAIAs are direct inhibitors of cyclooxygenase (COX) and cause reduced production of prostaglandins and thromboxane. Some NSAIAs are reported to be more COX-2 selective; COX-2 is induced during tissue injury and inflammation. However, it is important to remember that at excessive dosages both COX-1 (constitutive/housekeeping form responsible for physiological functions) and COX-2 inhibition is likely.

NSAIAs are generally readily absorbed following oral exposure. Metabolism is usually hepatic. In dogs, a number of NSAIAs undergo enterohepatic circulation. Adverse effects of NSAIAs have been reported to involve predominantly the gastrointestinal tract, the kidneys, coagulation, and the liver.

Gastrointestinal tract

Gastrointestinal injury is the most common adverse effect associated with excessive NSAIA exposure in dogs and cats. These agents have ulcerogenic effects in the stomach and duodenum as a result of both impaired synthesis of prostaglandins that are important in mucosal cytoprotection and local topical mucosal irritation.

Kidneys

Under normal conditions prostaglandins are of little importance in maintaining renal blood flow. However, they exert a compensatory vasodilatory effect to maintain renal perfusion and function in conditions that cause renal vasoconstriction. Thus nephrotoxicity and consequent renal insufficiency may occur in animals that are exposed to NSAIAs while in a state of volume depletion or hypotension, as well as following exposure to massive overdose.

Coagulation

NSAIAs can induce coagulopathy by inhibiting COX within platelets and thereby impairing the production of thromboxane. Among other functions thromboxane facilitates platelet aggregation.

Adverse effects associated with NSAIAs are more likely to occur in animals exposed to excessive dosages as well as in those with volume depletion, hypotension or pre-existing gastrointestinal or renal disease. Bleeding tendency may be more common in animals with other concurrent coagulation abnormalities (e.g. von Willebrand's disease). Hepatic injury is not a prominent feature of acute NSAIA intoxication.

Clinical signs

Early clinical signs of NSAIA intoxication in dogs are likely to reflect gastrointestinal complications and include vomiting, with or without haematemesis, and diarrhoea, with or without melaena (or haematochezia); inappetence, lethargy, depression, weakness and possible abdominal pain may occur. Dehydration and potentially hypovolaemia may be present. Cats may show gastrointestinal signs less frequently but tachypnoea may be more common than in dogs. In severe cases gastrointestinal perforation may occur with subsequent peritonitis that may be accompanied by abdominal pain and severe cardiovascular compromise.

Animals may also present with oliguric or polyuric acute renal failure.

Laboratory and other tests

Depending on the time elapsed since ingestion, clinicopathological findings may reflect gastrointestinal blood loss, with anaemia and possible panhypoproteinaemia. Anaemia may be preregenerative or regenerative (see Ch. 3). Prerenal azotaemia may be identified and urea may be disproportionately elevated compared to creatinine due to gastrointestinal haemorrhage. Renal insufficiency will likely manifest as azotaemia, hyperphosphataemia, possible hypercalcaemia and isosthenuria. Proteinuria may also be detected.

If gastrointestinal perforation and peritonitis are suspected, additional testing is mandatory. Abdominal radiography may show loss of serosal detail due to free peritoneal fluid, and free peritoneal gas. Abdominal ultrasonography may reveal free peritoneal fluid and may be used to guide abdominocentesis (see p. 293). Alternatively, blind abdominocentesis may be performed. Any fluid obtained should be examined cytologically and will typically be consistent with a purulent exudate if perforation has occurred.

Treatment

Depending on the time elapsed since ingestion, routine GID including the use of activated charcoal may be indicated to minimize further drug absorption. Intravenous fluid therapy using an isotonic crystalloid solution is indicated to correct hypovolaemia or dehydration and recurrence must be prevented to minimize the risk of nephrotoxicity.

Medical therapy designed to minimize further gastrointestinal compromise and to promote ulcer healing should be provided (Table 30.3). Routine use of antiemetics may be required.

Surgical intervention is required in animals with gastrointestinal perforation and standard management of

Table 30.3 Medical therapy for nonsteroidal antiinflammatory agent (NSAIA) intoxication

Drug	Dose	Comments
Misoprostol	D: 2–5 µg/kg p.o. q 8–12 hr	Synthetic prostaglandin analogue Highly effective; treatment of choice Contraindicated in pregnant animals Not recommended for cats Wear gloves; women of childbearing age to take extra precautions
Omeprazole	D, C: 0.5–1 mg/kg slow i.v., p.o. q 24 hr	Proton pump inhibitor thereby suppressing gastric acid production Maximum 3 days i.v. use recommended
Histamine (H_2) receptor antagonists	Doses as per Appendix 1	e.g. famotidine, ranitidine, cimetidine Less effective than misoprostol and omeprazole
Sucralfate	D: 0.5–2 g p.o. q 8–12 hr C: 0.25 g p.o. q 8–12 hr	Coats ulcerated/exposed mucosa and promotes re-epithelialization Less effective than misoprostol and omeprazole Administration 30–60 minutes before food is recommended Tablets can be crushed and mixed with water

C, cats; D, dogs; i.v., intravenous; p.o., per os.

acute renal failure (see Ch. 36) is indicated in appropriate cases. NSAIA-mediated acute renal insufficiency is often reversible with adequate supportive care.

Aspirin

Toxic dose

In dogs, aspirin administration at 50 mg/kg q 12 hr has been reported to cause vomiting, and haematemesis and gastric ulcer perforation have been reported at 100–300 mg/kg/day for 1–4 weeks. Due to deficiencies in aspirin metabolism, cats are more susceptible and the toxic dose is lower than for dogs.

Toxicokinetics, mechanism of toxicity, clinical signs

Aspirin (acetylsalicylic acid) is a synthetic NSAIA. Following ingestion, aspirin is readily absorbed and is then metabolized in the liver to salicylic acid. Some local hydrolysis to salicylic acid also occurs in the gastrointestinal tract. Salicylic acid is the active form and the form that is absorbed into the circulation. Elimination from the circulation depends on conjugation with glucuronic acid. At high dosages this conjugation becomes overwhelmed, resulting in delayed clearance and accumulation of the active drug. Cats have a defective glucuronic acid conjugation system that results in prolonged drug elimination compared to dogs and an increased susceptibility to aspirin poisoning.

Gastrointestinal irritation and injury are the most common adverse effects of aspirin ingestion and nephrotoxicity is also reported. Metabolic acidosis is responsible for the majority of clinical signs. The metabolic acidosis in salicylate poisoning is a high anion gap acidosis. Severe and fatal acidaemia may occur within a few hours of aspirin ingestion.

Salicylates also have toxic effects in the CNS although the exact mechanism of toxicity is not known. Seizures have been reported in both dogs and cats secondary to salicylate toxicity. Noncardiogenic pulmonary oedema is the most common cause of major morbidity in people and might be related to a salicylate-induced increase in the permeability of the pulmonary vasculature. Salicylates inhibit vitamin K-dependent synthesis of coagulation factors (II, VII, IX and X), leading to a prolonged prothrombin time, and also inhibit prostaglandin-dependent platelet aggregation. Aspirin-induced hepatitis has been reported in cats following excessive exposure.

Treatment

Treatment of aspirin poisoning is the same as described for other NSAIAs earlier in this chapter.

Paracetamol (acetaminophen)

Theory refresher

Paracetamol (acetaminophen in the USA) is used extensively by people and is widely available over the counter. It is contained in a variety of preparations, either solely or in conjunction with other drugs, including aspirin and opioids. It is an antipyretic and analgesic agent. Paracetamol has been used therapeutically in dogs but should not be administered to cats.

> **CLINICAL TIP**
>
> - Excessive canine and feline exposure to paracetamol typically occurs either as a result of accidental ingestion (most common in dogs) or due to misguided 'therapeutic' administration by owners (most common in cats).

Toxic dose

A dosage of 100–200 mg/kg has been reported to cause clinical signs in dogs although higher dosages may be required and occasionally signs are seen with lower dosages. Cats are much more sensitive and signs of poisoning are generally seen at 50–100 mg/kg but may occur with dosages as low as 10 mg/kg.

Toxicokinetics

Paracetamol is rapidly and almost completely absorbed from the gastrointestinal tract and undergoes hepatic metabolism. In dogs, low doses of paracetamol are predominantly metabolized via capacity-limited glucuronidation and sulphation. This produces nontoxic metabolites that are excreted in bile and urine. However, any metabolism (oxidation) via the cytochrome P450 pathway produces N-acetyl-para-benzoquinoneimine (NAPQI) that is highly reactive and toxic.

NAPQI is usually conjugated with cellular glutathione to produce nontoxic metabolites that are excreted in urine. As the dosage of paracetamol increases, a greater proportion undergoes metabolism via the cytochrome P450 pathway (due to saturation of the glucuronidation and sulphation pathways), resulting in greater production of NAPQI. Glutathione stores, especially in the liver and red blood cells, are subsequently exhausted, resulting in higher concentrations of toxic unconjugated NAPQI. At higher doses paracetamol also inhibits glutathione synthesis, further compromising this metabolic pathway.

Cats are less able to metabolize paracetamol via glucuronidation (and sulphation) and the end result is greater metabolism via the cytochrome P450 pathway and an increased susceptibility to poisoning compared to dogs.

Mechanism of toxicity

Glutathione is important in protecting cells from oxidative injury and depletion of glutathione by conjugation with NAPQI makes cells susceptible to oxidative damage. In dogs, hepatocellular oxidative injury and necrosis are most common, with consequent liver failure possible.

In cats, red blood cells are most susceptible, with Heinz body formation, methaemoglobinaemia and haemolytic anaemia possible. Feline haemoglobin is more prone to oxidation than canine haemoglobin. As methaemoglobin is unable to transport oxygen, methaemoglobinaemia compromises oxygen-carrying capacity, causing tissue hypoxia and characteristic muddy brown mucous membranes. Glutathione, deficient in these cases, is also required to reduce methaemoglobin to haemoglobin.

Clinical signs

In dogs, clinical signs usually relate to hepatotoxicity and include vomiting, anorexia, abdominal pain and icterus. Methaemoglobinaemia may be seen with higher exposures, resulting in muddy/chocolate brown or cyanotic mucous membranes. It is unusual for methaemoglobinaemia to occur in dogs without subsequent signs of hepatotoxicity but this has been reported. Mucous membranes may also be pale due to anaemia secondary to intravascular haemolysis. Oedema of the face and/or paws may also be identified. Neurological signs may be present with severe liver dysfunction and hepatic encephalopathy and are also potentially associated with severe methaemoglobinaemia.

In cats, the most common clinical signs are muddy brown, cyanotic or pale mucous membranes, oedema of the face (especially mandibular region) and/or paws, and respiratory compromise; vomiting, depression, hypothermia and pruritus may also occur. Neurological signs may be present with severe methaemoglobinaemia and coma is associated with poor prognosis. Icterus may occur and at lower exposures is predominantly the result of red blood cell lysis. Clinically significant hepatotoxicity may be seen at higher exposures.

CLINICAL TIP

- Both hepatic and erythrocyte-associated poisoning syndromes have been reported in both dogs and cats. Clinical signs usually develop within 4–24 hr of exposure.

Antidote therapy

Paracetamol is one type of poisoning for which specific antidote therapy is available and treatment is recommended even if there is a significant delay in institution as a successful clinical outcome may still be obtained. N-acetylcysteine is rapidly hydrolysed to cysteine in vivo that is required for intracellular glutathione synthesis. N-acetylcysteine administration thus attempts to address cellular glutathione deficiency. Glutathione itself cannot be used therapeutically as it is not readily taken up by cells. N-acetylcysteine also acts directly on NAPQI, facilitating its excretion, and is oxidized to sulphur in the liver, increasing the capacity of the sulphation pathway.

If N-acetylcysteine is not available, or in severe cases of poisoning, additional sources of sulphur donors may be used. S-adenosylmethionine (SAMe) is one such product that may also have other additional beneficial effects (see Appendix 1 for protocol). The use of cimetidine has been recommended in paracetamol poisoning. This agent can inhibit cytochrome P450-mediated oxidation and may therefore reduce the formation of NAPQI. Given this mechanism of action, cimetidine would need to be given very early on to be effective and is considered an adjunctive therapy only.

Methaemoglobin reduction

In addition to the above therapy, treatment designed to reduce methaemoglobin to haemoglobin may be administered. Methylene blue has been employed here but is typically not readily available. However, ascorbic acid (vitamin C) may be used and oral preparations can usually be easily obtained. Poor compliance may preclude administration in cats. The author has administered ascorbic acid in drinking water to dogs that were not vomiting. Preparations of ascorbic acid for intravenous use are available and the treatment regimen is the same as for oral preparations (see Appendix 1).

Case example 4

PRESENTING SIGNS AND CASE HISTORY

A 3-year-old male neutered Beagle was presented as an emergency for suspected paracetamol poisoning. The owners had been out that evening and had returned to find the dog ataxic with evidence of probable ingestion of a large number of paracetamol tablets.

Major body system examination

On presentation the dog was ambulatory but depressed. Tachycardia (heart rate 130 beats per minute) and brown mucous membranes were identified but the rest of the examination was unremarkable.

Emergency database

An intravenous catheter was placed in a cephalic vein and blood obtained via the catheter for an emergency database that was found to be unremarkable.

Case management

Additional venepuncture was performed and the dog's blood was confirmed to be dark brown in colour, suggestive of methaemoglobinaemia (Figure 30.4). An in-house coagulation analyser was available and prothrombin time (PT) and activated partial thromboplastin time (APTT) were found to be within normal limits.

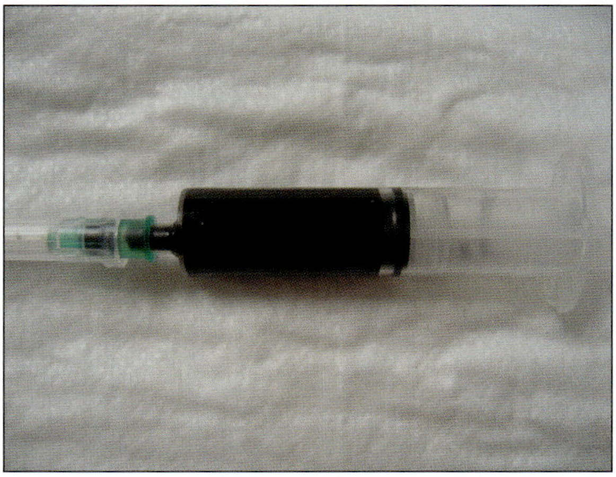

Figure 30.4 Dark brown blood from a dog with paracetamol intoxication.

CLINICAL TIP

- Methaemoglobinaemia is confirmed definitively by measurement using cooximetry. However, this is not widely available. Nevertheless, its presence can be inferred by putting a drop of the blood on filter paper; the filter paper stains brown and does not change colour. Alternatively, oxygen can be bubbled through a tube of the blood; if significant methaemoglobinaemia is present, oxyhaemoglobin does not form and the blood will not turn red.

Emesis was induced using apomorphine (0.02 mg/kg s.c.) and the vomitus contained a minimum of 30 paracetamol tablets (500 mg per tablet). The dog's body weight was 20 kg and an exposure of 750 mg/kg was therefore possible, although it was not clear exactly how many more tablets, if any, the dog had ingested. In addition, the degree of absorption prior to emesis could not be known.

CLINICAL TIP

The aims of treatment for paracetamol poisoning are:

- Minimize further paracetamol absorption
- Promote elimination of unmetabolized paracetamol
- Minimize NAPQI formation
- Supplement glutathione precursors to protect cells and encourage NAPQI elimination
- Provide oxygen supplementation
- Provide supportive therapy as required.

Initial therapy consisted of intravenous N-acetylcysteine (initial loading dose of 140 mg/kg i.v.; further five doses of 70 mg/kg i.v. q 6 hr) and oral ascorbic acid (vitamin C) (30 mg/kg p.o. in drinking water q 6 hr for five doses). Isotonic crystalloid intravenous fluid therapy was provided using compound sodium lactate at 4 ml/kg/hr and oxygen supplemented via an oxygen cage.

Twenty-four hours following presentation clotting tests were prolonged and moderate elevations in serum alanine aminotransferase (ALT) and bilirubin were detected. Mild anaemia was also identified (manual packed cell volume 30%, reference range 37–55%). A type-specific fresh whole blood transfusion (15 ml/kg over 4 hr) (see Ch. 40) was administered for the coagulopathy and anaemia, and additional therapy with S-adenosylmethionine (40 mg/kg p.o.) was commenced.

The dog continued to deteriorate, however, with evidence of haemolysis in the form of severe haemoglobinaemia and haemoglobinuria, with worsening anaemia despite blood transfusion, and with progressive severe dyspnoea. A haemoglobin-based oxygen-carrying solution (Oxyglobin®, Biopure Corporation; see Ch. 4) was administered (6 ml/kg i.v. over 1 hr) with no obvious clinical effect and the dog was euthanased approximately 36 hours after ingestion of the paracetamol tablets. A presumptive diagnosis of fulminant acute hepatic failure and severe haemolysis due to paracetamol poisoning was made.

CLINICAL TIP

- The prognosis in paracetamol poisoning depends on the dosage of paracetamol absorbed and the delay before institution of therapy. Aggressive early intervention is recommended.

Anticoagulant rodenticides

Anticoagulant rodenticides usually contain derivatives of either 4-hydroxycoumarin (e.g. brodifacoum, bromadiolone, difenacoum) or indane-1,3-dione (e.g. diphacinone, chlorophacinone). These preparations have a variable potency and duration of action that may be related to the generation type of the constituent compound. Second generation compounds are typically longer acting and have largely replaced older first generation ones. A variety of different commercial preparations are available.

CLINICAL TIP

- Anticoagulant rodenticide poisoning in dogs is usually primary (direct ingestion of rodenticide) but clinically significant secondary poisoning due to ingestion of poisoned rodents has also been reported. Cats are presented only rarely with rodenticide intoxication.

Toxic dose

Given the large number of anticoagulant rodenticide substances in use it is beyond the scope of this chapter to detail toxic doses for each individual substance and the reader is recommended to consult other texts or a veterinary poisons database.

Toxicokinetics

Anticoagulant rodenticides are generally absorbed slowly but substantially from the gastrointestinal tract. A long plasma half-life potentially of a number of days is typical, and the duration of action can be very prolonged – even up to several weeks in some cases. These compounds undergo slow metabolism by hepatic microsomal mixed-function oxidases to form inactive metabolites that are excreted in urine or bile.

Mechanism of toxicity

Vitamin K_1 hydroquinone is required for the conversion of inactive precursor coagulation factors to their active forms. During this conversion vitamin K_1 hydroquinone is oxidized to vitamin K_1 epoxide. Following absorption, anticoagulant rodenticides inhibit hepatic vitamin K_1 epoxide-reductase which is responsible for the conversion of vitamin K_1 epoxide back to vitamin K_1 hydroquinone. Anticoagulant rodenticides therefore impair vitamin K_1 'recycling' by the liver, leading to its depletion as existing stores are exhausted; they thereby prevent conversion of several inactive coagulation factors to their active forms. The vitamin K_1-dependent coagulation factors are factors II (prothrombin), VII, IX and X.

CLINICAL TIP

- Anticoagulant inhibition of vitamin K_1 epoxide-reductase is essentially competitive and reversible; therefore administration of exogenous vitamin K_1 acts therapeutically to reduce inhibition.

A delay in the onset of clinical signs following anticoagulant rodenticide ingestion is usually seen. This is due to the presence of circulating active vitamin K-dependent coagulation factors that must be exhausted for clinical signs to become apparent. Of the vitamin K-dependent factors, factor VII has the shortest plasma half-life. This factor is traditionally classified as part of the extrinsic coagulation pathway that is evaluated using the prothrombin time (PT). This explains the early clinical usefulness of measuring PT in cases of suspected anticoagulant rodenticide poisoning. Activated partial thromboplastin time (APTT) and activated clotting time

(ACT) are used to evaluate the intrinsic (includes factors II, IX and X) coagulation pathway and are expected to become prolonged subsequently also.

Clinical signs

Clinical signs usually develop from 3–5 days after exposure and may persist for more than 2 weeks without intervention. Clinical signs reflect bleeding tendency as described above and may be accompanied by a variety of nonspecific signs such as lethargy, depression and reduced appetite. Anticoagulant rodenticide poisoning may manifest with signs of respiratory distress, most commonly due to haemothorax but also secondary to pulmonary haemorrhage, and coughing (including haemoptysis) is reported. Bleeding into the peritoneal cavity and mediastinum is also reported. There may be evidence of external bleeding (e.g. nasal or gingival) and gastrointestinal haemorrhage may manifest as melaena, haematemesis and abdominal pain. Petechiae, ecchymoses and excessive bleeding at venepuncture sites may be identified. Bleeding in other sites will manifest with expected clinical signs (e.g. lameness secondary to bleeding into joints or neurological signs secondary to CNS haemorrhage).

In animals that have become anaemic secondary to blood loss, anticipated physical examination findings such as pale mucous membranes, tachycardia and hyperdynamic pulse quality will be present. If blood loss is considerable and rapid, evidence of hypoperfusion secondary to hypovolaemic shock may be identified.

Laboratory and other tests

In any animal presenting following suspected anticoagulant rodenticide ingestion a baseline minimum database should be established. This should include manual packed cell volume, plasma total solids, peripheral blood smear, and coagulation profile (in particular PT) taken before initiation of therapy (see below). PT is prolonged first in poisoned patients as factor VII becomes depleted earliest but prolongation of APTT and ACT usually also occurs before the onset of clinical signs.

A peripheral blood smear should be evaluated for platelet count and, where anaemia is identified, for evidence of regeneration. Mild to moderate thrombocytopenia is a common finding. Lack of a regenerative red blood cell response may represent preregenerative (as opposed to nonregenerative) anaemia (see Ch. 3). Blood typing may also be appropriate. Low serum total solids are expected in anaemia secondary to blood loss.

Thoracic and abdominal diagnostic imaging may identify major sites of haemorrhage, with the thoracic cavity being the most common site of bleeding. Thoracocentesis and abdominocentesis will likely reveal a nonclotting sanguineous effusion with packed cell volume similar to that of the patient's peripheral blood.

Treatment

Treatment of anticoagulant rodenticide poisoning is dependent largely on whether the patient is showing evidence of bleeding at the time of presentation. Routine GID, including the use of activated charcoal, is indicated in asymptomatic patients presenting within an appropriate timeframe. PT should be measured and no additional therapy is required if PT is within normal limits. Repeat testing of PT should be performed within 2–3 days. If a significant delay in obtaining the results of this test is unavoidable, it may be appropriate in individual cases to commence antidotal therapy with synthetic vitamin K_1 (phytomenadione) once blood sampling has been performed and to discontinue therapy if normal results are subsequently obtained. Guidelines for vitamin K_1 therapy in anticoagulant rodenticide intoxication are summarized in Box 30.8.

If vitamin K_1 therapy is commenced a significant period of time prior to sampling for testing of PT, subsequent results may be affected and a definitive diagnosis of coagulopathy secondary to rodenticide poisoning cannot be established. Subsequent vitamin K_1 therapy in these cases should then be managed as recommended for animals presenting with clinical signs of haemorrhage or with prolongation of PT.

CLINICAL TIP

- Animals with evidence of haemorrhage at presentation secondary to rodenticide ingestion will have PT prolongation. Nevertheless, it is essential to test PT at presentation, both to support the presumptive diagnosis and to allow monitoring of response to therapy.
- As with any severe coagulopathy, animals showing signs of haemorrhage secondary to suspected rodenticide poisoning should be handled gently, subjected to minimum stress and undergo exercise restriction. Venepuncture should only be performed using peripheral veins and with the smallest needle possible; adequate prolonged pressure should be applied to the site following sampling.

BOX 30.8 Guidelines for vitamin K_1 therapy in anticoagulant rodenticide intoxication

If symptomatic at presentation or prothrombin time (PT) prolonged (or significant delay anticipated in obtaining PT), administer vitamin K_1 2–5 mg/kg s.c. at multiple sites using the smallest possible needle. Preferably continue parenteral administration until PT normalizes, then change to oral administration at same daily dose, i.e. 2–5 mg/kg daily divided into two or three administrations.

Vitamin K_1 therapy should typically be continued for 2–6 weeks depending on the type of anticoagulant ingested (second generation compounds typically require a longer course of vitamin K_1 therapy). If the type of anticoagulant is unknown, a 2-week course of treatment is reasonable. After this time PT is rechecked and treatment discontinued as long as PT is normal. Prothrombin time is rechecked 2–3 days after stopping treatment:

- No further treatment is required if PT is normal.
- If PT is prolonged, vitamin K_1 therapy should be restarted and continued for a further 7 days before repeating the above process.
- Persistent PT prolongation or recurrence of spontaneous haemorrhage may suggest repeat exposure.

If asymptomatic at presentation and PT within normal limits, withhold treatment; recheck PT within 3 days.

Replacement of clotting factors may be performed in symptomatic patients by administering appropriate blood products. This is typically achieved through the use of fresh frozen plasma but fresh whole blood may be used to treat severe anaemia as well as coagulopathy in appropriate cases. Alternatively, a combination of fresh frozen plasma and packed red blood cells may be employed in these cases (see Ch. 40).

Prognosis

Prognosis is generally good with adequate and timely treatment but is partly dependent on site and severity of haemorrhage at the time of presentation.

Rodenticides containing vitamin D

Some rodenticide preparations contain calciferol (vitamin D_2) or cholecalciferol (vitamin D_3), either alone or together with anticoagulant agents. Calciferol/cholecalciferol is metabolized to calcitriol (1,25-dihydroxycholecalciferol) which induces hypercalcaemia via increased intestinal absorption, increased renal reabsorption and enhanced bone resorption. Hyperphosphataemia is also consistently present.

Clinical signs of hypercalcaemia are most commonly associated with the neurological, cardiovascular and gastrointestinal systems and with the kidneys. Depending on the preparation consumed, signs may be seen 8–48 hours post-ingestion. Treatment of hypercalcaemia involves: promoting calciuresis using intravenous 0.9% sodium chloride (normal saline) and furosemide; corticosteroid therapy to suppress bone resorption, reduce intestinal calcium absorption and promote calciuresis; possible additional use of salmon calcitonin; and, more recently, treatment with a bisphosphonate drug. Animals poisoned with anticoagulant rodenticides containing vitamin D may have severe morbidity.

Chocolate (theobromine)

Theobromine is a methylxanthine-derived alkaloid occurring naturally in cacao beans and found in chocolate, cocoa powder and other products produced from these beans. In addition, chocolate contains a lesser amount of caffeine, also a methylxanthine.

CLINICAL TIP

- The concentration of theobromine varies in different sources, with cocoa powder and plain (dark) chocolate generally containing significantly more than milk chocolate. The theobromine content of white chocolate is considerably lower. The literature contains reports of death in dogs following consumption of chocolate, cocoa powder, cacao bean shells and cocoa bean mulch.

Toxic dose

Fatal doses of theobromine are reported to be in the range of 90–250 mg/kg in dogs and 80–150 mg/kg in cats.

Toxicokinetics

Absorption of theobromine from the gastrointestinal tract is relatively slower in dogs compared to people, with complete absorption potentially taking up to 10 hours. Metabolism is primarily hepatic and enterohepatic circulation occurs. Excretion is considerably slower than in people.

Mechanism of toxicity

Methylxanthines inhibit cyclic nucleotide phosphodiesterases and also act as adenosine receptor antagonists. As with other methylxanthines, theobromine (and caffeine) causes CNS stimulation with consequent cardiac and respiratory effects. It directly stimulates the myocardium and skeletal muscle causing increased contractility and competitively inhibits cerebral benzodiazepine receptors. Theobromine also causes smooth muscle relaxation, especially of the bronchi, and renal diuresis.

Clinical signs

Clinical signs usually develop within 24 hours of ingestion and typically much sooner. Signs may persist for 48–72 hours in some cases. Commonly reported clinical signs include vomiting, abdominal discomfort, restlessness, excitability and hyperactivity, ataxia, tachycardia, and tachypnoea or panting. In more severe cases muscle rigidity, muscle tremors, hyperthermia, seizures and dysrhythmias have been reported. Urinary incontinence, polyuria and polydipsia may also occur. Severe seizures and/or cardiovascular compromise are typically reported in fatal cases.

Laboratory and other tests

An emergency database including electrocardiogram is recommended.

Treatment

Routine GID is indicated in appropriate cases. As theobromine is absorbed slowly in dogs, induction of emesis may be appropriate even after a significant delay; however, it may be best avoided in animals that are very hyperactive. Theobromine undergoes enterohepatic circulation so repeated use of charcoal may enhance elimination. There is no specific antidote for theobromine poisoning and therapy is otherwise symptomatic. This may include intravenous fluid therapy, antiemetic administration, sedation if excitability is excessive, and routine treatment of seizures. Antidysrhythmic therapy may also be indicated in some cases.

Prognosis

Prognosis is generally good with appropriate treatment but may be worse for animals showing marked cardiovascular or neurological signs at presentation.

Xylitol

Xylitol is a naturally occurring sugar alcohol found in low concentrations in a variety of fruits and vegetables. It is extracted commercially and used as a sweetener, being popular for use for example by diabetics and in low-carbohydrate diets. The use of xylitol has also been increasing due to its effects in reducing the formation of dental caries (anticariogenic effect) that has led to its inclusion in a number of products including chewing gum, sweets, toothpaste and other oral care products. Xylitol is also found in proprietary baked goods and is commercially available as a powder for baking. Manufacturers are not obliged to specify the xylitol content of products in all cases and sometimes only the total sugar alcohol content (including e.g. sorbitol, isomalt) is listed.

CLINICAL TIP

- Xylitol poisoning has been reported in dogs but no information is available at the time of writing regarding cats. Despite increasing awareness about xylitol intoxication in dogs, and uncertainty regarding the mechanism of toxicity, this substance is found in some well-known proprietary canine oral hygiene products.

Toxic dose

Hypoglycaemia has been reported to occur in dogs at dosages greater than 0.15 g/kg and a dosage of 0.5 g/kg has been associated with hepatic failure. However, it remains unclear whether the hepatotoxic effect of xylitol is dose-related or idiosyncratic, and the possibility of hepatic injury at doses less than 0.5 g/kg cannot therefore be excluded.

Toxicokinetics

Xylitol is a normal intermediate product in the glucuronic acid cycle but excessive exposure occurs through ingestion. Subsequent absorption varies between species but is rapid and almost complete in dogs. Slow release from ingested foodstuffs may delay absorption and explain the potentially sustained hypoglycaemia seen in dogs.

Metabolism is predominantly hepatic and occurs rapidly. Virtually no ur nary excretion occurs.

Mechanism of toxicity

In dogs xylito acts as a potent and dose-dependent stimulator of pancreatic insulin release (this effect is negligible or only mild in people). It also causes hepatic injury and probable acute hepatic necrosis by a currently unknown mechanism. Hypoglycaemia may occur as a result of the insulin release and may be both severe and sustained. Hypokalaemia may also result from insulin release. Clinically significant coagulopathy is one potential consequence of hepatic injury and consequent dysfunction. Hepatic failure may also contribute to hypoglycaemia and is thought to be responsible for this finding in dogs that do not show earlier evidence of hypoglycaemia attributable to insulin release.

Clinical signs

Clinical signs associated with hypoglycaemia often develop within an hour of exposure but may be delayed. Signs include lethargy, weakness, vomiting, ataxia, altered mentation from depression through to coma, and seizures. Signs associated with liver failure are more delayed in onset (up to 72 hours after exposure) and may occur with or without earlier signs of hypoglycaemia. Coagulopathy may manifest as petechiae/ecchymoses, haemorrhagic faeces, and excessive bleeding from venepuncture sites.

Laboratory tests

Blood glucose should be evaluated as part of the emergency database and may be normal or mildly to severely reduced. Occasionally dogs will present with hyperglycaemia that then progresses to hypoglycaemia. Regular monitoring is recommended even in dogs that are normoglycaemic at presentation. Electrolyte screening may reveal hypokalaemia that is usually mild or perhaps moderate.

If hepatic injury has occurred, a serum biochemistry profile may reveal a marked increase in serum alanine transaminase (ALT) activity, a mild to moderate increase in serum alkaline phosphatase (ALP) activity, and hyperbilirubinaemia. Prolongation of PT and APTT may be detected in coagulopathic animals, and mild to moderate thrombocytopenia is commonly reported. Regular monitoring of these parameters is recommended for 3–4 days following exposure to a toxic dosage, including in dogs that are normoglycaemic at presentation.

Treatment

CLINICAL TIP

- Given the potential for fatal acute hepatic failure following xylitol ingestion in dogs, the author recommends treating all cases.

Routine GID is indicated in appropriate cases. Emesis should not be induced in dogs with marked neurological compromise secondary to hypoglycaemia. Activated charcoal should be administered empirically but may have limited benefit due to low binding of xylitol (demonstrated in an in vitro study).

Hypoglycaemia is treated using standard parenteral and possibly oral glucose supplementation therapy that may need to be both aggressive and prolonged. Regular small meals and possible oral sugar supplementation may be sensible in asymptomatic dogs. Coagulopathy secondary to hepatic dysfunction may necessitate fresh frozen plasma (FFP) administration (see Ch. 40) and vitamin K_1 should be administered. As with any severe coagulopathy, animals should be handled gently, subjected to minimum stress and undergo exercise restriction. Venepuncture should only be performed using peripheral veins and with the smallest needle possible; adequate prolonged pressure should be applied to the site following sampling.

Empirical use of antioxidant hepatoprotectants such as SAMe, N-acetylcysteine and silymarin is reasonable. In cases of severe hepatic failure, treatment for possible hepatic encephalopathy may need to be instituted. Therapy is otherwise supportive and symptomatic.

Prognosis

The prognosis associated with hypoglycaemia alone from xylitol poisoning is good with timely and appropriate management. The prognosis for animals with evidence of hepatic dysfunction is guarded to poor, and grave for acute hepatic failure. Survival from xylitol poisoning may not be correlated with exposure dosage.

31 Cardiovascular emergencies

ACUTE DECOMPENSATED HEART FAILURE

Progressive heart disease results in failure of the heart to pump adequately and this may manifest as low-output heart failure, where sufficient blood is not pumped into the aorta or pulmonary artery, or congestive heart failure (CHF). In CHF, there is inadequate emptying of blood from the venous system: left-sided CHF results in congestion of the pulmonary circulation with pulmonary oedema; right-sided CHF causes congestion of the systemic circulation with ascites and pleural effusion. Bilateral heart failure presents with a combination of both types of signs.

Failure of the heart to pump adequately may result from systolic dysfunction, i.e. the heart is physically unable to eject enough blood, or from diastolic dysfunction, i.e. the ventricles are unable to fill properly. Both mechanisms are often involved and the end result is reduced cardiac output and a lowering of arterial blood pressure. Systolic dysfunction may result from failure of the myocardium itself (e.g. dilated cardiomyopathy), from an increase in ventricular pressure (pressure overload; e.g. pulmonic stenosis, subaortic stenosis) or from volume overload (e.g. atrioventricular valve disease). Diastolic dysfunction (impaired ventricular filling) may result, for example, from ventricular hypertrophy, dilated cardiomyopathy, atrioventricular valve stenosis or pericardial effusion (cardiac tamponade).

Compensatory mechanisms during heart disease include mechanisms relating to the heart itself, such as tachycardia, increased inotropy (force of contraction) and myocardial hypertrophy, and peripheral compensation involving vasoconstriction and sodium and water retention. In time these compensatory mechanisms become detrimental.

Treatment

Although signalment and history may help to some small degree, emergency treatment of animals with acute decompensated heart failure often needs to be performed without a definitive diagnosis of the nature of the underlying heart disease. Management of such cases may involve:

- Oxygen supplementation in all cases (see Ch. 6); minimum stress and intervention
- Reduction of pulmonary venous pressure (hence left ventricular preload), typically through the use of furosemide to promote diuresis and natriuresis
- Glyceryl trinitrate (2% topical preparation): primarily a systemic venodilator reducing preload and potentially therefore alleviating pulmonary oedema
- Anxiolysis and sedation using an opioid, preferably morphine (also causes vasodilation)
- Enhancing systolic function (positive inotropy) using pimobendan
- Emergency treatment of severe dysrhythmias (see Ch. 12), although the emphasis is very much on treatment for congestion in the first instance.

The use of additional agents such as sodium nitroprusside or dobutamine may be indicated in some cases but is likely to be restricted to referral institutions.

Canine chronic mitral valve insufficiency

Theory refresher

Chronic mitral valve insufficiency is usually the result of progressive valvular myxomatous degeneration and has a high prevalence in older dogs, especially of small to medium size. The most commonly affected breeds include the Cavalier King Charles spaniel, terrier breeds and poodles. The disease usually progresses over a period of years and is the most common cause of CHF in dogs.

In the long term, mitral regurgitation results in tachycardia, myocardial hypertrophy and reduced myocardial contractility; left atrial size and pressure increase, and pulmonary venous congestion and oedema may occur.

Coughing may be the result of left main stem bronchus compression by the enlarged left atrium and/or pulmonary oedema.

Acute severe decompensated heart failure may occur in dogs with mitral valve insufficiency due to:

- Chorda tendinae rupture
- Onset of atrial fibrillation
- Inadequate therapy of existing heart failure
- Overexertion.

Case example 1

PRESENTING SIGNS AND CASE HISTORY

An 11-year-old male neutered Norfolk terrier presented following an episode of collapse and onset of severe respiratory distress. The dog had had a number of similar episodes in the 2 weeks prior to emergency presentation but none had been as severe as the most recent one. He had a history of chronic mitral valve insufficiency and CHF for which he was receiving furosemide, pimobendan and benazepril. The owner reported a variable appetite recently and admitted that she had not managed to administer all of the dog's medications as directed. No other significant preceding history was reported.

Major body system examination

On presentation the dog was alert but clearly in respiratory distress. Flow-by oxygen supplementation was commenced while a major body system examination was performed. Cardiovascular examination revealed a heart rate of 160 beats per minute with a grade VI/VI left apical systolic murmur that had wide radiation. Femoral and dorsal pedal pulses were very weak but pulse deficits were not detected. The jugular veins did not appear distended. Mucous membranes were hyperaemic with a fast capillary refill time.

Respiratory rate was 60 breaths per minute and there was a notable increase in effort. Lung sounds were diffusely harsh bilaterally and focal patches of crackles were audible. The dog's abdomen was distended with a fluid thrill and rectal temperature was within normal limits. Blood pressure via Doppler sphygmomanometry was within normal limits at 130 mmHg.

Assessment The dog's cardiovascular examination revealed tachycardia and marked hypoperfusion as well as a maximal grade heart murmur. Putting this together with the respiratory findings and the dog's history, a diagnosis of decompensated CHF was most likely. The possible pulmonary oedema suggested left-sided heart failure, and the fluid thrill may have suggested a degree of right-sided failure as well.

Emergency database

As the dog remained tolerant and compliant with the flow-by oxygen supplementation, an intravenous catheter was placed in a cephalic vein and blood obtained via the catheter for an emergency database. This revealed mild hyponatraemia (137.0 mmol/l, reference range 140.0–153.0 mmol/l) and a mild increase in blood urea nitrogen (13.0 mmol/l, reference range 3.0–10.0 mmol/l) but was otherwise unremarkable.

Case management

Glyceryl trinitrate 2% paste (18 mm) was applied to the inner aspect of the dog's right pinna and he was then placed into an oxygen cage with continuous electrocardiographic monitoring; this showed the dog to be in sinus tachycardia. Furosemide (4 mg/kg i.v.) and morphine (0.1 mg/kg slow i.v.) were administered via an extension line exiting the oxygen cage. Ad lib water was provided.

CLINICAL TIP

- Glyceryl trinitrate paste can be absorbed through human skin and it is therefore important to take certain precautions. These include wearing gloves to apply the paste, and making sure that there are signs on the kennel and kennel sheet alerting personnel that paste has been applied to the patient. The site used must also be clearly identified; the paste is typically applied to clipped or hairless skin, such as the inner aspect of the pinna, and the site used is rotated between applications.

One hour later the dog's respiration had improved to some extent and he had also urinated. As he was compliant, thoracic radiographs were performed with flow-by oxygen supplementation throughout (Figure 31.1). These findings were consistent with the suspected

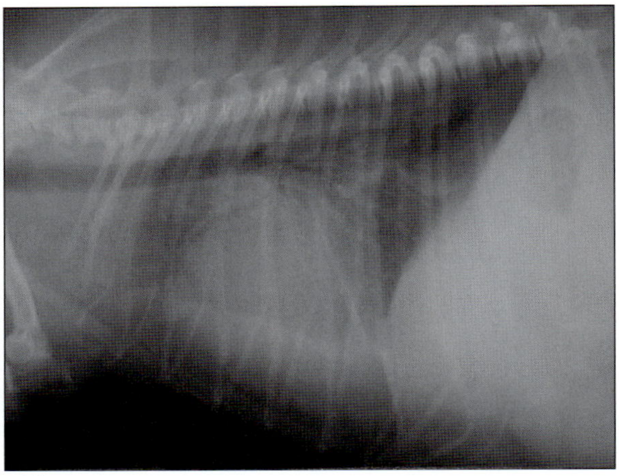

(a)

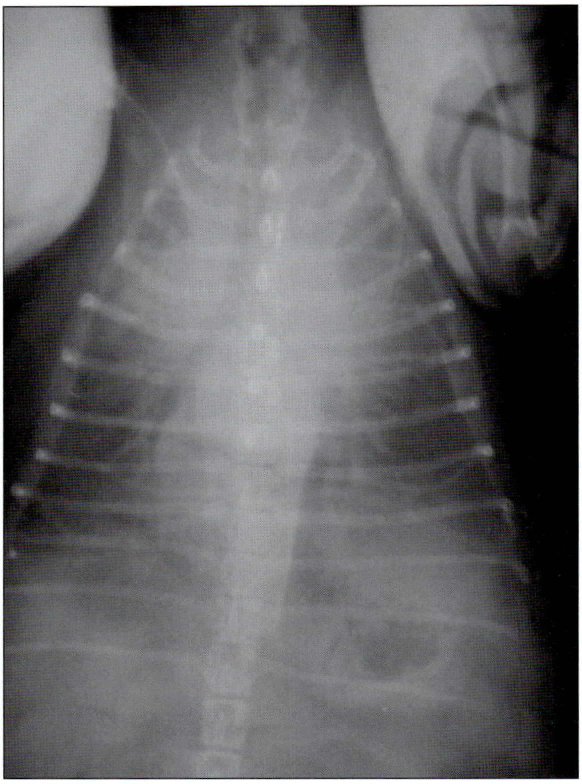

(b)

Figure 31.1 (a) Right lateral and (b) dorsoventral thoracic radiographs of a dog with end-stage mitral valve disease showing cardiomegaly with left atrial enlargement and dorsal displacement of the caudal part of the trachea, an alveolar lung pattern affecting mainly the cranial lung lobes with air bronchograms, mild bilateral pleural effusion and hepatomegaly.

diagnosis of decompensated left-sided CHF secondary to probable mitral valve insufficiency but there was also evidence of right-sided heart failure.

CLINICAL TIP

- Right-sided heart failure is relatively common in dogs with chronic mitral valve insufficiency. This is presumed to be due to concurrent tricuspid valve insufficiency as a result of myxomatous degeneration and/or pulmonary hypertension due to persistently elevated left atrial and pulmonary venous pressures.

The dog was returned to the oxygen cage and continued to be treated with intermittent intravenous boluses of furosemide (2–6 mg/kg q 1–2 hr, prn) and morphine (0.1 mg/kg slow i.v. q 6 hr). Glyceryl trinitrate paste (18 mm q 8 hr) was also applied and the dog was continued on oral pimobendan and benazepril.

Although the dog showed some early improvement, his clinical condition deteriorated again. The owners were offered the option of an emergency referral to a hospital with a cardiologist and facilities to offer more intensive management but decided instead to have the dog euthanased which was therefore done in their presence as soon as possible.

Canine tricuspid valve insufficiency

Tricuspid valve insufficiency is often an incidental finding in dogs and cats. Clinically significant tricuspid valve insufficiency may be seen with:

- Chronic mitral valve insufficiency
- Biventricular or right-sided dilated cardiomyopathy
- Bacterial endocarditis
- Chorda tendinae rupture
- Right ventricular dilation due to increased right ventricular pressure – e.g. secondary to pulmonary hypertension or pulmonary thromboembolism (PTE).

Right atrial enlargement may result in supraventricular tachydysrhythmias, and increased right atrial pressure may result in ascites, pleural effusion, pericardial effusion, hepatomegaly and splenomegaly. From an emergency perspective, animals with tricuspid valve insufficiency are more likely to require treatment for a concurrent disorder than for primary right-sided heart failure.

Canine dilated cardiomyopathy

Theory refresher

Dilated cardiomyopathy (DCM) is a primary myocardial disease characterized by enlargement of the heart, reduced systolic function and possible impaired diastolic function. The disease is seen most commonly in adult large and medium size dogs, with some breeds being over represented (e.g. the Great Dane, the Doberman Pinscher, the Irish Wolfhound, the Cocker Spaniel). There is significant variation between breeds with respect to both historical and clinical findings, and rate of disease progression.

DCM is definitively diagnosed by echocardiography that shows left (and perhaps bilateral) atrial and ventricular enlargement, and evidence of reduced left ventricular systolic function. Mitral regurgitation may be identified in association with the dilated left ventricle.

Case example 2

PRESENTING SIGNS AND CASE HISTORY

A 6-year-old male neutered Great Dane presented with a 10-day history of inappetence and retching that was worse when the dog was lying down. There had been some noticeable exercise intolerance on daily walks and the owner had noticed that the dog had a very fast heart rate prompting emergency presentation. The dog had had surgical treatment of gastric dilatation/volvulus syndrome 2 years previously but no other significant history was reported.

Major body system examination

On presentation the dog was ambulatory but quiet. Cardiovascular examination revealed an irregularly irregular heart rhythm with a left apical grade II/VI systolic heart murmur. Femoral pulses were weak and there were marked pulse deficits: heart rate 240 beats per minute, pulse rate 114 per minute. Mucous membranes were hyperaemic with a fast capillary refill time.

The dog was panting but it was decided not to stop this in order to auscultate the lung fields at initial presentation. Abdominal palpation was unremarkable but there was a mild increase in rectal temperature (39.5°C). Blood pressure via Doppler sphygmomanometry was within normal limits at 160 mmHg.

Assessment The dog's cardiovascular examination was highly suggestive of atrial fibrillation and the history of inappetence and exercise intolerance most likely suggested a degree of CHF. Given the dog's breed, there was a high index of suspicion for DCM. The mild increase in rectal temperature was suspected to represent hyperthermia rather than pyrexia.

Emergency database

An intravenous catheter was placed in a cephalic vein and blood obtained via the catheter for an emergency database. This was essentially unremarkable. Electrocardiography confirmed the presence of atrial fibrillation (see Ch. 12) with a ventricular response rate of approximately 220 beats per minute.

Case management

The dog was suitably compliant (a gentle giant!) so thoracic radiographs were taken to look for evidence of CHF and evaluate the size of the cardiac silhouette (Figure 31.2). The dog was subsequently started on furosemide (2 mg/kg p.o. q 12 hr) and digoxin (0.1 mg/m^2 p.o. q 12 hr) and referral arranged to a cardiologist for echocardiography and implementation of further management. This confirmed the suspicion of DCM with left atrial enlargement and pimobendan (0.125 mg/kg p.o. q 12 hr, 1 hour before feeding) and benazepril (0.25 mg/kg p.o. q 24 hr) were dispensed. The dog's ventricular response rate had reduced to 160 beats per minute when he was seen at the referral centre (5 days after digoxin was commenced) and additional antidysrhythmic therapy was not therefore indicated.

CLINICAL TIP

- Most dogs with atrial fibrillation have severe heart disease involving left atrial enlargement, and are in CHF of variable severity. Unless the dysrhythmia is very severe, the emphasis in these cases is very much on treating the CHF with furosemide and digoxin. Additional antidysrhythmic therapy is only indicated if treatment of congestion fails to reduce the ventricular response rate satisfactorily (conversion to sinus rhythm is very difficult and not necessarily of benefit).

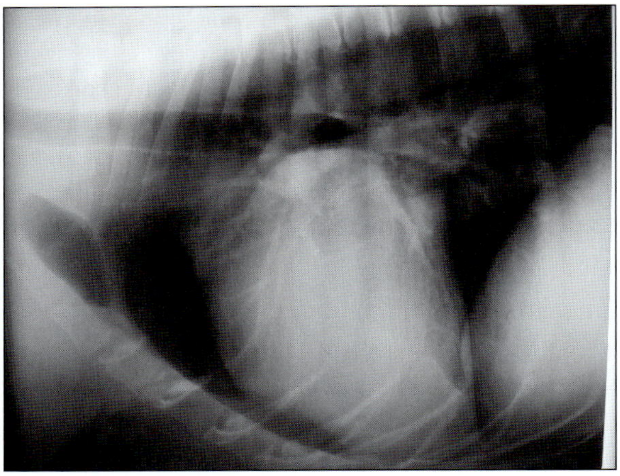
(a)

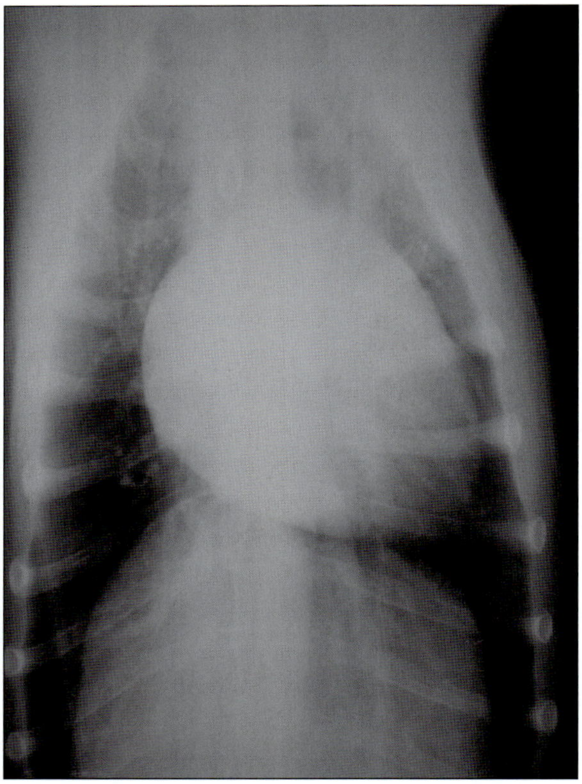
(b)

Figure 31.2 (a) Right lateral and (b) dorsoventral thoracic radiographs of a dog with dilated cardiomyopathy and mild pulmonary oedema. Peribronchial infiltrates are present throughout the lung, with patchy alveolar infiltrate in the caudoventral lung field.

Feline cardiomyopathies

Cardiomyopathy (i.e. primary disease of the myocardium rather than valvular disease) is the main form of heart disease in cats and is classified as follows:

- Hypertrophic cardiomyopathy (HCM)
- Dilated cardiomyopathy (DCM)
- Restrictive cardiomyopathy
- Unclassified cardiomyopathy
- Arrhythmogenic right ventricular cardiomyopathy (ARVC).

HCM is the most commonly diagnosed feline heart disease and is inherited in some breeds (e.g. the Maine coon). The disease is associated with ventricular thickening and in some cats systolic anterior motion of the mitral valve is identified on echocardiography (so-called hypertrophic obstructive cardiomyopathy). Systemic thromboembolism is a potential and very serious consequence of HCM in cats (see below).

CLINICAL TIP

- Heart failure (or sudden death) may be triggered in a cat with subclinical HCM by significant stress, general anaesthesia, or surgical intervention.
- In addition, ketamine increases sympathetic tone and may precipitate heart failure in such cats.

Feline DCM may be caused by taurine deficiency (predominantly nutritional but there may be genetic involvement) but idiopathic feline DCM is now the most common form. Severe myocardial failure may exist for a prolonged period before signs of heart failure are seen.

Congestive heart failure in cats

Due to the difference in lifestyles between the species, cats are more likely than dogs to present for veterinary attention only when they are in severe heart failure; cats are not usually exercised directly by owners and often have a more sedentary existence, therefore clinical abnormalities may be hidden for some time. It is nevertheless important to remember that the underlying cardiomyopathy will most likely have been chronically

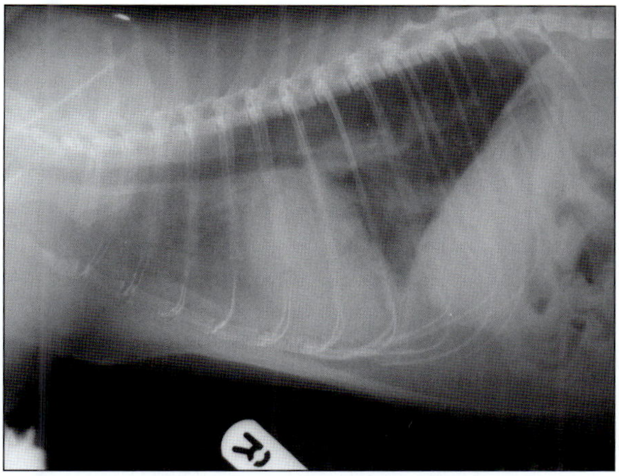

Figure 31.3 Right lateral thoracic radiographs of a cat with congestive heart failure; cardiomegaly and pulmonary oedema are present.

progressive and that subtle signs of heart failure may have been present for some time.

Pleural effusion is common in cats with CHF but this is rarely due to right-sided failure alone and the exact mechanism remains unclear. The nature of the pleural effusion may vary (modified transudate, pseudochylous, chylous) and heart failure is the most common cause of chylothorax in cats. Most cats have bilateral or left-sided disease and pulmonary oedema is usually present, even if it is harder to detect due to the pleural effusion (Figure 31.3).

In the nonreferral setting, treatment of acute decompensated CHF in cats is similar to that in dogs, namely oxygen supplementation, furosemide, glyceryl trinitrate and possibly morphine. Thoracocentesis is often required and a diagnostic procedure based on a sufficient index of suspicion is preferable to subjecting the cat to the stress of radiography; ultrasonography is a much less stressful way to identify pleural effusion, especially if a mobile machine is available (see Ch. 32).

CLINICAL TIP

- Cats with acute decompensated CHF are invariably even more susceptible to stress than their canine counterparts. Minimal stress and intervention and gentle handling are essential.

CLINICAL TIP

- Animals with acute CHF are frequently anorexic initially and may also not drink. These animals may be dehydrated, and potentially hypokalaemic, at the time of presentation and are at risk of further exacerbation as a result of aggressive diuretic therapy.
- While dogs often start to drink and perhaps eat as their clinical condition improves, in the author's experience it is very common for cats to remain anorexic. A balance is then required between the desire to withhold fluid therapy due to CHF and the morbidity and risks associated with worsening dehydration and electrolyte abnormalities, especially hypokalaemia. In such cases conservative use of fluid therapy may be required – e.g. 0.45% sodium chloride (half-strength, not 0.18% sodium chloride) given intravenously at 0.5 ml/kg/hr with potassium chloride supplementation, or daily subcutaneous administration (10 ml/kg).

FELINE AORTIC THROMBOEMBOLISM (SADDLE THROMBOEMBOLISM)

Theory refresher

The majority of cats with aortic thromboembolism (ATE) have cardiomyopathy, often HCM, which most commonly includes left atrial enlargement. Spontaneous echo contrast may be seen in the left atrium suggesting an increased risk of thromboembolism. Feline ATE may also occur with other forms of heart disease as well as in association with hyperthyroidism (potentially independently of the cardiac effects of this disorder) and neoplasia. ATE is more common in male cats, predominantly due to their greater predisposition to HCM.

Thrombi usually form in the left atrium, become dislodged, and then cause occlusion at a distal systemic site. Thrombi may also form in the other cardiac chambers. Clinical signs associated with systemic thromboembolism in general depend on:

- The site at which the embolus lodges
- Whether complete or only partial obstruction occurs
- The duration of obstruction
- The extent and diameter of any collateral circulation.

CLINICAL TIP

- In the majority of cases the thromboembolus lodges at the aortic trifurcation, i.e. where the terminal abdominal aorta divides into the external iliac arteries supplying the pelvic limbs and the source of the main arterial supply to the tail. In some cases a smaller clot may instead cause occlusion of one external iliac artery with less severe unilateral clinical signs. Thromboembolism of a brachial artery and consequent thoracic limb signs may occur and visceral and cerebral arterial thromboembolism have also been reported.

Treatment

CLINICAL TIP

- In the author's opinion, thrombolytic agents available at the time of writing should not be used for feline ATE. If they are used, this should only be done where facilities for intensive monitoring and aggressive intervention are available, and owners must be adequately counselled regarding the associated risks and high financial costs.

Thrombolysis

Definitive therapy of ATE has been attempted using exogenous thrombolytic agents (e.g. tissue-plasminogen activator (t-PA), streptokinase). However, no consistently successful results have been reported and complications include excessive haemorrhage, reperfusion syndrome with severe hyperkalaemia and metabolic acidosis, and sudden death. Mortality rates associated with treatment are high and in the author's opinion currently available thrombolytic agents should not be used. Mortality and complication rates are also high for balloon embolectomy, rheolytic thrombectomy and surgical thrombus removal. In all cases recurrent thrombosis may occur.

Anticoagulation

Although there is no evidence for a beneficial effect in feline ATE, aspirin (acetylsalicylic acid), unfractionated heparin, and more recently low molecular weight (fractionated) heparins (e.g. dalteparin) are agents commonly employed to try to prevent further thrombus formation. Other agents such as clopidogrel have also been used.

Vasodilation

Vasodilatory agents are also often employed in the acute stages in an attempt to improve perfusion to the affected limbs. Acepromazine is commonly chosen and may also help to reduce anxiety by providing sedation. Given the potential for this agent to cause hypotension, careful rational dosing is mandatory.

Heart disease and failure

Medical therapy for heart disease, including appropriate treatment of heart failure, should be provided as indicated (see above). Initial stabilization in cats suffering from acute decompensated CHF must take priority over therapy for aortic thromboembolism.

NURSING ASPECT

Cats with ATE require intensive nursing and suitable husbandry. Bedding should be clean, dry and well padded. Physiotherapy of the pelvic limbs is essential to minimize the effects of disuse. These cats may also be anorexic and placement of a nasooesophageal feeding tube may be required. Placement of other types of feeding tube will necessitate general anaesthesia which is undesirable in cats with heart disease. As the majority of cats with ATE have heart disease, minimum stress is important. That said, these cats may also be anxious and distressed by virtue of their predicament and regular fuss and attention are likely to prove beneficial.

Prognosis

In some cats limb sensation and function return rapidly (within several hours to a few days) following ATE due to intrinsic thrombolysis. Other cases may regain complete or partial limb sensation and motor function in time (often weeks to months) with adequate care. Finally, in a few cats, changes are irreversible, and cutaneous and muscular ischaemic necrosis develops. This variability in progression makes reliable prognostication with respect to pelvic limb compromise difficult in individual cases. Partial obstruction is likely to have a better prognosis than complete obstruction.

The high likelihood of underlying cardiomyopathy, the need for on-going medical therapy, and the possibility of recurrent ATE must be borne in mind. Nevertheless, a proportion of cats go on to enjoy an acceptable quality of life for several months (and occasionally longer) following an initial episode of ATE.

Case example 3

PRESENTING SIGNS AND CASE HISTORY

A 13-year-old male neutered domestic short hair cat presented for acute onset bilateral pelvic limb paralysis. The cat was an indoor cat and had seemed normal when last seen by the owner several hours earlier. The owner's attention had been drawn by the cat's vocalization and the cat had subsequently been found recumbent next to the chair in which he had been sleeping. The cat was distressed and was thought to have fallen off the chair.

CLINICAL TIP

- Although most cats that suffer ATE have heart disease, in a significant proportion there is no consistent preceding history. Adult cats of all ages may be affected. Especially in cats with outdoor access, ATE may be mistaken by owners for traumatic injury.

Major body system examination

Major body system examination revealed the cat to be vocalizing and distressed. Heart rate was elevated at 260 beats per min and a gallop sound was audible; a murmur could not be detected. Mucous membranes were pale pink with normal capillary refill time. The cat was tachypnoeic (respiratory rate 40 breaths per min) but lung field auscultation was appropriate for the rate and effort. Rectal temperature was reduced at 37.0°C. Abdominal palpation was unremarkable.

Femoral pulse was absent in both pelvic limbs and both paws were cold with pale digital pads. The quicks appeared purple in colour. Bilateral paralysis was present and the muscles of the right pelvic limb were swollen and severely painful on palpation. Pain sensation was absent from the left pelvic limb. An ultrasonic Doppler device for measuring blood pressure failed to detect blood flow in either pelvic limb and no active bleeding was detected when a nail in the left pelvic limb was cut back to its quick.

CLINICAL TIP

- Obstruction of blood flow to the pelvic limbs is likely to cause ischaemic injury to both the skeletal muscles and peripheral nerves. Ischaemic myopathy is typically very painful but the pain should alleviate as limb sensation is lost.
- A diagnosis of ATE is usually made on the basis of consistent clinical signs. In some cases, however, primary neurological disease can be mistaken for ATE; cutting through the quick in limbs without pain sensation and using an ultrasonic Doppler device help to increase the certainty of the diagnosis.

Case management

An intravenous catheter was placed immediately in a cephalic vein and analgesia provided (methadone 0.5 mg/kg i.v.) to alleviate the cat's pain while the examination findings, presumptive diagnosis and prognosis were discussed with the owner. The owner was very distressed, especially given the peracute clinical deterioration without any premonitory signs, but eventually opted for euthanasia to be performed without further intervention.

CLINICAL TIP

- Analgesia is paramount in cats presenting with pain and a pure opioid (e.g. morphine, methadone) is most appropriate initially. At recommended dose rates these agents have minimal cardiorespiratory effects. Buprenorphine may be a reasonable alternative in cats but its longer onset of action must be borne in mind in animals that present in severe pain.
- In the author's opinion analgesia should not be withheld while the presumptive diagnosis is discussed with the owner; immediate alleviation of suffering must be paramount regardless of whether euthanasia is subsequently performed.

CANINE PERICARDIAL EFFUSION

Theory refresher

Pericardial effusion is an abnormal accumulation of fluid in the pericardial sac. The haemodynamic consequences of this fluid accumulation depend on the rate of accumulation, the volume of fluid and the compliance of the pericardium. Fluid accumulation results in an increase in intrapericardial pressure that compromises ventricular filling. The right side of the heart is typically affected more than the left initially as the myocardium is thinner and intraventricular pressure is lower on the right side. The most severe clinical manifestation of this cardiac tamponade is cardiogenic shock characterized by low cardiac output failure and systemic hypotension. With more chronic effusion, signs of right-sided CHF usually predominate.

Causes

The two most common causes of canine pericardial effusion are neoplasia and idiopathic pericarditis. Intrapericardial tumours include haemangiosarcoma and heart base tumours. Echocardiographic findings may be highly suggestive of tumour type but histopathology is needed for definitive diagnosis; this is not realistic antemortem.

Haemangiosarcoma is the most commonly diagnosed canine cardiac tumour and arises most often from the wall of the right atrium or auricle. It is the most common cause of canine pericardial effusion and is assumed to have metastasized in virtually all cases at the time of diagnosis; prognosis is very poor. Surgical resection and adjuvant chemotherapy are offered by some referral centres.

The most common heart base tumours in dogs are aortic body tumours (chemodectomas). Mesothelioma is a diffuse neoplasm affecting serosal surfaces including the serous pericardium and does not cause obvious pericardial thickening on echocardiography. Pericardial fluid cytology is unable to differentiate effusion secondary to idiopathic pericarditis from effusion secondary to mesothelioma, and pericardial histopathology may also not be able to differentiate the two causes. Mesothelioma should therefore always be considered a differential diagnosis for presumed idiopathic pericardial effusion. Although pericardial fluid analysis is of limited benefit in most cases, cardiac lymphoma may be diagnosed in this way and is potentially responsive to chemotherapy.

Other causes of pericardial effusion include coagulation disorders, CHF, trauma, infectious causes and uraemia, although clinically significant effects with respect to tamponade are unlikely in these cases. Pericardial effusion and cardiac tamponade secondary to anticoagulant rodenticide toxicity have been reported in a dog and, if facilities allow, evaluation of coagulation is recommended prior to pericardiocentesis.

Constrictive and effusive-constrictive pericarditis

In some dogs historical and clinical findings are consistent with tamponade secondary to pericardial effusion but little or no effusion is subsequently identified. A diagnosis of constrictive or effusive–constrictive pericarditis due to fibrosis should be considered in such cases.

Left atrial rupture

Left atrial rupture and consequent haemopericardium are uncommon but may occur in dogs with chronic mitral valve disease. Associated clinical signs include collapse as well as coughing and dyspnoea, and physical examination findings include a heart murmur, poor peripheral pulses and muffled heart sounds. Dogs that suffer left atrial rupture are typically much smaller than those that present with pericardial effusion of other aetiologies and the presence of an audible heart murmur is another distinguishing feature.

Only partial drainage of the pericardial effusion is recommended as thorough drainage may exacerbate bleeding. Regardless of intervention, the prognosis is very poor with this condition.

Case example 4

PRESENTING SIGNS AND CASE HISTORY

A 4-year-old male neutered Saint Bernard dog presented with a 2-week history of lethargy, exercise intolerance, variable appetite and progressive abdominal distension.

CLINICAL TIP

- Pericardial effusion is seen most commonly in older large-breed dogs and especially in golden retrievers.
- In addition to the clinical signs in this case, weakness, episodic collapse, polydipsia, gastrointestinal signs, coughing and dyspnoea were also reported.

Major body system examination

Major body system examination revealed the dog to be anxious but ambulatory. Heart rate was elevated at 170 beats per minute and heart sounds were muffled. Peripheral pulses were weak but dorsal pedal pulses remained palpable and pulse deficits were not suspected. Mucous membranes were pale pink with a prolonged capillary refill time. Neither jugular venous distension nor *pulsus paradoxus* could be readily appreciated. The dog was panting continuously but lung auscultation was assessed as unremarkable. Marked abdominal distension with a palpable fluid thrill was detected.

CLINICAL TIP

- *Pulsus paradoxus* is a decrease in pulse strength during inspiration, reflecting a decrease in systemic arterial blood pressure. Pulse quality varies during respiration in normal dogs, becoming weaker on inspiration and stronger on expiration. However, this normal variation is exaggerated in cardiac tamponade and may be clinically detectable.

Case management

An intravenous catheter was placed into a cephalic vein and blood obtained via the catheter for an emergency database that was unremarkable. Continuous electrocardiogram monitoring was commenced and sinus tachycardia identified. Echocardiography confirmed the clinical suspicion of pericardial effusion (Figure 31.4).

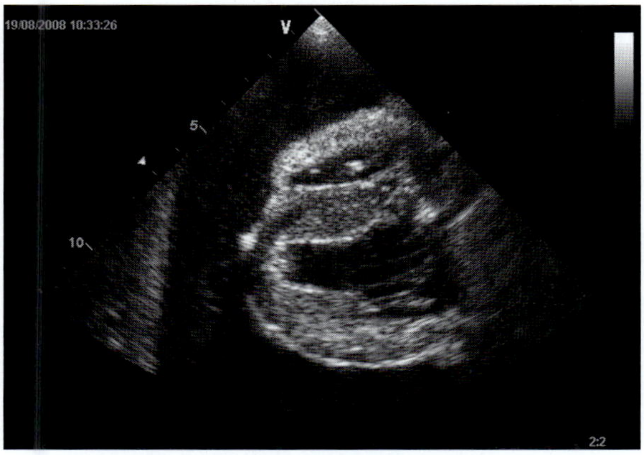

Figure 31.4 Echocardiogram image of pericardial effusion visible as an anechoic space around the heart; both a collapsed right ventricle and the left ventricle are also visible. (Photograph courtesy of Tobias Wagner)

CLINICAL TIP

- Many dogs with pericardial effusion are found to be in sinus tachycardia. Low voltage QRS complexes are relatively common and electrical alternans may also be seen. Electrical alternans is alternate-beat variation in the direction, amplitude or duration of any component of the ECG waveform, most obviously the QRS complexes (Figure 31.5). Swinging of the heart in the fluid-filled pericardial sac is one of the causes of this phenomenon.
- In addition to sinus tachycardia, ventricular dysrhythmias (see Ch. 12) are relatively common in dogs with pericardial effusion and may require specific therapy. Supraventricular dysrhythmias are identified less frequently.

CLINICAL TIP

- If available, echocardiography is the imaging modality of choice for confirming pericardial effusion. It is relatively easy to detect pericardial effusion as an anechoic space around the heart and ultrasonography is both more sensitive and specific and less stressful to the patient when compared to thoracic radiography.
- An enlarged globoid cardiac silhouette and an enlarged caudal vena cava may be identified radiographically but changes may be more subtle, especially in more acute cases. Thoracic radiography is usually indicated at some point during management of a dog with pericardial effusion, in particular to evaluate the lung field for neoplastic metastases.

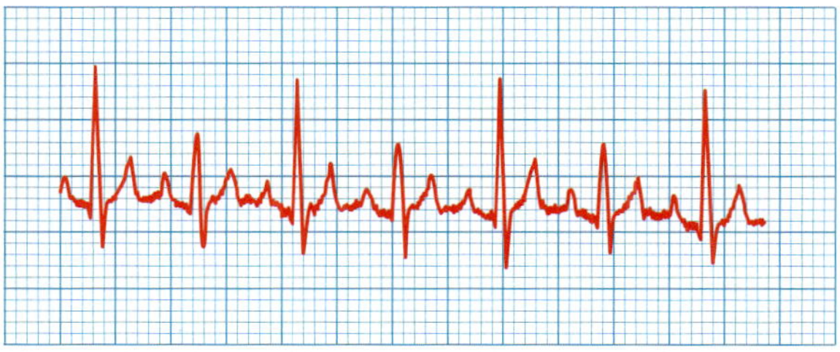

Figure 31.5 Electrical alternans in a dog with pericardial effusion showing alternate-beat variation in QRS amplitude. (Photograph courtesy of Adrian Boswood)

The dog was sedated using butorphanol (0.2 mg/kg i.m.) and midazolam (0.2 mg/kg i.m.) and pericardiocentesis successfully performed (see p. 293). One litre of sanguineous pericardial fluid was removed and the dog's cardiovascular status improved notably. Samples of the fluid were kept in appropriate containers for cytology. Ultrasonography showed only minimal residual pericardial effusion.

CLINICAL TIP

- Pericardiocentesis is the treatment of choice for pericardial effusion and diuresis or other medical therapy should be avoided.
- Not all dogs suffering from pericardial effusion require immediate pericardiocentesis. Fluid in the pericardial sac increases the sensitivity for detecting intrapericardial masses; in dogs that are relatively stable with only mild cardiovascular compromise it may be possible to delay drainage until comprehensive echocardiography can be performed.

The dog was kept on continuous electrocardiogram monitoring for several hours but only occasional ventricular premature complexes (VPCs) were noted. Repeat ultrasonography showed no recurrence of pericardial effusion. The dog was then referred (along with the fluid samples) for further investigations that failed to reveal an underlying cause for the effusion. A presumptive diagnosis of idiopathic pericardial effusion was made.

FELINE PERICARDIAL EFFUSION

Pericardial effusion is much less common in cats and typically occurs as part of a generalized systemic disorder, in particular CHF. Clinical signs specifically resulting from pericardial effusion and tamponade are unusual in cats and signs are more commonly associated with concurrent pulmonary oedema or pleural effusion. Tachypnoea and other respiratory signs are reported most frequently.

To the author's knowledge a comparable syndrome to that resulting from idiopathic pericardial effusion in dogs has not been reported in cats. Neoplasia is recognized as a cause of pericardial effusion in cats. Lymphoma is the most common feline cardiac neoplasm and usually causes pericardial effusion, cytological examination of which often provides the diagnosis. Pericardial effusion secondary to feline infectious peritonitis (FIP) has also been reported and a variety of other causes may be identified.

The procedure for pericardiocentesis in cats is similar to that in dogs. Sedation and ultrasound-guided aspiration are recommended.

32 Respiratory emergencies

FELINE PLEURAL EFFUSION

Theory refresher

Pleural effusion is a relatively common cause of severe respiratory distress in cats. A rational and considered approach to the stabilization of these cats is essential as they are typically critical and very susceptible to stress. In many cases, the pleural effusion would have been present for some time with little or no clinical manifestation; eventually a point is reached where the ability of the lungs to expand becomes so compromised that the cat is no longer able to cope. In addition, depending on the underlying cause, there may also be other pathological abnormalities compromising respiration (e.g. pulmonary oedema in congestive heart failure).

Causes

Causes of pleural effusion in cats include:

- Neoplasia
- Congestive heart failure
- Idiopathic chylothorax
- Feline infectious peritonitis (FIP)
- Haemothorax, traumatic or nontraumatic
- Pyothorax.

In the author's experience, neoplasia and congestive heart failure (see Ch. 31) are the two most common causes identified in cats (see Figures 32.1–32.4).

Case example 1

PRESENTING SIGNS AND CASE HISTORY

A 4-year-old male neutered domestic short hair cat presented with acute respiratory distress. The owner reported that the cat had a several day history of lethargy and inappetence, and that there may have been some weight loss in the preceding weeks. When the owner returned from work that evening she had found the cat to be dyspnoeic and arranged an emergency consultation. The cat had not previously been tested for feline leukaemia virus (FeLV) or feline immunodeficiency virus (FIV). No other significant history was reported.

CLINICAL TIP

- While awaiting the arrival of a cat reported to have respiratory distress, it is important to make preparations in advance to ensure that oxygen therapy can be provided upon arrival, potentially indicated drugs and approximate dose rates are to hand, and that equipment for performing thoracocentesis is readily available.

Observation

The cat was initially briefly observed in his carrier. He appeared alert and pupils were not mydriatic. Respiratory rate was increased with a moderate mixed increase in respiratory effort (including increased abdominal effort). The cat was not obviously cyanotic and was sitting in sternal recumbency with no obvious evidence of trauma.

Brief examination

It was possible to remove the top of the cat's carrier and as he appeared relatively calm, a brief examination was performed while he remained sitting in the same position. Flow-by oxygen supplementation had been started

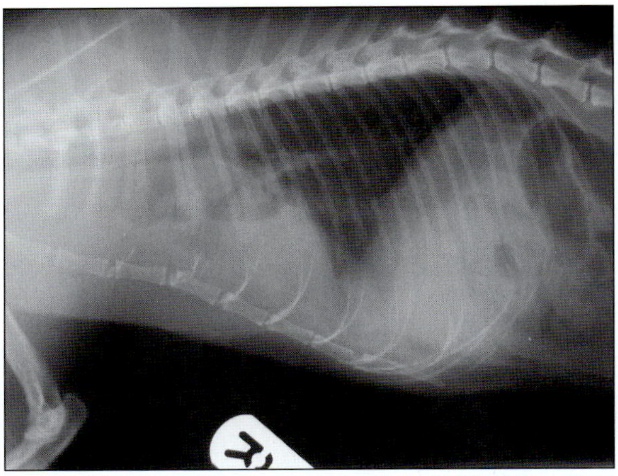

Figure 32.1 Right lateral thoracic radiograph of a cat with pleural effusion secondary to a cranial mediastinal mass.

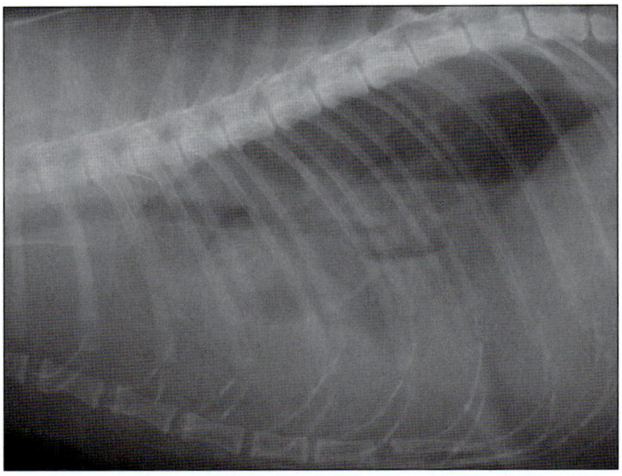

Figure 32.2 Right lateral thoracic radiograph of a cat with severe pleural effusion (diagnosis not made).

already. Sternal cardiac auscultation revealed a subjectively normal heart rate and neither a gallop sound nor a cardiac murmur could be heard. However, the heart sounds appeared muffled. Lung sounds were very dull ventrally and this appeared bilaterally symmetrical. Femoral pulses were normal.

Assessment

The brief examination performed thus far was consistent with pleural effusion. Both the lack of a gallop sound or heart murmur and the presence of normal femoral pulses suggested that the cat was not in congestive heart failure but this had to be interpreted with caution.

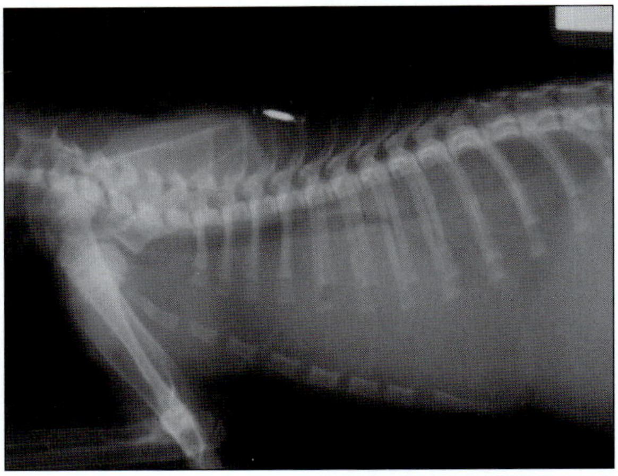

Figure 32.3 Right lateral thoracic radiograph of a cat with pleural effusion secondary to feline infectious peritonitis (FIP).

Oxygenation and client discussion

Following the brief examination, the cat was placed in an oxygen cage, still in his carrier with the top off, and kept under close observation. As the cat was readily compliant, morphine (0.1 mg/kg i.m.) was administered at this point in anticipation of thoracocentesis. The owner was advised that it was suspected that the cat had a pleural effusion for which the two most common causes in cats are neoplasia, especially lymphoma, and congestive heart failure; other possibilities in this case included pyothorax and an idiopathic effusion. The owner was keen to persevere with trying to stabilize the cat with a view to achieving a definitive diagnosis.

Further case management

The cat's respiration had improved to some extent following initial oxygen therapy but there was still a marked increase in respiratory effort. Given the suspicion of pleural effusion, it was decided to perform thoracocentesis for diagnostic and potentially therapeutic purposes (see p. 291). The procedure was only performed on the right side as a large volume of pleural fluid was removed (250 ml, approximately 50 ml/kg) and the cat's breathing improved significantly almost immediately. The cat was returned to the oxygen cage following thoracocentesis after clipping the fur over both cephalic veins and applying topical local anaesthesia (EMLA® cream 5%, AstraZeneca – see Ch. 5) to both sites. The pleural effusion was grossly milky in appearance. In-house cytology revealed that more than half of the cells present were small lymphocytes, and no bacteria were seen. It was

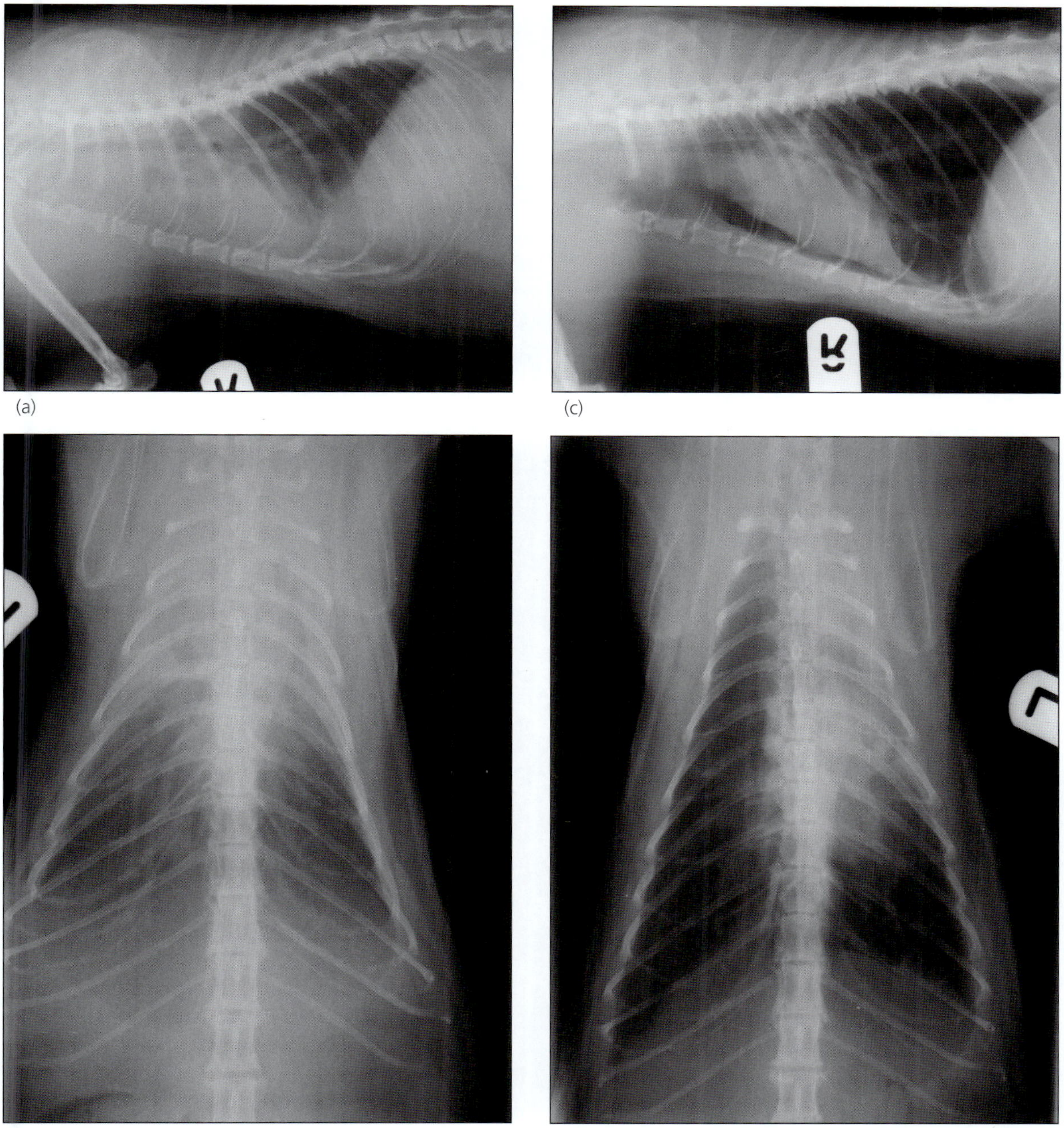

(a) (b) (c) (d)

Figure 32.4 Right lateral and dorsoventral thoracic radiographs of a cat with idiopathic chylothorax (a, b) before and (c, d) after thoracocentesis. The post-drainage films were taken the day after under general anaesthesia; an oesophageal stethoscope is visible.

therefore presumptively classified as a chylous effusion but samples had also been collected into additional sterile containers for submission to an external laboratory.

The cat remained comfortable in the oxygen cage and a cephalic intravenous catheter was placed later using minimal restraint and gentle handling. Blood was obtained via the catheter for an emergency database to be performed that was essentially unremarkable. As congestive heart failure remained a possibility, the cat was not started on intravenous fluid therapy at this time and the catheter was kept patent by regular flushing. Morphine (0.1 mg/kg slow i.v. q 6 hr) was continued but no other medications were indicated at this stage.

The cat remained stable overnight and it was possible to wean him off oxygen therapy. He was referred the next morning for further investigations which revealed a cranial mediastinal mass that was confirmed to be due to lymphoma. The cat was started on chemotherapy and was doing well at his most recent follow-up examination.

FELINE BRONCHIAL DISEASE (ASTHMA)

Theory refresher

Feline bronchial disease is the result of inflammation of the lower airways without an identifiable cause. A number of different terms have been used in the literature to refer to the same syndrome, including feline lower airway disease, feline allergic airway disease and feline asthma. The disease occurs most commonly in young to middle-aged cats and Siamese cats are overrepresented. Allergens or nonspecific airway irritants are likely to be involved in initiating or at least exacerbating airway inflammation. The relationship between respiratory infection and feline bronchial disease remains to be clarified.

Clinical signs are due to obstruction of the lower airways as a result of bronchial inflammation and subsequent smooth muscle constriction, oedema, mucous gland hypertrophy and excessive mucus secretion, and airway hyperactivity. In some cats, these changes are reversible, while in others chronic inflammation results in irreversible fibrosis and emphysema. Eosinophils are typically the primary inflammatory cells involved in the pathophysiology.

Clinical signs most commonly include coughing, and variable degrees of tachypnoea or dyspnoea. Severe obstruction of the lower airways prevents cats from exhaling completely, resulting in air trapping and hyperinflation of the lungs; this is identified radiographically as increased pulmonary radiolucency and a flattened, caudally displaced diaphragm.

Case example 2

PRESENTING SIGNS AND CASE HISTORY

A 6-year-old female neutered Siamese cat presented with acute onset respiratory distress.

PRESENTING SIGNS AND CASE HISTORY—cont'd

The owner reported that over the preceding 2 months the cat had been heard to cough occasionally, typically at night, but there was no other significant history. The cat was kept exclusively indoors, was fully vaccinated, and had previously been found to be negative for feline leukaemia virus (FeLV) and feline immunodeficiency virus (FIV).

CLINICAL TIP

- While awaiting the arrival of a cat reported to have respiratory distress, it is important to make preparations in advance to ensure that oxygen therapy can be provided upon arrival, potentially indicated drugs and approximate dose rates are to hand, and that equipment for performing thoracocentesis is readily available.

Observation, brief examination

On presentation the cat was in lateral recumbency with dilated pupils, open-mouth breathing and showing paradoxical abdominal movement. This is an ominous sign and the cat was therefore immediately started on oxygen supplementation. Very brief examination was performed that revealed a mild subjective bradycardia with no gallop sound or heart murmur heard; femoral pulse quality was unremarkable. Lung sounds were diffusely harsh with some wheezes.

Assessment

The respiratory findings were most consistent with feline lower airway disease, diffuse cardiogenic pulmonary oedema or pulmonary contusions. However, the cardiovascular examination was less suggestive of congestive heart failure and crackles would most likely be expected in a cat with such severe dyspnoea. The cat was an indoor cat and there was no history or other suggestion of blunt trauma. Both the history of coughing and signalment were also supportive of lower airway disease being the most likely diagnosis.

Case management

The cat was immediately administered dexamethasone (0.25 mg/kg i.m), terbutaline (0.01 mg/kg i.m.) and

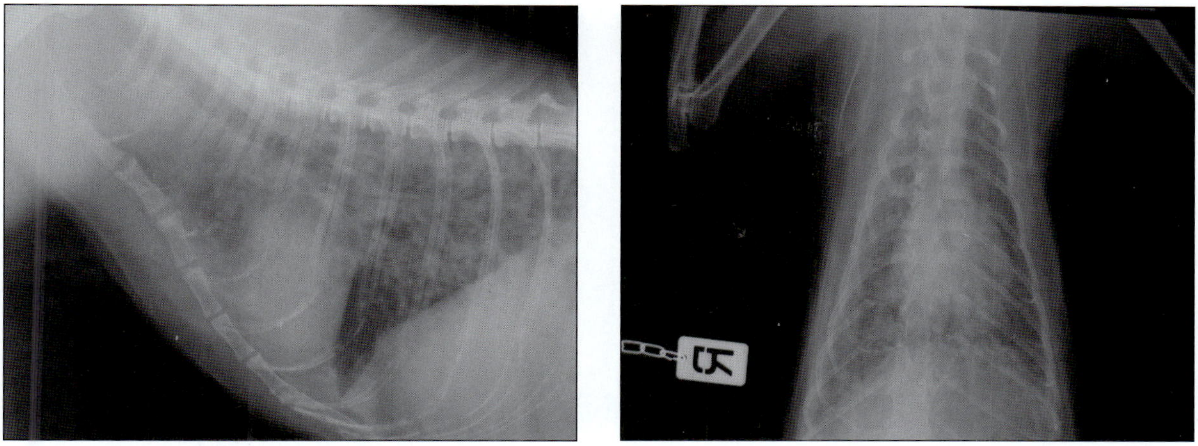

Figure 32.5 (a) Right lateral and (b) dorsoventral thoracic radiographs of a cat showing a severe diffuse bronchointerstitial lung pattern.

furosemide (2 mg/kg i.m.). Despite the suspicion of lower airway disease, furosemide was included in the initial therapy as a single dose is unlikely to be especially harmful in the absence of hypoperfusion or significant dehydration, and could potentially be life-saving if significant pulmonary oedema was in fact present. An intravenous catheter was placed into a cephalic vein and blood obtained via the catheter for an emergency database to be performed which was essentially unremarkable.

Oxygen supplementation was continued and the cat monitored closely, and she slowly began to show improvement. At the appropriate time, thoracic radiographs were taken under mild sedation (butorphanol 0.2 mg/kg i.v.) and revealed a severe diffuse broncho-interstitial lung pattern (Figure 32.5). A diagnosis of chronic bronchial disease with acute exacerbation was made.

The cat was maintained on oxygen supplementation, dexamethasone (0.25 mg/kg i.v. q 24 hr), terbutaline (0.01 mg/kg s.c. q 4 hr) and maintenance intravenous isotonic crystalloid therapy (buffered lactated Ringer's solution at 2 ml/kg/hr). She made a slow but steady recovery and was eventually discharged on oral prednisolone (1 mg/kg p.o. q 12 hr) and inhaled bronchodilator therapy (albuterol). A plan for ongoing management, including tapering of oral prednisolone and switching to inhaled fluticasone, was agreed with the owner. The owners were questioned at length and advised extensively about possible allergens (e.g. cat litter, cigarette smoke, carpet cleaners, air fresheners) in the home and the importance of minimizing the cat's exposure to them.

CANINE UPPER RESPIRATORY TRACT OBSTRUCTION

In the author's experience, upper respiratory tract obstruction is one of the most common causes of acute respiratory distress in dogs, especially in warmer weather following exercise. The two most common disorders are laryngeal paralysis and brachycephalic airway obstruction syndrome (BAOS). The initial approach to the stabilization of these dogs involves common interventions that centre on:

- Oxygen supplementation
- Sedation, usually acepromazine
- Intravenous access
- Cooling
- Minimal stress and intervention
- Possible corticosteroid administration, usually dexamethasone.

Occasionally dogs with chronic tracheal collapse present in an acute respiratory crisis.

Laryngeal paralysis

Theory refresher

Laryngeal paralysis is the result of dysfunction of the recurrent laryngeal nerves that supply the muscles which move the arytenoid cartilages. It may be congenital or acquired, and is almost always filateral in clinically symptomatic dogs.

In most cases acquired laryngeal paralysis is presumptively diagnosed as idiopathic; it may be that some of these cases are in fact due to an otherwise subtle generalised polyneuropathy. Acquired laryngeal paralysis may also be traumatic or iatrogenic in orgin.

There is a high incidence of megaoesophagus amongst dogs with laryngeal paralysis and these animals are also at risk of aspiration pneumonia. Thoracic radiographs are therefore indicated in all cases and can be taken while the patient is intubated if applicable. Non-cardiogenic pulmonary oedema may also be identified following upper respiratory tract obstruction, typically in the caudodorsal lung field.

Case example 3

PRESENTING SIGNS AND CASE HISTORY

A 9-year-old male neutered chocolate Labrador retriever presented with severe respiratory distress. The dog had been out exercising a few hours prior to presentation and had developed respiratory distress that had progressed since returning home. Subsequent questioning of his owner after stabilization revealed that he had a chronic history of intermittent coughing.

CLINICAL TIP

- Idiopathic laryngeal paralysis is seen most commonly in larger breed dogs and especially in Labrador and golden retrievers. Clinical signs are usually noted in older dogs although younger dogs may also be affected.
- A chronic history of exercise intolerance, excessive panting, louder breathing, coughing, and a change in the bark may be present. Dysphagia may also be reported.
- Some dogs present in acute respiratory distress.

Major body system examination

On presentation the dog was cyanotic, recumbent and extremely anxious. Loud inspiratory stridor was obvious and there was marked inspiratory effort. Respiratory rate was 60 breaths per minute. The dog was tachycardic (heart rate 150 beats per minute) but cardiovascular examination was otherwise unremarkable. Rectal temperature was elevated at 40.5°C and was interpreted as hyperthermia (as opposed to pyrexia; see Ch. 16).

Assessment Initial assessment was that the dog's most serious abnormality was upper respiratory tract dyspnoea that was most likely secondary to laryngeal paralysis.

CLINICAL TIP

- Laryngeal paralysis is a familiar cause of upper respiratory tract dyspnoea. Marked respiratory effort in the face of laryngeal dysfunction can result in hyperthermia that may be extreme. Hyperthermia and progressive laryngeal swelling contribute to the cycle of respiratory distress seen in an acute crisis.

Case management

Flow-by oxygen supplementation was commenced immediately. An intravenous catheter was placed (with collection of blood at the time of placement for an emergency database) and acepromazine (0.02 mg/kg) and butorphanol (0.3 mg/kg) administered intravenously. The dog was wetted with cool water and a fan applied, and he was then subjected to minimal stress

The cyanosis resolved quickly and 20 minutes after sedation there had been some improvement in respiratory status. Rectal temperature had reduced to 39.5°C and cooling was therefore stopped to avoid rebound hypothermia. Oxygen supplementation was discontinued and dexamethasone (0.25 mg/kg i.v.) administered. Intravenous isotonic crystalloid fluid therapy (3 ml/kg/h^{-}) was provided early on and repeat sedation performed as required until the dog's respiratory status had normalized. Subsequent referral for suspected laryngeal paralysis was arranged.

CLINICAL TIP

- On occasion dogs suffering an acute crisis will not respond to the management provided in this case and endotracheal intubation may prove necessary. In such cases laryngeal fold function should be evaluated under a suitably light plane of anaesthesia first before deeper anaesthesia is provided and intubation performed.

CLINICAL TIP—cont'd

- The laryngeal folds should abduct during inspiration and it may be helpful to have an assistant calling out each time inspiration occurs sc that laryngeal function can be correlated with respiration. If significant laryngeal oedema is identified, dexamethasone should be administered while the patient remains intubated.
- Emergency tracheostomy may be required but in the author's experience this is rarely the case.

Brachycephalic airway obstruction syndrome (BAOS)

Brachycephalic airway obstruction syndrome (BAOS) is the result of poor conformation that predisposes certain dogs to airway obstruction. Breeds affected by this condition include bulldogs, the Pekingese, pugs and the Boxer. Components of BAOS include:

- Elongated soft palate
- Stenotic nares
- Everted laryngeal saccules.

Affected dogs often also have a degree of tracheal hypoplasia. Following emergency stabilization as required, surgical intervention is usually necessary to improve the dog's clinical status long-term.

FELINE UPPER RESPIRATORY TRACT OBSTRUCTION

Although much less common than in dogs, occasionally cats present with severe upper respiratory tract dyspnoea. This is most commonly the result of a mass lesion (e.g. laryngeal lymphoma, nasopharyngeal polyp), although laryngeal paralysis has also been reported in cats. Although brachycephalic cats may have severe conformational abnormalities, the author has not seen one of these cats present with an associated primary acute respiratory crisis. However poor conformation will execerbate the effects of other disorders such as upper respiratory tract infection.

33 Haematological and haemostatic emergencies

CANINE IMMUNE-MEDIATED HAEMOLYTIC ANAEMIA (IMHA)

Theory refresher

Immune-mediated haemolytic anaemia (IMHA) is the result of red blood cell destruction by the immune system. Red blood cell destruction is initiated by the binding of immunoglobulin G (IgG) or IgM antibodies and complement to their surface. Both extravascular (reticuloendothelial system) and intravascular (causes haemoglobinaemia, haemoglobinuria) haemolysis may occur.

IMHA is generally classified into primary (idiopathic) IMHA, in which no inciting cause is identified, and secondary IMHA, which is associated with an underlying condition (Box 33.1). Primary IMHA is typically diagnosed in young or middle-aged adult dogs but can occur in older dogs too. IMHA is especially common in certain breeds (e.g. English springer spaniel, American Cocker Spaniel). These dogs were previously classified as having primary IMHA although this classification may no longer be appropriate given their genetic predisposition. In dogs with secondary IMHA, the underlying condition may or may not persist at the time of presentation, and may or may not be amenable to specific therapy. In the absence of useful historical information (e.g. with respect to drug administration or vaccination), thorough physical examination, thoracic and abdominal diagnostic imaging, urine microbiology and additional investigations as appropriate are required to rule out an underlying trigger for IMHA.

BOX 33.1 *Underlying conditions potentially associated with immune-mediated haemolytic anaemia*

- Drugs – especially antibiotics (e.g. penicillins, cephalosporins, sulphonamides); also nonsteroidal anti-inflammatory agents, methimazole (cats)
- Vaccines – generally within 30 days of injections
- Infection:
  - Viral (e.g. FeLV, FIV)
  - Bacterial (e.g. leptospirosis, mycoplasmosis), various acute and chronic infections, especially of urinary tract
  - Parasitic (e.g. babesiosis, ehrlichiosis)
- Neoplasia

FeLV, feline leukaemia virus; FIV, feline immunodeficiency virus.

Hereditary erythrocyte enzyme defects should be kept in mind as possible differential diagnoses in dogs of affected breeds presenting with evidence of haemolytic anaemia. Phosphofructokinase (PFK) deficiency occurs especially in the English springer spaniel, Cocker Spaniel breeds, and mixed breed dogs. Pyruvate kinase (PK) deficiency is most commonly reported in the Basenji as well as in several other breeds including the Beagle, the West Highland White terrier, the Cairn terrier and the miniature poodle.

Treatment

Medical therapy to decrease erythrocyte phagocytosis, complement activation and anti-erythrocytic antibody production is essential for primary IMHA and glucocorticoids are the mainstay of acute therapy. Other immunosuppressive agents may be used in addition to, but not instead of, glucocorticoids (Box 33.2). Immunosuppressive therapy is typically also required for secondary IMHA although success is significantly dependent on

BOX 33.2 Immunosuppressive agents that may be considered in addition to glucocorticoids in canine immune-mediated haemolytic anaemia (IMHA)

Although there is limited evidence for their efficacy in IMHA, the author typically uses one of these agents in all dogs with primary IMHA in an attempt to allow prednisolone therapy to be tapered more quickly, thereby minimizing side effects. Azathioprine is the cheapest option and is therefore used where possible. However, it likely has the slowest onset of action with a lag of 7–14 days and is therefore started as early as possible. Mycophenolate mofetil and especially ciclosporin are more expensive but may have a quicker onset of action. They are therefore typically only used in cases in which response to glucocorticoids is inadequate.
The author has no experience with the use of cyclophosphamide.

- Azathioprine: 2 mg/kg p.o. q 24 hr for up to 7–10 days, then q 48 hr long term; monitor for myelosuppression and hepatotoxicity
- Mycophenolate mofetil: 10–15 mg/kg p.o. q 12–24 hr
- Ciclosporin: 5–10 mg/kg p.o. q 12–24 hr; monitor trough blood concentrations intermittently to achieve effective but safe levels

whether the underlying condition persists and, if so, whether or not it is amenable to treatment. Clearly with neoplastic conditions in particular, it may not be possible or appropriate to treat the patient.

Dogs with IMHA are at increased risk of thromboembolic complications, especially pulmonary thromboembolism (causes dyspnoea, tachypnoea, cyanosis). Anticoagulant therapy is therefore used in addition to the immunosuppressive therapy. However, there remains much to be clarified with respect to both coagulation abnormalities in IMHA and the most effective preventative and therapeutic treatments. At the time of writing, ultralow dose (0.5 mg/kg p.o. q 24 hr) aspirin therapy is most widely recommended and discontinued at the same time as glucocorticoid administration ceases.

Case example 1

PRESENTING SIGNS AND CASE HISTORY

A 4-year-old female neutered English springer spaniel dog presented with a 2-day history of progressive lethargy, exercise intolerance and inappetence. The owner had noticed the dog passing grossly discoloured urine (pigmenturia), prompting emergency presentation. The dog had last received routine annual vaccination 6 months prior to presentation, and there was no recent history of drug administration. There was no notable history of travel and no other significant history was reported.

Major body system examination

On presentation the dog was ambulatory but weak and depressed. Cardiovascular examination revealed a heart rate of 136 beats per minute with no murmur or gallop sound heard. Peripheral pulses were hyperdynamic in quality without deficits, and mucous membranes were very pale with a rapid capillary refill time. Respiratory rate was 40 breaths per minute with a shallow pattern and lung auscultation was appropriate for the rate and effort. Abdominal palpation was unremarkable and the dog was mildly pyrexic (rectal temperature 39.3°C). Digital examination per rectum revealed normal faeces without evidence of melaena or fresh haemorrhage. Peripheral lymph nodes were normal, and no other abnormalities were detected; in particular, there was no evidence of jaundice.

Assessment

The tachycardia in this case may have been the result of mild hypovolaemia but mucous membranes were much paler than would be expected in such cases; mild hypovolaemia is associated with normal or pinker than normal mucous membranes. Very pale mucous membranes are associated with severe hypovolaemia but the dog's heart rate, peripheral pulse quality and mentation were not consistent with this. It was therefore suspected that the pallor was predominantly related to anaemia. Peripheral pulses have a fairly characteristic quality in anaemia and were consistent with anaemia in this case. The dog was therefore suspected to be showing signs of cardiorespiratory compensation for severe anaemia and, given her breed, there was a high index of suspicion for primary (idiopathic) IMHA. Mild pyrexia is a relatively common finding in such cases.

Emergency database

An intravenous catheter was placed in a cephalic vein and blood obtained via the catheter for an emergency database to be performed. This revealed severe anaemia (manual packed cell volume (PCV) 14%, reference range 37–55%) with raised plasma total solids (78 g/l, reference range 49–71 g/l); however, the serum was icteric in appearance. These findings were consistent with the suspicion of haemolytic anaemia. An in-saline agglutination test was performed (Box 33.3) and found to be strongly positive (Figure 33.1). Peripheral blood smear examination revealed a strongly regenerative anaemia with marked polychromasia and anisocytosis and an increase in nucleated red blood cells; marked spherocytosis was also identified. Platelet numbers were adequate, and a moderate subjective left-shifted neutrophilia and a monocytosis were suspected (see Ch. 3).

BOX 33.3 In-saline agglutination test for autoagglutination

One or more drops of fresh blood (or blood from an EDTA tube) are placed on a glass slide and an equal volume of normal saline added. The slide is gently rotated and then examined for evidence of macroscopic agglutination after approximately 1 minute. The slide is then examined microscopically as well (Figure 33.1). Saline is added to differentiate true agglutination from rouleaux formation. Rouleaux are chains of red blood cells stacked like coins, and are especially common in cats and animals with inflammation. They should be dissipated by the addition of saline.

CLINICAL TIP

- In addition to documenting haemolytic anaemia, definitive diagnosis of IMHA requires marked spherocytosis, spontaneous autoagglutination or a positive direct Coombs test to be identified. In the author's experience, most dogs presenting as emergencies with clinically significant IMHA have autoagglutination and/or marked spherocytosis at the time of presentation. The diagnosis can usually therefore be made on an emergency basis without the delay involved in awaiting the results of a Coombs' test.

In addition to the emergency database, an in-house biochemistry profile was performed that revealed hyperbilirubinaemia (total bilirubin 45 μmol/l, reference range 2–10 μmol/l) and a mild increase in liver enzymes. Free catch urinalysis revealed a specific gravity of 1.050 and dipstick analysis showed 3+ bilirubin and 2+ haemoglobinuria; no bacteria were seen and there was a normal

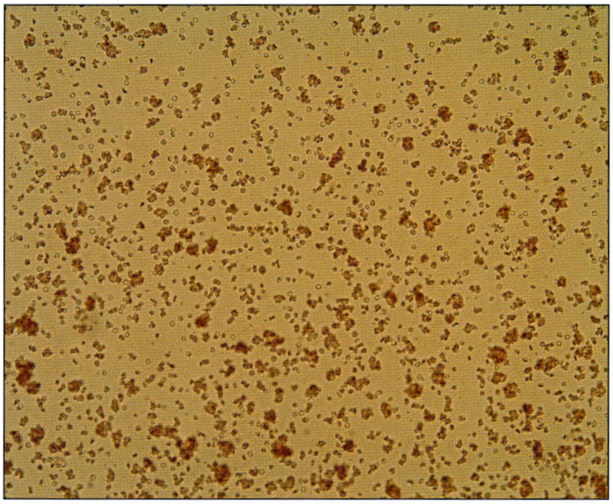

(a)

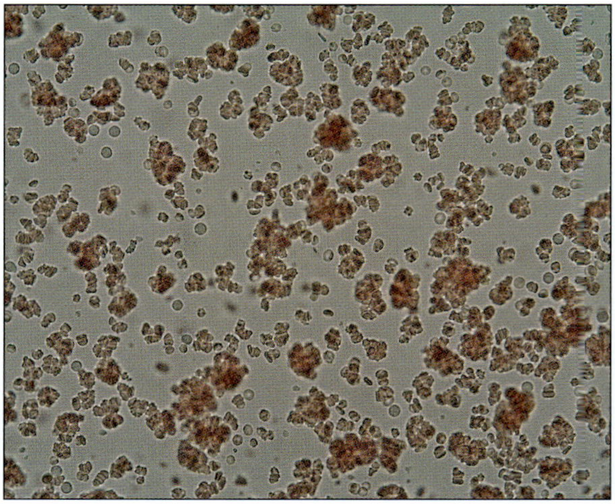

(b)

Figure 33.1 Microscopic in-saline agglutination (a) ×100 and (b) ×200 magnification. (Photographs courtesy of Kate English) number of white blood cells on sediment examination. In-house blood typing was performed (RapidVet-H Canine DEA 1.1®; DMS Laboratories, New Jersey, USA) and the dog was successfully typed as DEA 1.1 positive.

CLINICAL TIP

- Autoagglutination may interfere with blood typing (and crossmatching) which may not therefore be possible. In such cases, packed red blood cells from a DEA 1.1 negative dog should ideally be administered (see Ch. 40).
- If a blood transfusion cannot be performed, Oxyglobin® (see Ch. 4) may be used instead to provide oxygen-carrying capacity and improve clinical signs while allowing time for medical therapy to take effect. Despite the small bag size of this product, low rates are used (1–2 ml/kg/hr in dogs) which make this a practical option in small and medium size dogs. A total dose of 15–30 ml/kg is administered depending on clinical response, resource availability and financial constraints.

Case management

A packed red blood cell transfusion was administered and the dog received a total of approximately 10 ml/kg over 6 hours. Minimum intervention was performed in the interim, and by the end of the transfusion the dog's cardiorespiratory and mental status had improved significantly and predictably. Thoracic and abdominal radiographs were then taken and found to be sterile.

The dog was started on immunosuppressive therapy as follows:

- Dexamethasone 0.5 mg/kg i.v. q 24 hr for 1 day; as the dog was appetent and not vomiting, she was then switched on to prednisolone 2 mg/kg p.o. q 12 hr
- Azathioprine 2 mg/kg p.o. q 24 hr; dosing interval increased to every other day after 7–10 days.

In addition, the dog was started on aspirin (0.5 mg/kg p.o. q 24 hr) in an attempt to reduce the risk of thromboembolic disease, and maintenance isotonic crystalloid (Hartmann's solution 2 ml/kg/hr) fluid therapy was provided initially.

The dog made good clinical progress and was discharged after 5 days of hospitalization at which time PCV was 29%, anaemia was moderately regenerative, in-saline agglutination remained mildly positive, and hyperbilirubinaemia had resolved. A comprehensive plan for on-going monitoring and adjustment of therapy was agreed with the owner.

FELINE IMMUNE-MEDIATED HAEMOLYTIC ANAEMIA (IMHA)

Primary (idiopathic) IMHA is reportedly much less commonly in cats than it is in dogs. No breed association has been reported and the possibility of PK deficiency as a differential diagnosis should be borne in mind. This red blood cell enzymopathy has been reported in Abyssinian, Somali and domestic short hair cats.

Diagnosis and treatment of IMHA in cats follow similar principles to those described for dogs although it is noteworthy that identification of spherocytes in cats is more difficult due to normal feline erythrocytes often lacking central pallor. Cats must be blood typed and given type-specific fresh whole blood (see Ch. 40). If this is not possible, Oxyglobin® (see Ch. 4) is especially useful as a substitute by providing oxygen-carrying capacity in severely anaemic cats. Cats in general, and especially anaemic cats, are prone to fluid overload and Oxyglobin® is typically administered at a conservative 0.5–1.0 ml/kg/hr for the treatment of anaemia in euvolaemic cats.

CLINICAL TIP

- As with all anaemic cats, cats with IMHA are likely to be highly susceptible to stress and excessive stress may cause marked clinical deterioration. These cats should therefore be handled and restrained gently by experienced personnel only, and should be subjected to minimum interventions.
- Topical local anaesthesia (see Ch. 5) should be used prior to venepuncture.

Glucocorticoid administration is the most important part of acute therapy. Azathioprine should not be administered to cats and chlorambucil (2 mg total dose p.o. q 24–72 hr) is the immunosuppressive agent of choice in this species in addition to glucocorticoid therapy.

Mycoplasma haemofelis

Mycoplasma haemofelis (previously *Haemobartonella felis*) infection is a cause of IMHA in cats which may be addressed specifically. Although treatment does not typically clear infection completely, parasitaemia resolves quickly and clinical improvement occurs within a few days. Diagnosis typically requires a blood sample to be submitted for polymerase chain reaction (PCR) assay with some delay before the results are received. The author therefore typically treats all cats with suspected primary IMHA for possible mycoplasmosis until the PCR results are received. Doxycycline (5–10 mg/kg p.o. q 12–24 hr for 10–21 days) is the preferred treatment but may be problematic to administer enterally in cats that are anorexic, especially as minimizing stress is essential in anaemic cats. If doxycycline is administered directly by mouth, a small amount (5 ml) of water must be syringed straight after to prevent the tablet becoming lodged in the oesophagus and causing a potentially serious oesophagitis. Parenteral enrofloxacin (5 mg/kg slow i.v. diluted, s.c. (or p.o.) q 24 hr) may be administered instead and is likely to be preferable in a number of these cats; the potential for enrofloxacin to cause retinal toxicity and permanent blindness in cats must not be overlooked but this has only been reported at higher doses. Immunosuppressive glucocorticoid therapy is required in the short term in cats found to have mycoplasmosis but can be tapered more quickly than for primary IMHA.

PRIMARY (IDIOPATHIC) IMMUNE-MEDIATED THROMBOCYTOPENIA (ITP)

Thrombocytopenia may be the result of an increase in platelet destruction or consumption, a decrease in platelet production, or sequestration. In many diseases, the actual platelet count reflects a combination of more than one of these processes occurring concurrently.

Causes

Infectious diseases

Infectious causes of thrombocytopenia are usually associated with systemic signs, physical examination findings and clinicopathological abnormalities beyond thrombocytopenia alone. Examples include leptospirosis, feline leukaemia virus (FeLV) infection, feline immunodeficiency virus (FIV) infection, ehrlichiosis, babesiosis and rickettsiosis.

Neoplasia

Thrombocytopenia may occur in association with a number of tumours but is most severe with tumour types that can affect haematopoiesis (e.g. lymphoma, multiple myeloma). Thrombocytopenia may also be the result of chemotherapeutic agents employed in the treatment of neoplasia.

Immune-mediated thrombocytopenia

ITP may be primary (idiopathic) or secondary to an infectious, inflammatory or neoplastic process, as well as to a variety of drug therapies. ITP occurs as a result of antibodies directed against platelet membrane antigens and subsequent phagocytosis or lysis. Primary (idiopathic) ITP is much more common in dogs than in cats, and especially occurs in females and certain breeds (e.g. the Cocker Spaniel, poodles, the Old English Sheepdog).

Clinical signs of ITP

Clinical signs of ITP are as expected with severe thrombocytopenia and include epistaxis, gingival bleeding, melaena, vomiting and possible haematemesis (see Ch. 21). Physical examination may reveal petechiae and ecchymoses, evidence of cardiorespiratory compensation for blood loss anaemia, and pyrexia. A variety of other nonspecific signs may be found.

Diagnosis of ITP

Animals with ITP typically have very severe thrombocytopenia; machine platelet counts are typically less than 10×10^9 platelets/litre, and peripheral smear examination may reveal no platelets at all or an average of less than 1 platelet per high-power (×100) field. The diagnosis of ITP is routinely made on the basis of identifying a thrombocytopenia of this severity in an animal with compatible clinical signs. Thereafter, investigations are performed to identify a primary cause and if one cannot be found, a presumptive diagnosis of ITP is made.

Occasionally dogs with ITP are also found to have evidence of immune-mediated red blood cell destruction and these dogs are therefore classified as having Evans' syndrome. Nevertheless, management of these cases is the same as for ITP and IMHA.

Treatment of ITP

Immunosuppressive therapy using corticosteroids is the mainstay of therapy for ITP and is similar to treatment for IMHA; additional immunosuppressive therapies may be included (see Box 33.2). Animals with secondary immune-mediated platelet destruction may also require more short-term corticosteroid therapy in addition to specific treatment for the primary disorder.

Vincristine may be used to promote the release of functional platelets from the bone marrow but the author typically only uses this agent in cases that fail to show signs of improvement on corticosteroid alone. Human intravenous IgG has also been used but is very expensive and has limited availability.

Packed red blood cell or fresh whole blood transfusions may be required in animals with sufficiently severe gastrointestinal haemorrhage. Platelet transfusions are often discussed and may be provided using fresh whole blood, platelet-rich plasma or platelet concentrates. The availability of the latter in particular is likely to increase with time. However, platelet transfusions are typically discouraged in dogs with ITP; the transfused platelets are also susceptible to antibody binding and will very likely have a short lifespan of less than 1 day and perhaps as short as a few minutes only. The use of platelet transfusions as a short-term, potentially life-saving measure in dogs with severe bleeding may become more practical in the future.

Supportive intravenous crystalloid therapy, gastroprotectants, antiemetics and other symptomatic treatments may be required in the early stages of treatment.

CLINICAL TIP

- Recovery in dogs with ITP is very much dependent on response to immunosuppressive therapy. Adequate oxygen-carrying support (red blood cells or potentially a haemoglobin-based oxygen-carrying solution) is provided, if required, to allow enough time for a response to occur (perhaps 2–7 days, can be longer).
- Owners must be warned that, although uncommon, dogs with ITP may suffer a bleed into a vital organ such as the brain or the lungs, following which the prognosis for recovery is likely to be grave.

CANINE *ANGIOSTRONGYLUS VASORUM* INFECTION

Theory refresher

Angiostrongylus vasorum (canine lungworm) is a metastrongylid helminth infecting domestic dogs as well as foxes. Molluscs (snails, slugs) act as intermediate hosts. Larvae ingested in molluscs generally migrate from the small intestine to the right ventricle and pulmonary vasculature where they mature to adulthood. However, extensive aberrant larval migration into many body organs and tissues has been documented. *Angiostrongylus vasorum* has a worldwide distribution, and infections are continuously being identified in new areas both within the United Kingdom and globally.

CLINICAL TIP

- It is becoming increasingly apparent that *Angiostrongylus vasorum* infection should not be excluded as a possible differential diagnosis on the basis of geographical location alone as infections are continuously being identified in new areas.

Clinical signs

A wide variety of clinical signs has been reported but most dogs diagnosed with clinically significant disease have respiratory signs, bleeding disorders or neurological signs. Ocular signs, including intraocular larval migration, have also been reported relatively frequently. However, aberrant systemic dissemination of the larvae means that additional syndromes as a result of haemorrhage, granulomatous inflammation or infarction at other sites may well be recognized more commonly in the future. Respiratory signs are the result of pulmonary inflammation secondary to both eggs and to larval migration through the parenchyma. Over time, pulmonary hypertension may develop, resulting in right-sided cardiac changes (*cor pulmonale*).

Neurological signs associated with angiostrongylosis may occur as a result of larval migration through, or bleeding into, the central nervous system; both abnormalities have been documented. Reported neurological signs include reduced mentation from depression through to coma, behavioural changes, seizures and loss of vision related to brain involvement; and spinal and neck pain, ataxia, and paresis or plegia related to spinal cord involvement.

The mechanism(s) of coagulation defects due to *Angiostrongylus vasorum* remain to be clarified. Although many dogs have variably abnormal coagulation tests, the author has certainly seen cases in which routinely available means of evaluating coagulation (platelet count, buccal mucosal bleeding time, prothrombin time, activated partial thromboplastin time) have been within normal limits despite clinical evidence of coagulopathy. The same is true for a small number of cases in which

D-dimers/fibrin degradation products (FDPs) and von Willebrand factor levels have been measured. A chronic intravascular consumptive coagulopathy (chronic disseminated intravascular coagulation (DIC)) has been suggested as a mechanism by some authors.

Angiostrongylosis has been diagnosed in dogs with a variety of clinical presentations of bleeding, including:

- Excessive bleeding following a surgical procedure – often an elective neutering procedure in a young dog
- Excessive bleeding following trauma or at venepuncture sites
- Ecchymoses/petechiae
- Haemoptysis
- Spontaneous subcutaneous haematomas
- Spontaneous intraocular, episcleral or subconjunctival haemorrhage
- Gastrointestinal haemorrhage
- Spontaneous haemoabdomen
- Spontaneous haemothorax (larvae may be identified in the pleural fluid).

Although neoplastic rupture is the most common cause of spontaneous haemoabdomen, this typically occurs in older dogs. Angiostrongylosis should therefore be considered especially in young dogs presenting with spontaneous haemoabdomen (as well as anticoagulant rodenticide intoxication for example, see Ch. 30).

Diagnosis

The diagnosis of canine angiostrongylosis is currently made most reliably by faecal analysis or cytology on airway samples (transtracheal wash, tracheal wash via endotracheal tube or bronchoalveolar lavage). In-house faecal smear examination (Box 33.4) allows diagnosis to be made on an emergency basis and, in the author's experience, the diagnosis can be made in most dogs with clinical angiostrongylosis on the basis of faecal smear examination, albeit that in some cases multiple smears may need to be examined (see Figure 33.2). Faecal analysis via Baermann faecal flotation is currently the most reliable method available although this clearly involves some delay before results are received. In the author's opinion, treatment should be implemented before results are received in cases in which there is a high index of suspicion for angiostrongylosis but faecal smear examination is negative or cannot be performed. Serology for detecting antibodies against *Angiostrongylus vasorum* antigen is now available and likely to become more widely used in the future.

BOX 33.4 Faecal smear preparation for detection of *Angiostrongylus vasorum* larvae

In an emergency scenario, faeces for examination is often obtained via manual removal from the rectum and as such, only a small amount may be available. In such cases, it is most appropriate to smear the faeces directly on to one or more slides, add a small amount of water to the slide, cover the slide with coverslips (if available), and examine microscopically using a low (×20) magnification with the condenser down.

If a larger amount of faeces is available, the faeces should be placed in a container to which water is then added. The solution is mixed thoroughly and multiple smears are then made for microscopic examination.

Angiostrongylus vasorum larvae have a characteristic appearance and should not be mistaken for hairs which are straight with a line down the middle (Figure 33.2).

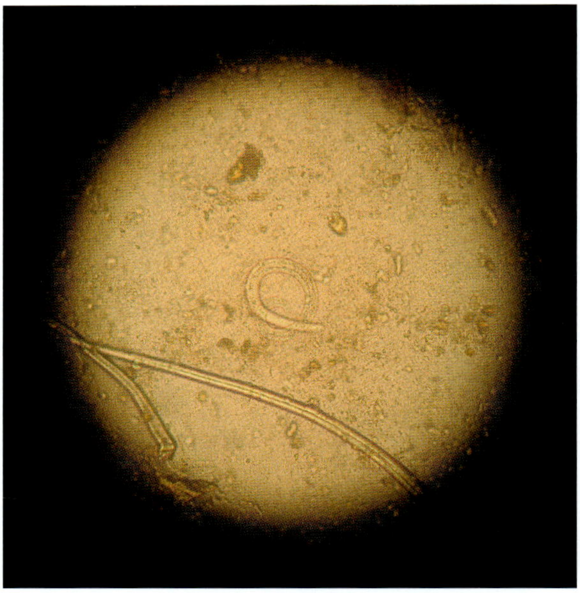

Figure 33.2 Curled up *Angiostrongylus vasorum* larva (centre), not to be confused with straight hairs with a line down the middle (lower down).

Treatment

Treatment of canine angiostrongylosis is described in Case example 2. In addition, both total and ionized hypercalcaemia have been reported in dogs with angiostrongylosis and may be sufficiently severe as to require specific intervention (0.9% sodium chloride diuresis, furosemide). Hypercalcaemia is thought to be due to granulomatous inflammation and should resolve fully with successful anthelminthic therapy.

Case example 2

PRESENTING SIGNS AND CASE HISTORY

A 2-year-old male neutered English Mastiff dog presented with a 3-day history of progressive respiratory distress, coughing (haemoptysis), excessive panting, exercise intolerance, lethargy and inappetence. The dog was known to be a scavenger but no other significant previous history was reported. Deworming therapy had not been administered since puppyhood.

CLINICAL TIP

- Although angiostrongylosis can be diagnosed in older dogs, the majority of dogs presenting with clinical disease are young adults. The disease has been diagnosed in dogs as young as a few months of age.
- There is no reported breed predilection although many of the reported cases in the United Kingdom have been in Staffordshire bull terriers.

Major body system examination

On presentation the dog was ambulatory but weak. Cardiovascular examination revealed a heart rate of 135 beats per minute with good peripheral pulses; heart sounds could not be reliably heard. Mucous membranes were pink with a normal capillary refill time. The dog was panting but there was also a notable increase in respiratory effort and lung sounds were diffusely harsh bilaterally. Abdominal palpation was compromised by the dog's size but no obvious abnormalities were detected. Rectal temperature was markedly elevated at 39.8°C but rectal examination was otherwise unremarkable. As much faeces as possible was removed manually at this time for further analysis. No other abnormalities were detected on physical examination. Pulse oximetry was attempted but a reliable measurement could not be obtained. Body weight was 75 kg.

Assessment

The dog was identified as being in respiratory distress and the degree of respiratory noise obscured auscultation of the heart sounds. However, it was not felt appropriate to stop the dog from panting. Systemic perfusion appeared normal on physical examination and it was therefore suspected that the dog's respiratory compromise was more likely to be of primary respiratory rather than cardiac origin. The history of haemoptysis provided further support for this assessment; while coughing is often the result of cardiac disease, haemoptysis would be considered unusual. The elevated rectal temperature could have been the result of both hyperthermia secondary to respiratory distress, especially given the dog's breed, and pyrexia resulting from the underlying disorder.

Emergency database

Flow-by oxygen supplementation was commenced and an intravenous catheter placed into one of the cephalic veins. Blood was collected via the catheter for an emergency database that revealed mild anaemia (manual PCV 32%, reference range 37–55%) with raised serum total solids (80 g/l, reference range 49–71 g/l). Peripheral blood smear evaluation was suggestive of a mildly regenerative anaemia (based on the degree of polychromasia and anisocytosis – see Ch. 3) and showed adequate platelet numbers, a subjective moderate mature neutrophilia and a subjective mild eosinophilia. The regenerative anaemia was suspected to be the result of blood loss, with serum total solids being increased as a result of hyperglobulinaemia, the latter being relatively common in angiostrongylosis. Facilities were not available to measure either clotting times or serum calcium concentration.

While the dog continued to receive oxygen supplementation, a direct faecal smear was examined and found to contain a large number of *Angiostrongylus vasorum* larvae (Figure 33.2). The remainder of the faecal sample was submitted for a Baermann faecal flotation to be performed; this was not to confirm the diagnosis that had already been made, but rather to assess more accurately the severity of the worm burden and provide a means of more reliably monitoring response to therapy.

Case management

A diagnosis of severe parasitic pneumonia secondary to *Angiostrongylus vasorum* infestation was made. As the dog was very amenable, thoracic radiographs were taken following administration of butorphanol (0.2 mg/kg i.v.) with oxygen supplementation throughout and revealed a generalized interstitial to alveolar lung pattern (Figure 33.3). The distribution of the lung changes was considered to be most consistent with parasitic pneumonia.

CLINICAL TIP

- Although there are no pathognomic radiographic changes for *Angiostrongylus vasorum* infection, peripheral and/or multifocal alveolar changes are highly suggestive, especially in a young dog with compatible clinical signs. The distribution of these changes is not a common feature of other causes of alveolar disease (e.g. pulmonary oedema).
- Bronchial thickening is also relatively common in dogs with angiostrongylosis.

The dog was maintained initially on nasal oxygen supplementation using bilateral indwelling nasal oxygen catheters (see Ch. 6). Given the severity of the parasite burden, he was treated with both milbemycin oxime/praziquantel (Milbemax®, Novartis Animal Health, Frimley, UK) at a dose of three tablets (approximately equal to 0.5 mg/kg milbemycin and 125 mg/kg praziquantel) as a single dose once weekly for 4 weeks, and imidacloprid/moxidectin (Advocate Spot-on solution®, Bayer plc, Newbury, UK) as a single dose of 7.5 ml (10 mg/kg imidacloprid and 2.5 mg/kg moxidectin) applied topically. Dexamethasone (0.1 mg/kg i.v. q 24 hr) was also administered for the first few days in an attempt to reduce the pulmonary inflammatory reaction associated with dying *Angiostrongylus vasorum* larvae.

The dog made gradual improvement and was weaned off oxygen supplementation over a period of 48 hours. He was eventually discharged after being hospitalized for 7 days with instructions to keep him strictly rested and to prevent scavenging, and went on to make a full recovery. His owner was advised both regarding on-going prophylaxis once treatment had been completed and with respect to treatment of the other dog in the household due to a high likelihood of infection in that dog as well.

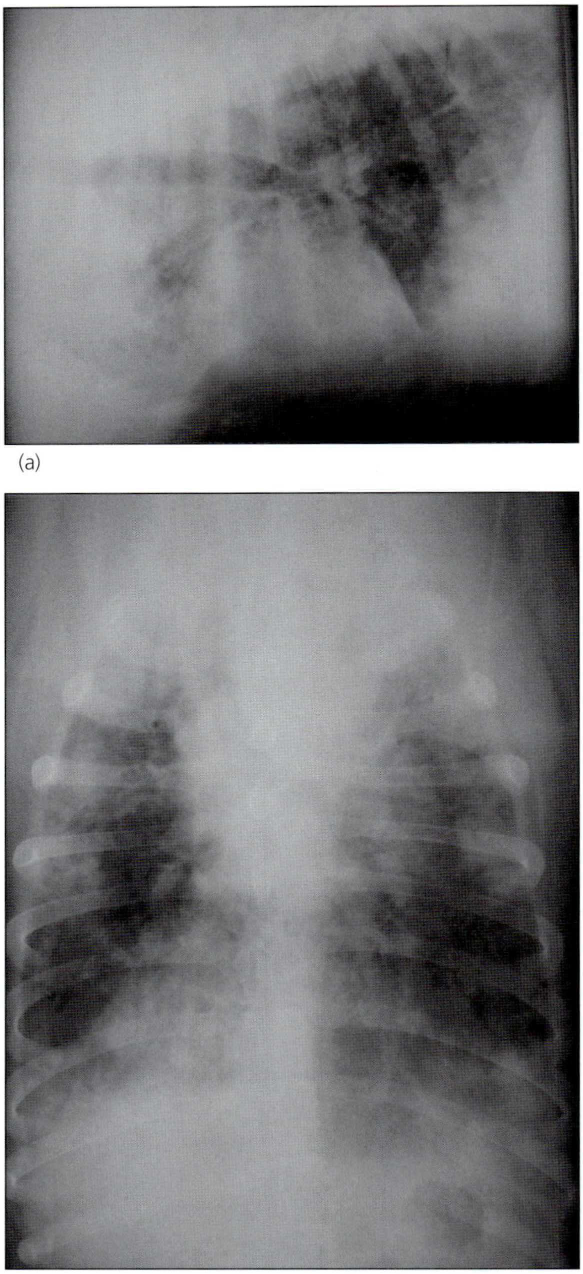

(a)

(b)

Figure 33.3 (a) Right lateral and (b) dorsoventral thoracic radiographs from a dog with *Angiostrongylus vasorum* infection; a generalized interstitial to alveolar lung pattern is present.

CLINICAL TIP

- Until relatively recently there were no licensed veterinary products for treatment of canine *Angiostrongylus vasorum* infection and the off-licence use of fenbendazole was common practice.
- Although licensed for other types of lungworm in dogs and other species, fenbendazole is not licensed at the time of writing for canine *Angiostrongylus vasorum* infection. However, two veterinary products (Milbemax®, Novartis Animal Health; Advocate Spot-on solution®, Bayer plc) are now licensed for the treatment of canine angiostrongylosis in the United Kingdom and should therefore be used instead of fenbendazole in accordance with the cascade for drug prescription.
- The author has on occasion continued to use fenbendazole off-licence with owner consent in dogs with heavy parasite burdens where a satisfactory response to a licensed product was not felt to be achieved.

CLINICAL TIP

- Administration of exogenous glucocorticoids is relatively common practice in the treatment of canine angiostrongylosis. Death of the worms in response to appropriate anthelminthic treatment may cause a temporary worsening of inflammation in affected tissues and associated clinical deterioration. Glucocorticoids are therefore typically administered to dogs in which an inflammatory reaction to the dying worms may be of particular concern – namely those with significant respiratory, neurological or intraocular signs – or in whom a heavy parasite burden is detected regardless of the primary syndrome.
- The author has most commonly administered parenteral dexamethasone (0.1 mg/kg i.v. q 24 hr) for example for 3–5 days, but oral prednisolone (0.7 mg/kg p.o. q 24 hr) has also been used. Longer courses may be required and a decision should be made on an individual case basis.

34 Endocrine emergencies

CANINE PRIMARY HYPOADRENOCORTICISM (ADDISON'S DISEASE)

Theory refresher

The adrenal cortex produces corticosteroid hormones, including mineralocorticoids (primarily aldosterone) and glucocorticoids (primarily cortisol). Naturally occurring primary hypoadrenocorticism in dogs and cats is thought to be the result of immune-mediated destruction of both adrenal cortices and is the focus of this discussion. Secondary adrenocortical failure may also occur, either naturally due to diseases of the brain or as a result of chronic exogenous corticosteroid administration (i.e. iatrogenic causes).

Primary hypoadrenocorticism classically manifests with signs of both mineralocorticoid and glucocorticoid deficiency. Lack of aldosterone results in hyponatraemia (and hypochloraemia) with concurrent extracellular fluid volume depletion. Reduced cardiac output, systemic hypoperfusion and hypotension may ensue as a result of chronic renal fluid loss, acute gastrointestinal fluid loss and inadequate dietary intake. Reduced glomerular filtration rate (GFR) results in prerenal azotaemia. The aetiology of hyperkalaemia in primary hypoadrenocorticism is multifactorial and the most deleterious effects occur on cardiac function.

Cortisol affects almost every tissue in the body, and is significantly involved in haemodynamics and the cardiovascular system, metabolism, inflammation and immunological function, and gastrointestinal integrity. Its production increases during times of physiological stress. Lack of secretion may result in gastrointestinal signs, reduced mentation and activity levels, reduced energy metabolism and fasting hypoglycaemia, and especially impaired tolerance to stress.

Some dogs have atypical primary hypoadrenocorticism with only glucocorticoid insufficiency.

Clinical signs

Clinical signs are nonspecific and variable in both nature and severity. Most dogs are chronically affected. However, owners may not have noticed more subtle abnormalities or may not have considered them significant. Thus some dogs are only presented for veterinary attention when they suffer an acute Addisonian crisis. Clinical signs reported in primary hypoadrenocorticism are listed in Box 34.1. These signs are vague and nonspecific and may also occur in a large number of other disorders. It is therefore essential to keep primary hypoadrenocorticism on the differential diagnosis list for all dogs presenting with any of these signs until a definitive diagnosis is made.

BOX 34.1 *Clinical signs reported in dogs with primary hypoadrenocorticism*

- Depression
- Inappetence/anorexia
- Lethargy
- Vomiting (regurgitation)
- Weight loss
- Weakness, usually episodic
- Diarrhoea (including possible haematochezia or melaena)
- Waxing and waning illness
- Polyuria, polydipsia
- Shaking, shivering or restlessness
- Episodic collapse or syncope
- Abdominal discomfort

Case example 1

PRESENTING SIGNS AND CASE HISTORY

A 4-year-old female neutered bearded collie dog presented with a 3-day history of lethargy that had progressed to noticeable weakness, and occasional vomiting. Her owners reported that her appetite had been variable over the preceding 3 months and that she had had occasional episodes of diarrhoea. No other significant history was reported.

CLINICAL TIP

- Primary hypoadrenocorticism is diagnosed most commonly in young to middle-age female dogs and breeds at increased risk include Poodle breeds, the Great Dane, the West Highland White terrier (and other terrier breeds), the bearded collie and the Rottweiler. Mixed breed dogs are most commonly affected.

Major body system examination

On presentation the dog was ambulatory but depressed. Cardiovascular examination revealed a heart rate of 80 beats per minute with mildly weak femoral pulses and even weaker dorsal pedal pulses. Mucous membranes were pink with a capillary refill time of 2 seconds, and the dog's extremities were cool to the touch. Respiratory examination and abdominal palpation were unremarkable. Rectal temperature was mildly reduced (37.3°C). Electrocardiography was performed and the dog was found to be in sinus rhythm.

Assessment

The dog's cardiovascular examination was suggestive of moderate hypovolaemia and her apparently normal heart rate was therefore considered to be an inappropriate bradycardia. Together with her signalment and history, this finding prompted a very high index of suspicion for hypoadrenocorticism (Addison's disease) with the bradycardia thought to be the result of hyperkalaemia and impaired response to endogenous catecholamines due to glucocorticoid deficiency.

Emergency database

An intravenous catheter was placed in a cephalic vein and blood obtained via the catheter for an emergency database. This revealed remarkable findings of moderate to severe hyponatraemia (128.5 mmol/l, reference range 140.0–153.0 mmol/l), moderate hyperkalaemia (7.0 mmol/l, reference range 3.6–4.6 mmol/l), mild hypoglycaemia (4.0 mmol/l, reference range 4.2–6.6 mmol/l), mild azotaemia (blood urea nitrogen 20 mmol/l, reference range 3–10 mmol/l; creatinine 250 μmol/l, reference range 50–140 μmol/l) and mild hyperphosphataemia (2.90 mmol/l, reference range 0.94–2.13 mmol/l). The sodium to potassium ratio was markedly reduced (18.4 : 1, normal range 27 : 1–40 : 1). Peripheral blood smear examination was considered remarkable due to an absence of a neutrophilia and lack of an obvious lymphopenia (i.e. absence of a stress leucogram); a subjective eosinophilia was not noted.

CLINICAL TIP

- Serum sodium to potassium ratio is often, but not always, reduced in primary hypoadrenocorticism. The majority of dogs presenting in an acute crisis will have electrolyte abnormalities but electrolytes are normal in a small percentage (atypical primary hypoadrenocorticism). Other causes of hyperkalaemia and/or hyponatraemia should also be considered as appropriate (see Ch. 3)
- Hypercalcaemia (typically mild) and hypoalbuminaemia are also reported in some cases.

CLINICAL TIP

- Many dogs with primary hypoadrenocorticism have isosthenuric urine (specific gravity 1.007–1.015). Increased urine specific gravity is usually expected in the face of prerenal azotaemia; however, chronic urinary sodium loss disturbs the normal medullary concentration gradient (renal medullary washout) and therefore impairs water reabsorption.

Although not identified in this case, bone marrow suppression due to hypocortisolism can result in anaemia that may be mild to moderate in severity. A normocytic normochromic non- or minimally regenerative anaemia is identified. However, manual packed cell volume (PCV) at presentation may also be affected by both haemoconcentration (increases PCV) and potentially also gastrointestinal blood loss (decreases PCV).

Case management

CLINICAL TIP

- An acute Addisonian crisis is one of the true canine emergencies with a very real risk of rapid deterioration and death. Death as a result of an acute Addisonian crisis is more likely to be due to hypovolaemia and cardiovascular collapse than the effects of hyperkalaemia. While hyperkalaemia may be common in dogs with Addison's disease, in the author's experience specific intervention beyond fluid therapy (causes dilution and promotes kaliuresis) is rarely indicated.
- Isotonic crystalloid fluid therapy for hypovolaemia is therefore the most important intervention. There is ongoing debate regarding the relative merits of 0.9% sodium chloride (normal, physiological saline) versus buffered lactated Ringer's solution (Hartmann's solution, compound sodium lactate). Ultimately which of these is chosen is likely to be inconsequential in the vast majority of cases and starting fluid therapy is the priority.

The findings of the emergency database strongly supported the suspected diagnosis of classic hypoadrenocorticism. The dog was started on intravenous 0.9% sodium chloride (normal, physiological saline). A conservative bolus of 20 ml/kg was administered over 20 minutes and a constant infusion of 6 ml/kg/hr was then provided. As the dog was clinically stable, an adrenocorticotrophic hormone (ACTH) stimulation test was performed over 1 hour prior to the administration of dexamethasone (0.5 mg/kg i.v. q 6). As hypoglycaemia was only mild, supplementation was not provided.

CLINICAL TIP

- A variety of exogenous glucocorticoid preparations may be used to treat an acute Addisonian crisis. Some authors prefer the use of hydrocortisone or prednisolone as these agents have some mineralocorticoid activity but their clinical superiority over dexamethasone remains controversial.
- Intravenous therapy is essential in these cases and injectable dexamethasone is the most widely available agent in general veterinary practice. There is usually time to perform an ACTH stimulation test prior to glucocorticoid administration but it is noteworthy that dexamethasone is the only routinely used agent that does not react with the cortisol assay, thereby increasing the measured concentration. Dexamethasone can therefore be administered before completion of the test.
- The recommended dose of dexamethasone is 0.5 mg/kg i.v. q 2–6 hr initially and then 0.05–0.1 mg/kg i.v. q 8–12 hr once the patient is stable and until oral medication is possible. Dose recommendations for other glucocorticoid preparations can be found in Appendix 1.

By the following day, the dog's serum potassium concentration was within normal limits and only mild hyponatraemia persisted. The dog had made good clinical progress, becoming noticeably brighter and eating well without vomiting. She was started on oral mineralocorticoid (fludrocortisone 0.01 mg/kg p.o. q 12 hr) and glucocorticoid (prednisolone 0.2 mg/kg p.o. q 24 hr) supplementation and the results of the ACTH stimulation test received subsequently confirmed the suspected diagnosis (cortisol concentration both prior to and following administration of synthetic adrenocorticotrophin was less than 27.6 nmol/l).

The dog was discharged 3 days after initial presentation on oral medication as above. A good deal of time was spent educating the owner on the disease, including provision of a client education leaflet, and a comprehensive plan for on-going management was agreed. The owner was advised that the dog had a good prognosis with normal life expectancy as long as lifelong appropriate management was provided.

CLINICAL TIP

- Thoracic radiography was not performed in the case described here. Changes secondary to severe hypovolaemia (especially microcardia and narrowed caudal vena cava) are relatively common in dogs presenting in an acute Addisonian crisis. However, these findings are not specific to this disorder and may also result from other causes of hypovolaemia.
- Megaoesophagus is occasionally identified and resolves quickly with stabilization. The exact pathogenesis remains unclear but may be related to muscle weakness.

FELINE PRIMARY HYPOADRENOCORTICISM

Both primary and secondary hypoadrenocorticism are considered rare in cats. Clinical signs and physical examination findings are nonspecific, and clinico-pathological findings are similar to those in dogs. An acute crisis is managed in the same way as it is in dogs; however, as is often the case, cats tend to take longer to show noticeable clinical improvement (3–5 days in cats versus a matter of hours often in dogs).

DIABETIC KETOACIDOSIS (DKA)

Theory refresher

Diabetes mellitus is due to relative or absolute insulin deficiency and results in persistent fasting hyperglycaemia and glucosuria. Lack of insulin means that tissues are unable to take up glucose and are therefore in a state of glucose deficiency. Ketone bodies (acetoacetate, β-hydroxybutyrate and acetone) are derived from hepatic oxidation of free fatty acids and used as an energy source by multiple tissues during periods of glucose deficiency. However, excessive ketone body production, as occurs in uncontrolled diabetes mellitus, results in hyperketonaemia, ketosis and metabolic acidosis. In addition to insulin deficiency and resistance, counter-regulatory hormones (e.g. adrenaline (epinephrine), noradrenaline (norepinephrine), glucagon, cortisol) may also play a role in the pathogenesis.

There is a spectrum from ketonuric animals that are otherwise relatively well, appetent and without metabolic acidosis (diabetic ketosis) to those with severe metabolic acidosis and signs of systemic illness (diabetic ketoacidosis (DKA)). The majority of dogs and especially cats with diabetic ketosis or ketoacidosis have another concurrent disorder (Box 34.2) that may potentially increase counter-regulatory hormone production in addition to other associated adverse effects. DKA is diagnosed most often in middle-aged to older male cats and female dogs.

BOX 34.2 Common concurrent disorders in small animals with diabetic ketoacidosis

- Acute/chronic pancreatitis
- Bacterial infection – especially urinary tract infection
- Viral infection (cats)
- Hepatic lipidosis (cats)
- Cholangiohepatitis (especially cats)
- Chronic renal insufficiency
- Other endocrine disorders – hyperadrenocorticism (especially dogs); hypothyroidism (dogs); dioestrus; acromegaly (cats)
- Exogenous glucocorticoid administration
- Neoplasia
- Pyometra

Obligatory osmotic diuresis, excessive renal and gastrointestinal water and electrolyte loss, severe metabolic acidosis, hyperosmolality, and dehydration and hypovolaemia are characteristic of DKA.

Treatment considerations

DKA is most often diagnosed in animals without a prior diagnosis of diabetes mellitus. These animals will have either been subclinical for the diabetes mellitus or tolerating their clinical signs until clinical decompensation occurs as a result of another disorder. Mortality is often related to the presence, nature and severity of a concurrent disorder.

The importance of having a very thorough and informed conversation with owners cannot be stressed enough following a diagnosis of DKA. Owners need to be made aware of the intensive and often prolonged management required in trying to stabilize patients with DKA. The clinical course can be highly unpredictable depending on the concurrent disorder and the cost implications of the management required should be stressed. Assuming it is possible to stabilize the patient, owners also need to be willing and able to provide lifelong care for a pet with diabetes mellitus, and again the practical and cost implications of this should be discussed, along with the possibility of recurrence of DKA; recurrence is more common in cats.

Animals with DKA require very comprehensive and intensive management and monitoring. These animals often have multiple metabolic, electrolyte and acid–base abnormalities, and frequently require not only insulin administration but also glucose, potassium and phosphorus supplementation. Multiple blood samples are required for regular monitoring and the use of a central venous catheter is often preferable both for patient welfare and ease of sampling. Prolonged inappetence is common and feeding tube placement may be necessary. Finally, extensive investigations may be required to identify any concurrent disorder(s).

With all of this in mind, the author is of the opinion that if finances allow, these cases should be referred for specialist care once the diagnosis is made. In the author's experience, it can end up costing much more in terms of both patient welfare and financial expenses by attempting to manage these cases without adequate facilities or expertise and then having to refer due to poor response to treatment.

Animals with diabetic ketosis that remain relatively well and appetent require less intensive management than those with DKA and may be satisfactorily managed without referral. The reader is directed to other texts for information regarding the management of these cases.

Case example 2

PRESENTING SIGNS AND CASE HISTORY

A 7-year-old male entire Miniature Doberman Pinscher dog presented with a several day history of vomiting, polyuria/polydipsia, anorexia and progressive weight loss. He had also started to tremble on the day of presentation. No other significant history was reported.

Major body system examination

On presentation the dog was ambulatory but markedly depressed. Cardiovascular examination revealed a heart rate of 160 beats per minute with no murmur heard. Femoral pulses were mildly hyperdynamic and dorsal pedal pulses were readily palpable; no pulse deficits were detected. Mucous membranes were pinker than normal with a capillary refill time of 1 second. The dog was panting but respiratory examination was appropriate for the rate and effort. Mild discomfort was detected on abdominal palpation and the urinary bladder was found to be small. The dog was mildly pyrexic (rectal temperature 39.4°C). Severe dehydration (estimated at 10%) was suspected on the basis of very dry oral mucous membranes and severely reduced skin turgor.

Assessment

The dog was assessed as being mildly hypovolaemic which was suspected predominantly to be the result of severe dehydration. The tachycardia was likely to be multifactorial in origin, representing a combination of hypovolaemia, pyrexia and abdominal discomfort.

Emergency database

An intravenous catheter was placed in a cephalic vein and blood obtained via the catheter for an emergency database that showed a number of abnormalities. Manual PCV was 39% (reference range 37–55%); however, plasma total solids (TS) were significantly elevated (85 g/l, reference range 49–71 g/l). It was therefore suspected that the dog was anaemic but PCV was increased at presentation due to haemoconcentration. The dog was also found to be severely hyperglycaemic (blood glucose 29.6 mmol/l, reference range 4.20–6.60 mmol/l). The serum from one of the haematocrit tubes filled for PCV/TS measurement was therefore used to measure serum ketones (see Ch. 3) with a urine dipstick and was found to be strongly positive.

Mild to moderate azotaemia was identified (blood urea nitrogen 25 mmol/l, reference range 3–10 mmol/l; creatinine 300 μmol/l, reference range 50–140 μmol/l) that was suspected to be predominantly prerenal in origin. Serum electrolytes were included in the emergency database and the dog was found to be moderately hyponatraemic (132.0 mmol/l, reference range 140.0–153.0 mmol/l) before correction for glucose (Box 34.3) with a mild corrected hypochloraemia. Serum potassium concentration was within the normal range at presentation. Peripheral blood smear examination revealed a neutrophilic degenerate left shift (i.e. increased number of band neutrophils despite a subjectively normal total neutrophil count) and no obvious red blood cell regeneration. A serum SNAP® cPL™ Test (Idexx Reference Laboratories, Wetherby, UK) was performed to measure canine pancreas-specific lipase and found to be abnormal, suggesting acute pancreatitis.

A urine sample was obtained prior to commencing fluid therapy via urethral catheterization performed using aseptic technique. Dipstick analysis revealed

BOX 34.3 Sodium in diabetic ketoacidosis

For several reasons, total body sodium content is almost always decreased in patients with DKA; however, serum sodium concentration is not representative of total body sodium.

In addition, insulin deficiency causes poor cellular uptake of glucose leading to increased extracellular (i.e. interstitial and intravascular) glucose concentration. This creates a transcellular osmotic gradient such that water moves out of the cells and causes a decrease in intravascular sodium concentration (pseudohyponatraemia). In general, for each 3.4 mmol/l increase in blood glucose concentration above the reference range, serum sodium concentration decreases by 1.0 mmol/l. Therefore, the corrected serum sodium concentration in this case example (Case example 2) was 132.0 + ((29.6 – 6.6)/3.4) = 138.7 mmol/l.

marked glucosuria and ketonuria, mild proteinuria and no haematuria. Urine specific gravity was found to be 1.060. Significant glucosuria will increase urine specific gravity measured using a refractometer (4+ glucosuria on dipstick analysis approximately increases specific gravity by 0.008 to 0.010) but even after correction for glucosuria, the specific gravity was still considered to be increased. This was consistent with prerenal azotaemia. Urinary sediment was considered benign but the sample was submitted for microbiology.

CLINICAL TIP

- Ideally urine specific gravity is measured prior to starting fluid therapy but fluid therapy should not be withheld if a urine sample cannot be obtained quickly – commencing treatment is the priority and urine output should increase as hypovolaemia and dehydration are corrected.

Case management

On the basis of the information available a diagnosis of DKA with acute pancreatitis was made. The dog was given a 10 ml/kg bolus of buffered lactate Ringer's solution over 30 minutes and the rate then reduced to 6 ml/kg/hr to correct dehydration over 24 hr. Buprenorphine (0.02 mg/kg i.v. q 6 hr) was also administered.

CLINICAL TIP

- Isotonic crystalloid fluid therapy is very much the first priority in the management of patients with diabetic ketoacidosis. Although insulin administration is ultimately essential, it should not be commenced until hypovolaemia is treated and preferably rehydration has been on-going for a period for time. Fluid therapy increases glomerular filtration rate and may therefore significantly reduce blood glucose concentration.
- It is not uncommon for insulin therapy to be withheld for several hours (2–6 hr) in appropriate cases. The choice of isotonic crystalloid is unlikely to make any significant difference clinically.

A lengthy discussion was had with the dog's owner about the diagnosis that had been made and the implications both in terms of short- and long-term management. The owner was both willing and felt able to provide lifelong management for the dog's diabetes mellitus and given the need for 24-hour intensive care and frequent monitoring, it was decided to refer the dog for specialist care shortly after presentation.

IATROGENIC HYPOCALCAEMIA FOLLOWING BILATERAL THYROIDECTOMY

Hypoparathyroidism is the most significant postoperative complication associated with bilateral thyroidectomy. It occurs if the parathyroid glands are either devascularized, or accidentally injured or removed. Mild postoperative hypocalcaemia is common following bilateral thyroidectomy but emergency treatment may be required if the cat becomes symptomatic.

CLINICAL TIP

- Maintenance of normal calcium homeostasis typically returns, although it can take several days to months. This may be through recovery of parathyroid function or via nonparathyroid hormone-related mechanisms.

BOX 34.4 Treatment of hypocalcaemia

Acute therapy

Calcium gluconate 10% solution (100 mg calcium gluconate/ml, approximately 9 mg elemental calcium/ml): give 0.5–1.5 ml/kg i.v. bolus over 5–20 minutes, repeat until signs resolve

- Equivalent to 50–150 mg calcium gluconate/kg (or 4.5–13.4 mg elemental calcium/kg)
- Monitor for bradycardia; electrocardiogram monitoring recommended

Subacute therapy

Calcium gluconate 10% solution: administer 0.3–0.6 ml/kg/hr constant rate infusion (CRI)

- Equivalent to 30–60 mg calcium gluconate/kg/hr (or 2.7–5.4 mg elemental calcium/kg/hr)
- Dilute with 0.9% sodium chloride (normal, physiological saline); using buffered lactated Ringer's solution for dilution may result in calcium precipitation

Chronic oral therapy

Calcium: 15–100 mg elemental calcium/kg q 24 hr (typically divided into 2–4 equal doses)

- Usually tapered while continuing with more long-term vitamin D therapy
- Calcium carbonate is preferred as it contains the highest concentration of elemental calcium, so reducing the number of tablets to be administered

Vitamin D

- Dihydrotachysterol: 0.01–0.03 mg/kg p.o. q 24–48 hr
- Alfacalcidol: 0.01–0.05 μg/kg p.o. q 24 hr
- Calcitriol: 0.01–0.03 μg/kg p.o. q 24 hr

Notes:

Serum calcium concentration should be monitored daily initially during hospitalization or more frequently as dictated by clinical status.

Calcium chloride can be used instead of calcium gluconate but carries a greater risk of significant tissue irritation if administered perivascularly and is therefore not preferred.

1 mg elemental calcium is equivalent to 11.2 mg calcium gluconate, 7.7 mg calcium lactate and 2.5 mg calcium carbonate.

Hypocalcaemia develops within 1–5 days following surgery and associated clinical signs may include anorexia, weakness, depression, vocalization, nervous/restless/aggressive behaviour, facial rubbing, ataxia, stiffness, muscle twitching or tremors, tetany and generalized seizures. Third eyelid prolapse may occur in cats and cardiovascular abnormalities may also be identified.

In the blood, calcium is found in three forms: ionized, protein bound and complexed (e.g. with phosphate, bicarbonate). Ionized calcium is the biologically active form and cats showing signs of hypocalcaemia will have reduced ionized calcium concentration. Clinical signs do not occur if ionized calcium concentration is normal. However, measurement of total rather than ionized calcium is more widely available. A correction formula involving albumin for conversion of total calcium to ionized calcium is no longer recommended for use and is definitely not valid in cats. Although total calcium may not reliably correlate with ionized calcium concentration, in a cat with appropriate clinical signs and measured total hypocalcaemia following bilateral thyroidectomy, it is reasonable to assume that ionized calcium will also be reduced and to instigate treatment immediately (Box 34.4). The severity of clinical signs should dictate the aggressiveness of the treatment provided.

35 Ocular emergencies

Ocular emergencies are relatively common and represent some of the conditions with which many clinicians are both least familiar and confident. Serious ocular disorders should be treated as true emergencies as delayed management may in some cases result in permanent loss of vision or of an eye; many of the emergency conditions are also associated with pain that is often severe and must be addressed as quickly as possible. Referral to a more highly qualified ophthalmologist is appropriate in many instances and part of the role of the primary clinician is to differentiate the cases that require urgent referral from those in which more delayed referral may be acceptable. The primary clinician should be familiar with appropriate stabilization and early treatment that may be required prior to referral.

CLINICAL TIP

- In the author's experience, it can be difficult to arrange emergency referral to an ophthalmologist in the evenings and on weekends. However, a number are happy to provide telephone advice and this may be facilitated to an extent by making use of increasingly available technologies to send high quality photographs.
- Ophthalmology is one of the medical disciplines where being practised at performing thorough examinations, having confidence in one's findings, and having access to adequate resources to refer to is essential.

CLINICAL TIP

- Many ocular emergencies are traumatic in origin. As always, it is essential to examine and stabilize the major body systems first before concentrating on the injured eye(s) (see Ch. 1). In particular, traumatic ocular injuries may be associated with significant additional head trauma and intracranial hypertension (see Ch. 28).
- Many animals with severe ocular injuries require sedation or general anaesthesia for proper examination and possible surgical intervention. These animals must be stabilized first, even if this requires a delay of 24–48 hours (or more); while delayed management of the eye may result in loss of vision or of the eye, inadequate stabilization of severe abnormalities of the major body systems may result in death.
- Topical anaesthesia can greatly facilitate conscious examination in some cases and suitable noninvasive interim measures (such as topical lubrication and antibiosis) should be implemented for the eye as appropriate.

An extensive discussion of the common ocular emergencies is beyond the scope of this book and the reader is referred to other more authoritative texts, including the ophthalmology book in this series. A summary of the findings and treatment for common ocular emergencies is provided in Table 35.1 and use of an Elizabethan collar is typically indicated.

Table 35.1 Summary of findings and treatment for common ocular emergencies

Disorder	Cause(s)	Examination findings	Emergency treatment and comments
Acute anterior uveitis	Traumatic injury Systemic infectious disease Lens-induced (cataract, luxation) Immune-mediated Neoplasia (e.g. lymphoma) Idiopathic	Painful red eye Miotic pupil (iridocyclospasm) Aqueous flare (causes loss of clarity of anterior chamber) Conjunctival hyperaemia Scleral or episcleral vascular congestion Abnormal iris ± Loss of vision ± Hypopyon, hyphaema Reduced IOP (<10 mmHg)	*Topical*: Corticosteroid (anti-inflammatory) Atropine (mydriatic, cycloplegic) Antibiosis *Systemic*: Possible corticosteroid or NSAIA Opioid if required Treatment of underlying cause if identified
Acute conjunctivitis	Allergic (especially dogs) Infectious disease (usual cause in cats) Keratoconjunctivitis sicca (KCS) in dogs Foreign body (e.g. grass awn, seed)	Red eye, variably painful Conjunctival hyperaemia Chemosis (conjunctival oedema) Ocular discharge No loss of vision Reduced STT in KCS	Topical: Corticosteroids if no ulceration and infection not suspected (therefore typically contraindicated in cats) Antibiosis (cover chlamydial infection in cats) Possible antiviral therapy (cats) Ciclosporin and artificial tears for KCS
Acute glaucoma	*Primary* (e.g. Cocker Spaniels, Basset Hound, Beagle) *Secondary* (especially cats): Anterior uveitis Lens luxation (e.g. terrier breeds) Cataract Hyphaema Intraocular neoplasia	Painful red eye Mydriatic nonresponsive pupil Corneal opacity Conjunctival hyperaemia Scleral or episcleral vascular congestion Iris normal Loss of vision Raised IOP (usually > 40 mmHg)	Rapid reduction of IOP essential to prevent permanent loss of vision *Systemic*: Intravenous mannitol Opioid analgesia *Topical*: Prostaglandin analogue (e.g. latanoprost) Carbonic anhydrase inhibitor (e.g. dorzolamide)
Corneal foreign body	e.g. plant material, wood or paint chips	Visible foreign body plus signs of irritation and inflammation	*Superficial*: Topical anaesthesia; gentle copious sterile saline lavage to try to dislodge ± lift off using 25-gauge needle or cotton-tipped applicator; corneal ulcer treatment once removed *Deep or full thickness*: Referral
Corneal laceration	Traumatic injury (especially cat scratch) Foreign body	Laceration surrounded by corneal oedema May be difficult to identify laceration if significant corneal oedema or hyphaema	Medical therapy if partial thickness *Topical*: Antibiosis Atropine if miosis Referral for surgery if deep or full thickness Injury to anterior lens capsule and leakage of lens material may trigger severe uveitis

Table 35.1 continued

Disorder	Cause(s)	Examination findings	Emergency treatment and comments
Corneal ulcer – superficial	Traumatic injury Infectious disease Topical irritation Exposure keratitis Keratoconjunctivitis sicca (KCS) Foreign body Entropion	Painful eye Conjunctival hyperaemia Ocular discharge (likely epiphora) Corneal oedema Miotic pupil (reflex uveitis) Fluorescein positive	*Topical*: Antibiosis Atropine if miosis Topical corticosteroid contraindicated (delay ulcer healing) *Surgical*: Cotton-tipped applicator debridement ± keratotomy (grid or punctuate) in dogs with indolent (nonhealing) superficial ulcer Referral for conjunctival graft (not third eyelid flap) for deeper noninfected stromal ulcer
Corneal ulcer – infected stromal (deep)	As for superficial ulcer	As for superficial ulcer but discharge may be mucopurulent Yellow-white stromal infiltrate seen around ulcer	*Topical*: Aggressive antibiosis – especially with fluoroquinolone against possible *Pseudomonas* infection Atropine Collagenase inhibitor (autologous serum, acetylcysteine) if rapidly progressive (melting ulcer) *Systemic*: NSAIA Opioid if required May perforate rapidly (see below) Surgery if progresses despite aggressive medical therapy
Corneal ulcer – descemetocele	As for superficial ulcer	As for deep infected stromal ulcer but Descemet's membrane is exposed and bulging forward; it does not retain fluorescein so typically see a corneal ulcer with a dark centre surrounded by a fluorescein-positive rim	Emergency referral for surgery; aggressive medical therapy as for infected stromal ulcer in interim but only if good compliance NB. Cage rest and minimal restraint or neck pressure (increasing IOP may induce corneal rupture)
Corneal ulcer – perforation	As for superficial ulcer	Painful eye Corneal oedema Misshapen cornea Misshapen pupil Possible fibrin clot over corneal defect (pink or red tissue) Possible iris prolapse	Emergency referral for surgery Otherwise as for infected stromal ulcer plus systemic antibiosis NB. Cage rest, minimal restraint, gentle handling
Hyphaema	Traumatic injury Uveitis Glaucoma Coagulopathy (e.g. thrombocytopenia, angiostrongylosis) Neoplasia Systemic hypertension Retinal detachment	Blood in anterior chamber ± painful eye Variable IOP	May be only sign of systemic coagulopathy Treatment of underlying cause; blood should reabsorb May require treatment for secondary uveitis

Continued

Table 35.1 continued

Disorder	Cause(s)	Examination findings	Emergency treatment and comments
Primary anterior lens luxation	Hereditary condition	Painful eye Epiphora Corneal oedema Consistent with secondary glaucoma or anterior uveitis Edge of lens may be visible	Treatment for glaucoma if indicated Referral for emergency surgery
Proptosis	Traumatic injury, especially in brachycephalic dogs	Forward displacement of globe outside orbital socket and entrapment of eyelids Encouraging signs with respect to sight preservation include consensual pupillary light reflex, miotic pupil and positive menace response	Stabilization of major body systems including intracranial hypertension first; topical sterile eye lubrication (q 1–2 hr) and antibiosis in interim General anaesthesia for globe replacement and tarsorrhaphy (or enucleation if injury too severe); postoperative topical and oral antibiosis, topical atropine, short course of corticosteroid

IOP, intraocular pressure, NSAIA, nonsteroidal antiinflammatory agent; STT, Schirmer tear test.
Normal IOP in dogs (and cats) is 15–25 mmHg. Normal STT in dogs is > 15 mm/min (wide variability in cats).

36 Urinary tract emergencies

URETHRAL OBSTRUCTION

FELINE

Theory refresher

Clinical signs associated with the lower urinary tract – in particular dysuria, stranguria, pollakiuria and haematuria – are a common reason for cats to be presented both as routine and emergency patients. Lower urinary tract disorders include urolithiasis, feline idiopathic cystitis, urinary tract infection, anatomical defects, behavioural disorders and neoplasia. An increased risk of lower urinary tract disease has been reported for example in cats confined indoors and those restricted to dry food diets with inadequate fluid intake, and signs are most commonly seen in 2- to 6-year-old cats.

Depending on the underlying disorder, complete urethral obstruction may or may not occur and this clearly has significant implications from an emergency perspective. Complete urethral obstruction almost exclusively occurs in male cats and is a potentially fatal condition (see below). Cats presenting with lower urinary tract signs but without obstruction usually have a small or empty bladder and require symptomatic medical therapy, analgesia in particular. Many of these cats will have idiopathic cystitis and will improve within 3–5 days. All these cats require appropriate analgesia but antibiosis should only be used in cases in which bacterial infection is documented by microbiology.

CLINICAL TIP

- Lower urinary tract signs typically suggest a degree of inflammation of the lower urinary tract with associated irritation and discomfort. However, it must be remembered that only a small proportion of cats with lower urinary tract signs have either a primary or a secondary infectious process and the empirical use of antibiosis is strongly discouraged. Antibiosis should ideally be administered only on the basis of confirmed infection and the choice of agent should be directed by sensitivity testing.

NURSING ASPECT

On an emergency basis, nurses are often the first members of staff to speak to owners ringing about cats with lower urinary tract signs. In the author's opinion, emergency consultation should be recommended for all cats showing dysuria, stranguria, pollakiuria or haematuria. Male cats in particular may have urethral obstruction which can be rapidly fatal. Both unobstructed male and female cats require analgesia as a minimum as these clinical signs are typically associated with varying degrees of pain.

In some cases of urethral obstruction owners report that their cat is straining nonproductively but are unable to distinguish stranguria from constipation. It is also noteworthy that not all cats with urethral obstruction show consistent urinary signs, at least earlier on. In some cases, owners ring to report an abnormal pelvic limb gait that is often presumed to be the result of trauma; alternatively, the cat may be showing nonspecific vocalization or apparent discomfort, especially when picked up. There is therefore perhaps an argument to examine all male cats with potentially compatible signs of obstruction. As a minimum, the author would strongly recommend examining all male cats with potential signs of obstruction that either have a history of lower urinary tract disease or that are confined indoors (at increased risk of urethral obstruction).

Mechanical urethral obstruction is much more common in male cats due to the narrow diameter of the penile urethra; it occurs very infrequently in females. Urethral plugs are the most common cause in male cats but uroliths may also cause obstruction, potentially in combination with a plug. Urethral strictures and rarely tumours are other possible causes. Urethral plugs are often made up of struvite material in a proteinaceous matrix. The most common uroliths in cats are made of struvite or calcium oxalate. Unlike in dogs, struvite urolithiasis in cats is not typically associated with urease-producing bacterial infection.

Prolonged urethral obstruction results in hypovolaemia and systemic hypoperfusion that may occur for a number of reasons, including the effect of hyperkalaemia and acidaemia on the cardiovascular system, and dehydration where this is a factor. In addition to azotaemia, urethral obstruction can result in profound electrolyte and acid–base disturbances including metabolic acidosis, hyperphosphataemia and hypocalcaemia. Hyperkalaemia occurs mainly due to impaired urinary excretion of potassium. The clinical manifestations of hyperkalaemia reflect alterations in cell membrane excitability and of greatest concern are the potentially life-threatening effects on cardiac conduction (Box 36.1).

BOX 36.1 Electrocardiographic findings associated with hyperkalaemia

- Sinus bradycardia (Figure 36.1)
- Prolongation of the PR interval
- Widening and bizarre appearance of the QRS complex, including sinoventricular rhythm
- Decreased amplitude, widening or complete absence (atrial standstill) of the P wave (Figures 36.2 and 36.3)
- Peaked/tall T waves (Figures 36.2 and 36.3)

CLINICAL TIP

- The severity of clinical signs resulting from hyperkalaemia does not necessarily correlate with the absolute increase in serum potassium concentration. The treatment required is therefore dependent not only on the cat's serum potassium level but also, very importantly, on whether the hyperkalaemia is assessed to be clinically significant.

Continued

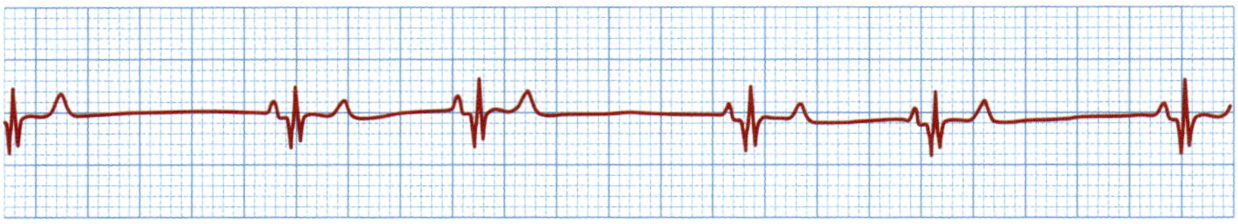

Figure 36.1 Sinus bradycardia in a cat. (Courtesy of Virginia Luis Fuentes)

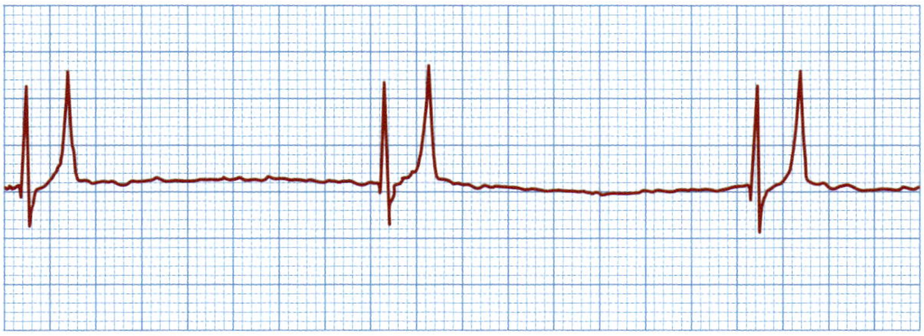

Figure 36.2 Atrial standstill in a cat with hyperkalaemia showing absence of P waves; peaked T waves are also present. (From Darke PGG, Bonagura JD, Kelly DK 1996 Color atlas of veterinary cardiology. Mosby-Wolfe, London, with permission.)

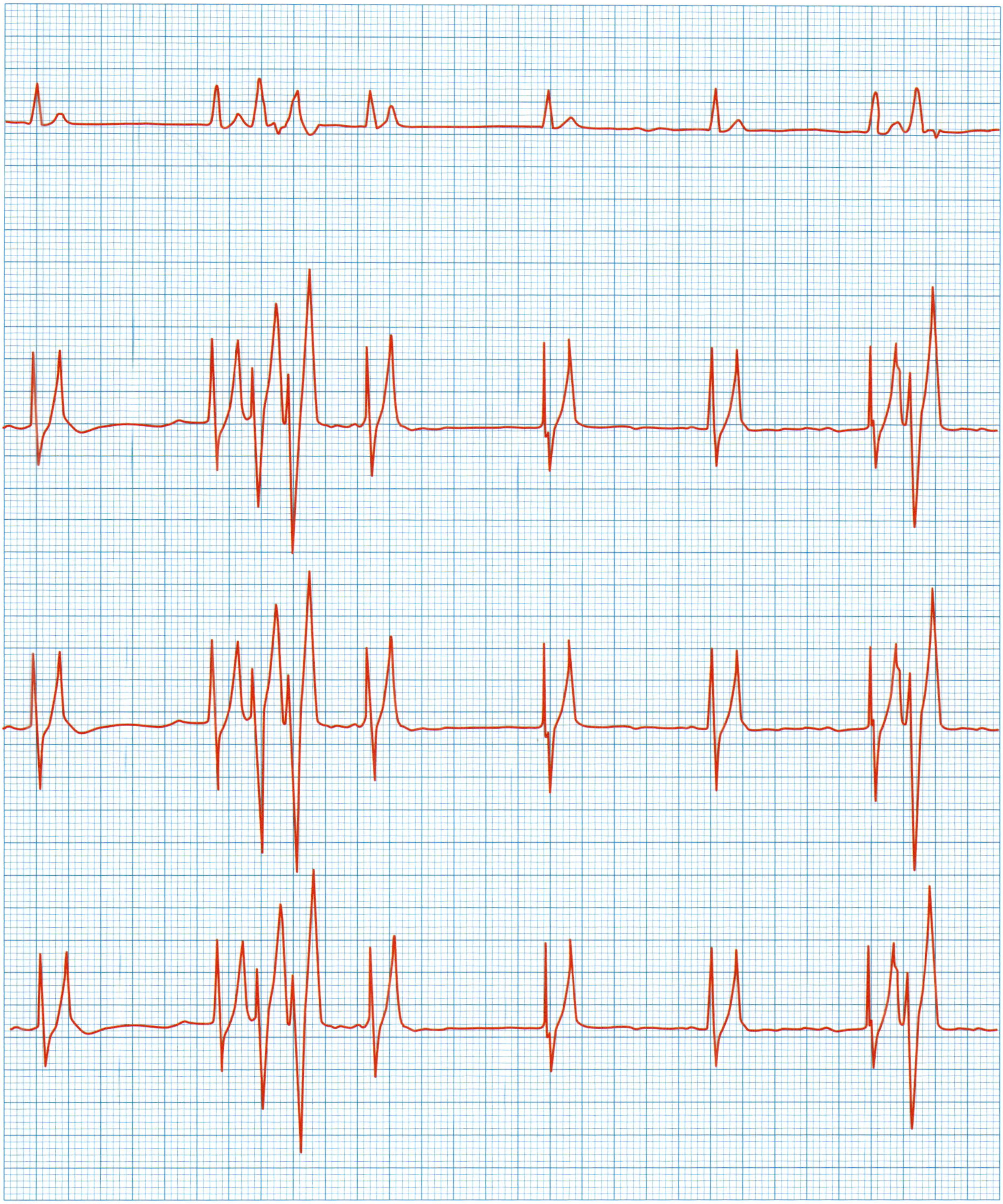

(a)

Figure 36.3 Electrocardiogram from a cat with severe hyperkalaemia (a) before and (b) shortly after administration of calcium gluconate. The pre-treatment strip shows atrial standstill with absence of P waves, as well as peaked T waves and ventricular premature complexes (VPCs). P waves are visible and there are no VPCs in the post-treatment strip.

Continued

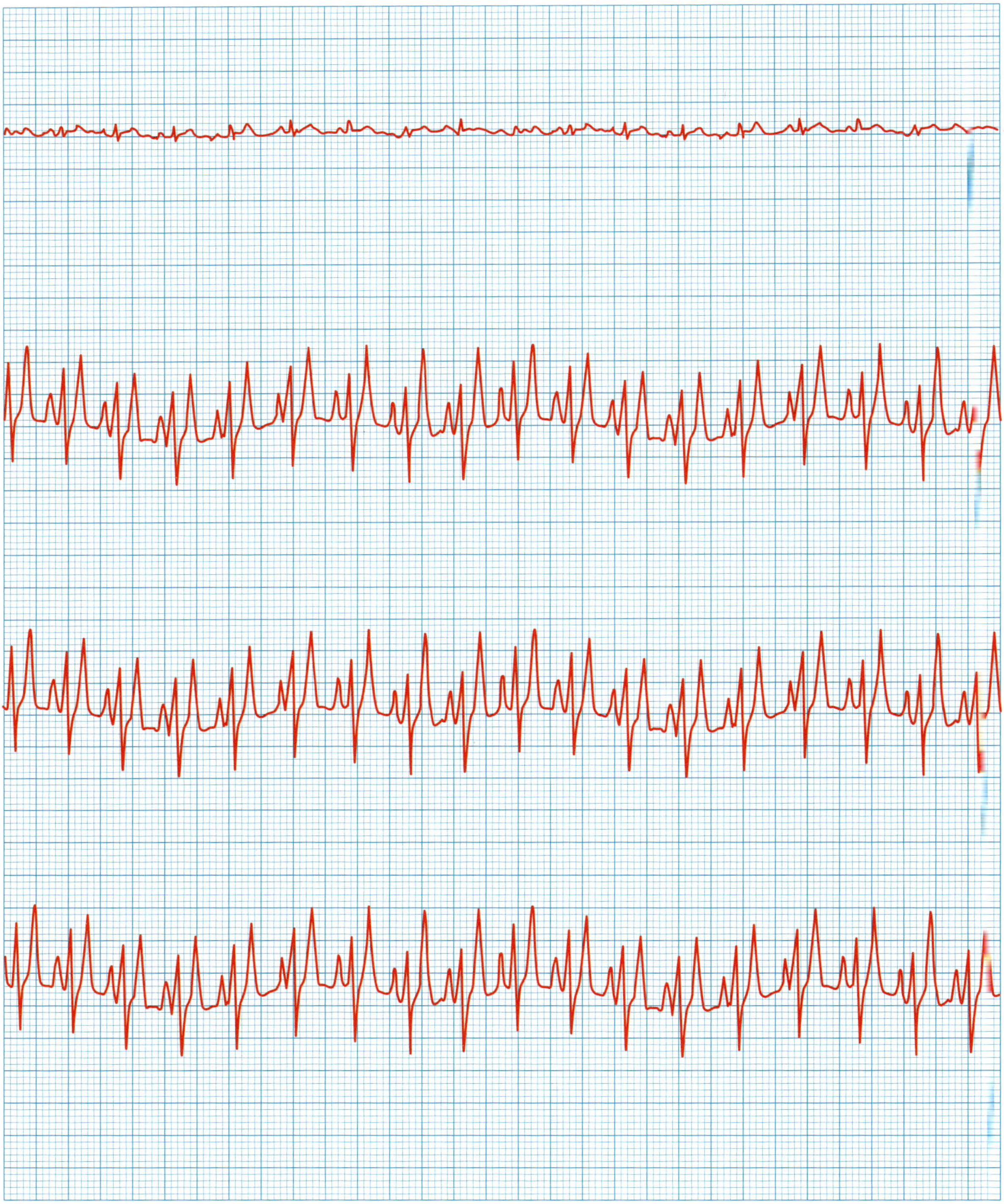

(b)

Figure 36.3 continued

CLINICAL TIP—cont'd

- If treatment is deemed necessary, it should be performed before urethral catheterization is attempted; treatment is directed at improving the cat's clinical status and not at the serum potassium concentration per se. In some cases, intravenous fluid therapy and restoring urine production and drainage is all that is necessary for hyperkalaemia to resolve. However additional therapy is required in cases in which hyperkalaemia is assessed to be having clinically significant effects on the cardiovascular system. Further treatment options for hyperkalaemia are summarized in Table 36.1.
- If serum electrolytes cannot be measured but clinically significant hyperkalaemia is suspected on the basis of electrocardiography or perhaps physical examination alone, the author firmly believes that empirical use of calcium gluconate, and potentially insulin with glucose, is appropriate. This treatment can be life-saving and is unlikely to cause any significant harm if not required.

Cats with urethral obstruction present with a spectrum of clinical compromise and, as always, the management provided should be appropriate to the individual case. With rational intensive management, even the most moribund of patients has an excellent prognosis for full short-term recovery. Long-term prognosis clearly depends on the underlying urinary tract disorder.

Case example 1

PRESENTING SIGNS AND CASE HISTORY

A 4-year-old male neutered domestic short hair cat presented collapsed. The owner reported that the cat may have been lethargic 24 hours prior to presentation and was inappetent on the morning of presentation. The owner was at work during the day and had returned to find the cat collapsed, at which point she contacted the practice for an emergency consultation. The cat had outdoor access and the owner had not noticed any clinical signs of lower urinary tract disease. No other significant preceding history was reported.

Major body system examination

On presentation the cat was obtunded. Cardiovascular examination revealed a heart rate of 60 beats per minute with no obvious murmur. Femoral pulses could not be

Table 36.1 Treatment of clinically significant hyperkalaemia

Agent	Dose/route	Comments
10% calcium gluconate	0.5–1.0 ml/kg i.v. bolus over 30–60 s	Rapid onset of action (can be a few seconds) and first line choice in a crisis Short duration of action (often 10–15 minutes) Monitor ECG during administration Does not lower serum potassium concentration but restores normal cell membrane excitability Will also address possible ionized hypocalcaemia Bolus can be repeated while other measures are used to reduce hyperkalaemia directly
Neutral (regular, soluble) insulin	0.1–0.5 IU/kg i.v.	Slower onset of action (can be more than 15 minutes)
Glucose solution	0.25–0.5 g/kg i.v.	Lowers serum potassium concentration by moving potassium into cells Intravenous glucose supplementation typically required for several hours (monitor and adjust accordingly)
Sodium bicarbonate	1–2 mmol/kg slow i.v. (repeat if necessary)	Also lowers serum potassium concentration by moving potassium into cells Effect can persist for several hours Access to on-site acid–base analyser much preferred

ECG, electrocardiogram; IU, international units; i.v., intravenous.

palpated and mucous membranes were very pale without a discernible capillary refill. Respiratory rate was 36 breaths per minute and lung auscultation was unremarkable. Abdominal palpation revealed a moderate to large rigid bladder, and rectal temperature was markedly lowered (33.0°C).

CLINICAL TIP

- Although rare, urinary bladder rupture may occur due to urethral obstruction and therefore the absence of a palpable bladder does not exclude this condition. Cats with urethral obstruction and bladder rupture are very likely to be moribund and severely azotaemic.

Assessment The cat was assessed as being severely hypovolaemic. While severely hypovolaemic cats are very often bradycardic and hypothermic, the degree of bradycardia in this case was inappropriately severe. Bladder palpation was suggestive of urethral obstruction and the severity of bradycardia was therefore suspected to be partly due to hyperkalaemia.

Emergency database

An intravenous catheter was placed in a cephalic vein and blood obtained via the catheter for an emergency database. The most significant findings of this were severe hyperkalaemia (10.1 mmol/l, reference range 3.6–4.6 mmol/l) and severe azotaemia (blood urea nitrogen 80.0 mmol/l, reference range 3.0–10.0 mmol/l; creatinine 1950 μmol/l, reference range 50–140 μmol/l). Facilities were not available to measure blood pH or ionized calcium.

Continuous electrocardiography was commenced that demonstrated atrial standstill with a wide-complex sinoventricular rhythm.

CLINICAL TIP

- Urethral obstruction is a major cause of postrenal azotaemia that frequently is (very) severe. However, in most cases the azotaemia fully resolves, often within 24 hours, if the obstruction is relieved so diuresis can occur and adequate fluid therapy is provided.
- Very occasionally, prolonged urethral obstruction and back pressure on the kidneys

CLINICAL TIP—cont'd

may result in sufficient renal injury as to cause a degree of renal azotaemia that may therefore persist long-term. However, in the author's experience this is rare in cats with feline urethral obstruction that are presented for treatment.
- The degree of azotaemia at presentation should not be used as a prognostic indicator and renal insufficiency must not be assumed until full treatment for urethral obstruction has been provided.

Case management

The cat was started on a 20 ml/kg bolus of 0.9% sodium chloride (normal, physiological saline) and treated immediately thereafter with 10% calcium gluconate (see Table 36.1) to which there was a rapid response with respect to heart rate and rhythm (see Figure 36.3). Neutral (regular, soluble) insulin and glucose were administered intravenously at this time. No warming measures were performed initially in order not to worsen hypoperfusion (see Ch. 17) but the cat was given a low dose of methadone (0.1 mg/kg i.v.). Another dose of calcium gluconate was also given, prompted by deterioration of the heart rhythm.

The cat was monitored very closely and continuously reassessed. Perfusion showed some improvement following the initial bolus, after which the cat was assessed to be mildly to moderately hypovolaemic. A further smaller bolus (10 ml/kg) of saline was administered. Serum potassium concentration was rechecked approximately 30 minutes after the initial emergency database and was improving in keeping with clinical progress.

CLINICAL TIP

- All cats with urethral obstruction will benefit from intravenous fluid therapy prior to catheterization. An isotonic replacement crystalloid is the fluid of choice to restore perfusion and enhance urinary potassium excretion. Normal saline (0.9% sodium chloride) has traditionally been recommended due to its lack of potassium. However, this

CLINICAL TIP—cont'd

fluid may contribute to existing metabolic acidosis and there is no clinically significant difference between the use of 0.9% sodium chloride solution and Hartmann's (buffered lactated Ringer's solution) which contains a small amount of potassium. The priority is very much to start the cat on one or other of these solutions at a rate that is appropriate for the degree of hypovolaemia (see Ch. 2).

- One of the concerns often raised with regard to fluid therapy prior to urethral catheterization is that of further filling a bladder that may already be quite distended. However, in cats in need of aggressive fluid therapy, urine production is likely to have decreased significantly and the bladder will be filling extremely slowly (if at all). This is due to the effects of back pressure transmitted from the urethral obstruction to the kidneys via the bladder and ureters. In addition, in a cat without preexisting renal disease, urine output is largely dependent on renal blood flow. In an obstructed cat with hypotension and consequent renal hypoperfusion, urine production may therefore be further compromised. There is little rationale in performing bladder drainage before adequate fluid resuscitation has been instituted.

Stabilization continued in this vain until the cat's clinical condition had markedly improved with a stable cardiovascular system and much more appropriate mentation. The cat was then sedated for urethral catheterization using ketamine (2 mg/kg i.v.), midazolam (0.2 mg/kg i.v.) and a further dose of methadone (0.1 mg/kg i.v.). Intravenous fluid therapy was continued at 6 ml/kg/hr in the interim. A further two boluses of ketamine were required subsequently to complete the procedure. Catheterization was performed using a 5-French MILA® Tomcat urethral catheter (MILA International, inc., Erlanger, Kentucky, USA) (Fig. App2.2) that was connected to a urine collection bag (Closed System Drainage Set (Drainset)®, Infusion Concepts, Halifax, UK) (Figure App2.3) in a closed system (see p. 296).

CLINICAL TIP

- With respect to chemical restraint for urethral catheterization, the author would caution against the use of medetomidine in all but the most stable of cats due to the potential for marked cardiorespiratory side effects.
- The author uses a combination of a pure opioid with ketamine and midazolam to good effect. Being a benzodiazepine, midazolam should promote urethral relaxation which is desirable. Ketamine predominantly undergoes renal excretion in cats and there is therefore the potential for this agent to accumulate in the occasional obstructed cat in which urinary drainage cannot be re-established in the short-term.
- Occasionally additional chemical restraint is required and in such cases propofol, alphaxolone or inhalant anaesthesia can be used. However, it is essential to ensure the patient is as stable as possible before this.

CLINICAL TIP

- Some clinicians prefer to perform cystocentesis very early on in the sickest cats with urethral obstruction in order to provide immediate urine drainage. Cystocentesis is a simple technique to perform, especially in a full bladder, and allows rapid bladder drainage; this can also facilitate urethral catheterization by relieving the pressure on the urethral obstruction in some cases. The procedure also provides uncontaminated urine samples for bacteriology. In a very small proportion of blocked cats, urethral catheterization is unsuccessful and cystocentesis is a convenient option pending further management.
- However, whenever cystocentesis is performed, there is a risk of subsequent urine leakage into the abdomen and uroperitoneum. When cystocentesis is performed on a hard tense bladder, the sudden release of pressure could potentially significantly increase the risk of urine leakage – the effect may be rather like popping a balloon. In addition, the integrity of the

Continued

CLINICAL TIP—cont'd

bladder wall may be compromised in obstructed cats, increasing the likelihood of bladder wall rupture following cystocentesis. Delayed urine leakage is more likely in animals in which dysuria and bladder distension recur following cystocentesis.

- The author has very successfully managed cats with very severe hyperkalaemia and acidaemia due to urethral obstruction without performing cystocentesis early on and would strongly recommend that cystocentesis is reserved for those cases in which urethral catheterization cannot be performed. If bacteriology is required, the first urine sample collected following urethral catheterization may be used.

Following urethral catheterization, the cat was maintained on a 2.5% glucose saline solution at an empirical rate of 8 ml/kg/hr initially with close monitoring of urine output and hydration parameters. Analgesia was continued in the form of buprenorphine (0.02 mg/kg i.v. q 6 hr) and potassium supplementation was provided as needed. Blood glucose, potassium, urea and creatinine concentrations were monitored intermittently and glucose supplementation stopped when appropriate. The urinary catheter was removed after being in situ for 36 hours, by which time the azotaemia had also resolved and the urine appeared grossly normal.

The cat was subsequently discharged approximately 24 hours later after he had demonstrated normal urination. Meloxicam (0.3 mg/kg s.c.) was administered prior to discharge, at which time the cat had been nonazotaemic for 48 hours.

CLINICAL TIP

- Intravenous fluid therapy must be continued following urethral catheterization using an isotonic replacement crystalloid at a rate that is adequate to keep up with urine output, provide for maintenance requirements and correct any existing dehydration. A postobstructive diuresis often occurs early on following urethral obstruction and can result in large volumes of urine being excreted (severity may correlate to severity of postrenal azotaemia). Dehydration

CLINICAL TIP—cont'd

will develop or worsen if adequate fluid therapy is not provided during this period. However, excessive fluid therapy is also to be avoided as it may promote renal medullary washout, with the cat temporarily losing the ability to concentrate its urine.

- Despite possible hyperkalaemia at presentation, cats with urethral obstruction may develop hypokalaemia following catheterization as a result of postobstructive diuresis and the likelihood of anorexia. Serum potassium should be monitored and supplementation provided as necessary. If insulin was administered prior to catheterization it is important to monitor blood glucose in the short term and provide intravenous supplementation (2.5–5%) if necessary.

CLINICAL TIP

- The routine use of antibiotics is contraindicated in the presence of an indwelling urethral catheter and this practice is likely to select positively for more resistant bacteria. Antibiosis should only be commenced if a urinary tract infection has been confirmed.

CLINICAL TIP

- Nonsteroidal anti-inflammatory agents should typically not be administered early on in cats with urethral obstruction. These agents are contraindicated in all hypovolaemic or dehydrated patients (see Ch. 5) and ideally should not be administered to cats with urethral obstruction until azotaemia has resolved.
- In addition, glucocorticoid administration may be considered during or following urethral catheterization if significant urethral mucosal inflammation is suspected, and the concurrent use of both types of agent is contraindicated.

NURSING ASPECT

Following urethral catheterization, cats require close attentive monitoring and nursing. With respect to feeding, the priority in the short term is to tempt them to eat and the author is happy to offer these cats highly palatable foods rather than attempt to enforce a prescription urinary support diet. However, these cats have many short-term reasons to be inappetent (hospitalization, indwelling urethral catheter, Elizabethan collar) and force-feeding is both unnecessary and likely to induce food aversion; it should therefore be avoided.

Indwelling urethral catheters and closed collection systems need to be checked regularly to ensure that they remain in place, are not leaking and have not become blocked or disconnected. In addition, usual standards of care with respect to TLC, clean dry bedding and gentle handling are important.

Canine urethral obstruction

Mechanical urethral obstruction is considerably less common in dogs than cats but the same principles apply with respect to management of the emergency patient. This section will highlight some notable features of the canine condition.

Canine urethral obstruction may occur due to urolithiasis, blood clots, strictures, neoplasia, severe urethritis or penile fractures. In male dogs the urinary bladder may also become trapped in a perineal hernia. Transitional cell carcinoma is the most common cause of urethral obstruction in female dogs, while obstructive urolithiasis is more common in males. Uroliths that become lodged in the urethra may be flushed into the bladder by retrograde hydropulsion for subsequent medical dissolution or removal (surgical or nonsurgical) (see p. 298); occasionally urethrotomy may be required.

Struvite (radioopaque) uroliths are the most common type in dogs in general, and occur more commonly in female dogs. Unlike cats, these stones are typically associated with urease-producing bacterial infections. Calcium oxalate (radioopaque) uroliths are more common in male dogs than females, especially if neutered or overweight. Canine breeds at increased risk of calcium oxalate urolithiasis include the Yorkshire terrier, the Lhasa Apso, the Miniature Schnauzer and the Shih Tzu, along with various other small breeds. It is noteworthy that many of these breeds also appear at increased risk of struvite urolithiasis although the latter is also seen for example in the Cocker Spaniel and mixed breed dogs.

Urate (radiolucent) uroliths are most often identified in the Dalmatian, but an increased incidence is also reported in the English Bulldog. Urate stones in other breeds may be secondary to a portosystemic shunt causing impaired uric acid and ammonia metabolism; this is especially common in the Yorkshire terrier. Cystine (radioopaque) uroliths are seen in young to middle-aged dogs and occur most commonly in the Dachshund, the Staffordshire bull terrier, the English Bulldog and the Newfoundland.

It should also be remembered that dysuria in dogs may also be the result of prostatic enlargement, for example due to acute bacterial prostatitis or abscessation. Haemorrhagic or purulent fluid may drip from the penis and defecatory tenesmus may occur. These dogs often have a stiff gait and may be painful on caudal abdominal palpation. Rectal examination reveals prostatomegaly and pain on palpation. Occasionally systemic signs of lethargy, pyrexia and even sepsis may be seen.

ACUTE RENAL FAILURE AND LEPTOSPIROSIS

Acute renal failure

Theory refresher Acute renal failure (ARF) refers to a rapid decrease in glomerular filtration rate (GFR), the consequences of which include accumulation of uraemic toxins and metabolic waste products, and dysfunctional fluid, electrolyte and acid–base homeostasis. The kidneys normally receive 20% of cardiac output, making them especially susceptible to ischaemic and toxic injury.

Causes

ARF may occur due to prerenal, postrenal or, most commonly, intrinsic renal causes.

Prerenal renal failure Prerenal disease is the result of decreased renal blood flow, usually due to generalized hypoperfusion resulting from severe dehydration, hypovolaemia from other causes, or other forms of shock. Prolonged prerenal azotaemia may result in structural injury and irreversible intrinsic renal failure. It is essential to correct prerenal azotaemia before performing interventions that may predispose patients to further renal injury (e.g. general anaesthesia, nephrotoxic drugs).

Intrinsic renal failure Intrinsic renal failure is the result of renal parenchymal injury. It may occur as a result of ischaemia, glomerular disease or tubular disease, and is characterized by azotaemia with isosthenuria (urine specific gravity 1.007–1.015). Toxins, including nephrotoxic drugs, are the most common cause in companion animals, although it is noteworthy that in most cases the diagnosis is one of association (i.e. between a compatible history and the development of ARF) without definitive proof. In some cases there is no compatible history and the diagnosis remains entirely presumptive.

Toxins associated with ARF in companion animals include grapes and raisins (dogs), lilies (cats), vitamin D (ARF due to hypercalcaemia) and ethylene glycol (see Ch. 30). Drugs with the potential for significant nephrotoxicity include nonsteroidal anti-inflammatory agents and aminoglycoside antimicrobials, although a large number of other drugs have been implicated. ARF may also occur as a result of primary traumatic injury (rare) as well as in syndromes such as heatstroke, sepsis and disseminated intravascular coagulation (DIC).

Leptospirosis (see below) is probably the most commonly recognized infectious cause of ARF. Pyelonephritis may also cause ARF and most commonly occurs as a result of ascending lower urinary tract infection secondary to bacterial cystitis. Clinical signs may include lethargy, inappetence, vomiting, pyrexia and renal pain. Pyelonephritis may also occur secondary to haematogenous spread of bacteria.

Postrenal renal failure Postrenal causes of ARF involve obstruction and/or rupture of the urinary tract. Although animals with postrenal abnormalities can have severe azotaemia, in most cases irreversible intrinsic renal injury does not occur if the cause is treated early. Ureteral obstruction due to calcium oxalate uroliths is increasingly recognized as a cause of ARF in cats.

Phases and progression

ARF is typically classified as being oliguric, anuric or polyuric based on the amount of urine being produced and this classification is important with respect to both management and potential prognosis. In an adult animal, oliguria is typically defined as urine output of less than 0.5–1 ml/kg/hr and polyuria as urine output of more than 2 ml/kg/hr. In general, a normal animal that suffers sufficiently severe renal injury will first become oliguric, which may or may not then progress to anuria. Conversion from oliguria or anuria to polyuria does not necessarily equate with recovery of the kidneys; however, it is an encouraging sign and also greatly facilitates patient management. In the author's experience, polyuria is associated with a better outcome, at least with respect to discharge from the hospital.

Polyuria must be treated with appropriate intravenous fluid therapy to match urine output; these animals are unable to concentrate their urine in the face of inadequate fluid intake and will become dehydrated. Once the patient is stable, fluid therapy can be tapered by 10–20% each day as long as urine output decreases at a similar rate and azotaemia does not worsen. Animals that survive to discharge are likely to retain a degree of azotaemia, which may or may not then fully resolve over the subsequent weeks.

Treatment

ARF carries a guarded prognosis but treatment is designed to support the patient in order to allow as much time as possible for the kidneys to recover. Management involves:

- Removing or providing specific therapy for the primary cause if applicable
- Minimizing the possibility of further renal injury
- Providing treatment for azotaemia and correcting fluid imbalances and electrolyte abnormalities
- Providing intensive supportive care and therapy for other clinical manifestations, such as vomiting and anorexia

Treatment of ARF is further described in Case example 2.

CLINICAL TIP

- At the time of presentation, animals with ARF will have already suffered renal injury about which nothing can be done; in a significant number of cases, recovery will not occur despite aggressive therapy that may or may not include dialysis. However, the chances of a successful outcome are maximized by early and intensive treatment and close monitoring; although not entirely essential, objective monitoring of urine output is invaluable in guiding therapy and maximizing the chances of optimal management.
- If not precluded by financial constraints, the author would strongly recommend the referral of dogs and cats with ARF for specialist care if optimal management cannot be provided within the primary clinic.

Leptospirosis

Theory refresher

Leptospires are filamentous spirochaete bacteria that are maintained in nature by subclinically infected wild and domestic reservoir hosts. Direct transmission occurs through contact with infected urine, venereal and placental transfer, bite wounds or ingestion of infected tissues; indirect transmission occurs through contaminated water sources, soil, food or bedding. Recovery from clinical disease depends on an appropriate antibody response but recovered dogs may excrete organisms intermittently in urine for months after infection (the organism does not replicate outside the host).

The incidence of classic canine leptospirosis caused by *Leptospira icterohaemorrhagiae* or *L. canicola* decreased dramatically with the widespread use of vaccination. However, the incidence of canine leptospirosis has risen again due to an increasing prevalence of serovars that are not commonly included in vaccinations. Clinical cases of leptospirosis in cats are reported infrequently as cats are resistant.

Clinical findings

Leptospirosis is a multisystemic disease with a wide variety of possible clinical signs and clinicopathological abnormalities that are likely to be related to the virulence of the specific serovar and the age and immune status of the host. Peracute infections may occur with massive leptospiraemia and possible death with minimal signs.

Acute and subacute infections may manifest with a variety of nonspecific clinical signs as well as one or more of the following:

- Renal injury and possible acute renal failure: azotaemia, possible oliguria/anuria
- Hepatic injury and jaundice; possible liver failure
- Coagulopathy: haematemesis, haematochezia, melaena, petechiae or ecchymoses; thrombocytopenia may be present
- (Vasculitis with associated tissue oedema)
- (Acute lung injury and possible pulmonary oedema)
- (Uveitis).

Diagnosis

Diagnosis of leptospirosis is typically made on the basis of compatible history and clinical findings, and demonstrating high initial or convalescent serum antibody titres. Titres (initial) can be negative in the first 7–10 days of acute illness and testing may need to be repeated once or twice, 2–4 weeks apart (convalescent). It is noteworthy that dogs with positive titres generally cross-react to a variety of serovars and the serovar with the highest titre is interpreted as belonging to the infecting serogroup. Polymerase chain reaction (PCR) analysis can be performed on urine collected prior to the instigation of treatment and may provide a more rapid diagnosis.

CLINICAL TIP

- Interpretation of *Leptospira* serology can be confusing in some cases and the reader is recommended to consult with the external laboratory used if there is any uncertainty about the results obtained; this is especially true in the context of animals presenting following recent vaccination.

Treatment

Treatment of leptospirosis involves appropriate supportive therapy for the individual patient (e.g. for dehydration, electrolyte abnormalities, renal failure or hepatic injury) and specific treatment of the infection. Treatment of leptospirosis is biphasic. Penicillin-derived antibiotics are used for 2 weeks to treat circulating leptospiral organisms; preparations for intravenous administration are readily available and are of use in the early stages when inappetence is likely. This phase of treatment is then followed by a 2-week course of a tetracycline-derived antimicrobial.

CLINICAL TIP

- Treatment for leptospirosis should be administered as soon as possible to maximize the chance of reversing tissue injury; this typically involves commencing treatment prior to confirming the diagnosis based on a sufficient index of suspicion.

CLINICAL TIP

- Leptospirosis is a potentially zoonotic disease and appropriate measures must be taken with respect to the handling of urine in any case in which this disorder is a possibility.

Case example 2

PRESENTING SIGNS AND CASE HISTORY

A 3-year-old female neutered Labrador retriever presented with a 2-day history of lethargy, depression, anorexia and vomiting. The owner was not sure how much the dog had been drinking; however, she reported that the dog appeared to be urinating less often. There was no known history of drug administration and the dog had received appropriate vaccination including against *L. icterohaemorrhagiae* and *L. canicola*. Scavenging was a possibility as the dog received daily walks during which she was often let off the lead and out of sight, and she also had free access to the owner's garden. No other significant history was reported.

Major system examination

On presentation the dog was depressed but ambulatory. Heart rate was increased (132 beats per minute) but cardiovascular examination was otherwise unremarkable. Mucous membranes were mildly hyperaemic and appeared jaundiced; capillary refill time was approximately 1 second. Respiratory rate was increased at 36 breaths per minute but there was only a mild increase in effort and auscultation was appropriate. Abdominal palpation was unremarkable and the bladder could not be palpated. Rectal examination was unremarkable but the dog was mildly hypothermic (37.0°C). Doppler (systolic) blood pressure was normal at 140 mmHg.

Assessment

The tachycardia, tachypnoea, mild hyperaemia and hypothermia in this case were suspected to be the result of a systemic inflammatory process but no further conclusions could be drawn.

Emergency database

An intravenous catheter was placed in a cephalic vein and blood obtained via the catheter for an emergency database. This revealed high-normal manual packed cell volume (PCV) (52%, reference range 37–55%) and serum total solids (TS) (66 g/l, reference range 49–71 g/l). Mild hyperkalaemia (5.8 mmol/l, reference range 3.6–4.6 mmol/l) and mild hyponatraemia (136.1 mmol/l, reference range 140.0–153.0 mmol/l) were identified. Peripheral blood smear examination revealed a moderate thrombocytopenia, unremarkable red blood cell morphology, and a subjective moderate mature neutrophilia. The dog was found to be severely azotaemic (blood urea nitrogen 60 mmol/l, reference range 3.0–9.1 mmol/l; creatinine 900 μmol/l, reference range 98–163 μmol/l) and moderately hyperphosphataemic (4.20 mmol/l, reference range 0.8–2.0 mmol/l) with marked hyperbilirubinaemia (95 μmol/l, reference range 0–2.4 μmol/l). Brief abdominal ultrasonography revealed a very small bladder and no free fluid was detected.

Case management

The severity of the azotaemia was consistent with either a severe renal or a postrenal azotaemia but there was no evidence to support the latter; a prerenal component was possible. In addition, the dog was not anaemic as would be expected if she had been suffering from chronic renal failure with an acute crisis. Given all the findings in this case, a diagnosis of ARF was made. There was no evidence of haemolysis and the hyperbilirubinaemia was presumed to be posthepatic or hepatic in origin. These two findings, in addition to the moderate thrombocytopenia, were suggestive of possible leptospirosis and a sample was submitted for serology.

A soft indwelling Foley urethral catheter was placed under sedation (butorphanol 0.3 mg/kg i.v., diazepam 0.2 mg/kg i.v.) using strict aseptic technique and barrier nursing, and the bladder emptied. The catheter was connected to a closed urinary collection system. Urinalysis revealed: isosthenuria (urine specific gravity 1.013); marked bilirubinuria with mild glucosuria, proteinuria and haematuria; and an increase in red and white blood cells on sediment examination. The dog was not felt to be hypovolaemic but moderate dehydration (7%) was suspected, and she was started on 0.9% sodium chloride (normal, physiological saline) at 10 ml/kg/hr to provide rehydration and maintenance requirements over approximately 8 hours (see Ch. 2). Amoxicillin/clavulanic acid (20 mg/kg i.v. q 8 hr) was started for possible leptospirosis, and antiemetic therapy (maropitant 1 mg/kg s.c.) and omeprazole (0.7 mg/kg slow i.v. q 24 hr) were administered.

After 10 hr of fluid therapy, there had been minimal urine production. The dog was therefore given a bolus of furosemide (4 mg/kg i.v.), and 1 hour later her urine output had increased to 1.0 ml/kg/hr. Mannitol (1 mg/

kg i.v over 30 minutes) was administered and the dog was started on a constant rate infusion of furosemide (0.3 mg/kg/hr). The dog was monitored closely for signs of fluid overload, in particular with respect to respiratory rate and effort, and regular monitoring of blood pressure and blood parameters performed.

Over the following 12 hours, the dog remained oliguric and despite appropriate tapering of fluid therapy and further diuresis, began to show signs of fluid overload in the form of chemosis and peripheral subcutaneous oedema. Her azotaemia and hyperbilirubinaemia also worsened. The dog's owners were advised at this point that she either needed to be referred for peritoneal dialysis (haemodialysis was not available) or sadly euthanased on welfare grounds, having failed to respond to medical management. The owners elected for the latter which was done without further delay. Postmortem was declined but the results of *Leptospira* serology were subsequently received and confirmed the suspected diagnosis (microagglutination test (MAT) positive for *Leptospira copenhageni* at 1/3200).

CLINICAL TIP

- Adequate fluid replacement is essential in managing ARF and it is not possible to draw reliable conclusions about either urine output or the true severity of azotaemia until this has been achieved. Initial fluid therapy should be aggressive if hypovolaemia is present and more conservative for rehydration (see Ch. 2).
- Some animals with ARF will be oliguric or even anuric at the time of presentation and there is therefore a very real risk of fluid overload, i.e. if fluid therapy is provided but urine is not produced. However, it is not possible to establish urinary status until adequate fluid replacement has been provided. Persistent dehydration is likely to exacerbate renal injury.
- Diuretics are only indicated if adequate fluid therapy fails to restore satisfactory urine output. Dialysis (peritoneal or haemodialysis) is indicated if fluid therapy and diuretic administration are unable to establish sufficient urine output such that evidence of fluid overload occurs.

37 Dystocia

Telephone enquiries regarding possible cases of dystocia are relatively common in companion animal emergency practice. Owners are often anxious and distressed at these times and veterinary staff must have a good understanding of normal gestation and parturition in order to provide sound logical advice.

THEORY REFRESHER

Normal gestation and parturition

The bitch

Normal gestation Average length is 65 days (range 56–72 days). This range reflects the variable correlation between copulation and actual fertilization in the bitch. Once fertilization actually occurs, the true gestation length is less variable.

Labour

Labour is divided into three stages.

First stage Stage one occurs 24–48 hours before parturition. Behavioural changes may include:

- Nesting behaviour
- Restlessness
- Panting
- Attention-seeking or being seclusive
- Shivering
- Inappetence
- Vomiting.

Physical changes may include:

- Mammary gland changes and lactation 1–7 days before parturition
- Marked decrease in body temperature 8–24 hours before parturition (typically found to be 35–37°C)
- Progressive cervical dilation and vaginal relaxation
- Initiation of subclinical uterine contractions (no abdominal straining).

Second stage Stage two occurs 3–24 hours before parturition. There are three cardinal signs indicating that the dam is in stage two although all three signs may not be present in any individual case.

- Body temperature increases to normal or slightly above normal
- Abdominal contractions begin (concomitant with strong uterine contractions)
- Clear fluid is discharged from the vulva – this is fluid from the ruptured chorioallantois and usually signifies delivery of the first neonate within 30 minutes to 4 hours. Allantoic fluid should precede each neonate.

A green vulval discharge is normal in the bitch as long as it is produced less than 2 hours before, with, or after foetal delivery. This discharge is due to placental separation. Following delivery the dam should remove the amniotic membranes, sever the umbilical cord, and clean and bond with the foetus.

Third stage Stage three represents expulsion of placental and foetal membranes and occurs concurrently with stage two in pluriparous dams. Expulsion usually occurs within 15 minutes of delivery but the dam may deliver two or more foetuses before any membranes are expelled. Maternal consumption of the membranes may induce gastrointestinal signs and should be discouraged. Discharge of residual foetal fluids and placental remains may persist for 3–6 weeks after parturition has ended. However failure to pass the majority of all placentas within 4–6 hours of the end of second stage labour should prompt veterinary attention.

The queen

Gestation and parturition in the queen are similar to the bitch with a few noteworthy exceptions.

- Normal gestation in the queen is 63–67 days. This narrower range reflects the induced ovulation that occurs in this species.

- It is not uncommon for a queen to disappear from the home during stage one labour, leaving owners unaware of the changes occurring.
- Body temperature may decrease in the 12 hours prior to parturition but this is a less consistent finding.
- In the queen normal vulval discharge due to placental separation is red-brown in colour (green in the bitch).

Dystocia

The incidence of dystocia in dogs and cats is reported to be approximately 5% and dog breeds that may be at increased risk include chondrodysplastic and brachycephalic breeds, especially Pugs and Bulldogs, as well as Scottish terriers, Boston terriers, Yorkshire terriers and the Chihuahua. Dystocia is most common in short-faced breeds as well as Devon Rex and Siamese cats. Primary uterine inertia is the most common cause of dystocia in dogs and cats and is a maternal cause. Other maternal causes include mechanical obstruction (e.g. due to narrowing of the pelvic canal secondary to healed fractures), maternal anxiety and systemic illness. Foetal malpresentation is the most common foetal cause of dystocia in dogs and cats. Others include foetal oversize, malformation and death.

CLINICAL TIP

- If a dam is in active labour the stress of transportation and veterinary examination may endanger the life of a foetus that is in the birth canal and undergoing normal parturition. Attempting to progress parturition at home must, however, be balanced with the realization that the sooner cases that require veterinary attention receive this treatment the more likely it is that a successful outcome will be achieved (see Box 37.1).

BOX 37.1 Indications for veterinary attention during parturition

- Prolonged gestation: due date (if known) reached without signs of labour
- A history of previous dystocia
- More than 24 hours of anorexia in the full-term queen
- No signs of labour more than 24 hours after the decrease in body temperature in the full-term bitch
- No signs of labour 12–24 hours after body temperature increases again in the full-term bitch
- More than 4 hours since the onset of second stage labour without a foetus being passed
- Strong active but nonproductive abdominal contractions for more than 30 minutes
- Flank biting or other signs suggesting severe abdominal discomfort in the dam
- A green (bitch) or brown (queen) vulval discharge without a foetus being born in the subsequent 2 hours
- Sanguineous or malodorous vulval discharge
- Weak irregular nonproductive straining for more than 2 hours
- More than 2–4 hours between foetuses being delivered
- Failure to deliver all foetuses within 24 hours (bitch) or 36 hours (queen) from the onset of second stage labour
- Signs of systemic compromise in the dam
- The presence of a foetus or foetal membranes protruding from the vulva for more than 15 minutes

Note that posterior presentation is considered to be a normal variation in dogs and cats.

Oxytocin

Oxytocin is a hormone that is released during labour and that causes uterine smooth muscle contraction as well as milk letdown. It is used to treat dystocia due to uterine inertia by increasing the frequency and strength of uterine contractions which it does by promoting calcium influx into myometrial cells. Oxytocin also promotes uterine involution after birth as well as reducing uterine haemorrhage and assisting in expulsion of retained placentas.

CLINICAL TIP

- The use of oxytocin is contraindicated in the presence of pelvic obstruction, inadequate dilation of the cervix, vaginal masses or strictures, and inguinal hernias.

Recommended dose rates traditionally have been 1–2 IU/kg i.m. (or s.c.), with a maximum dose of 20 IU in the bitch and 2–4 IU total dose i.m. (or s.c.) in the queen. More recently, however, it has been suggested that lower doses than those quoted here may be as effective but with less risk of inducing uterine tetany. Repeated doses may be given every 20–30 minutes if required but failure to respond to two or three doses is usually considered an indication for surgical intervention. The period of time in between oxytocin doses can be used to prepare for caesarean section.

General anaesthesia

Pregnant animals have various physiological and pharmacokinetic differences that make them more sensitive and vulnerable to all aspects of general anaesthesia. Furthermore, most injectable and inhalational agents used for general anaesthesia cross the placental barrier and thereby affect the foetuses. Foetuses may also be adversely affected by cardiovascular compromise or hypoxia in the dam or by analgesic agents administered to the dam. The aim therefore when selecting a drug protocol for caesarean section is to choose a protocol that minimizes compromise of the dam and the foetuses while ensuring that the dam receives adequate analgesia. Numerous protocols are recommended. Familiarity with the drugs being used is perhaps one of the most important factors in protocol selection. Regardless of the drug protocol selected, efficient induction and neonate delivery are essential (see also Ch. 39).

CLINICAL TIP

- Due to both pressure on the stomach from the enlarged uterus and delayed gastric emptying and reduced gastrooesophageal sphincter tone secondary to increased progesterone levels, animals undergoing caesarean section are at increased risk of vomiting and subsequent aspiration. It is sensible to minimize the amount of time these animals spend in dorsal recumbency and to ensure that a cuffed endotracheal tube is used during general anaesthesia. The use of metoclopramide as part of the premedication may be rational.

Ovarohysterectomy

In cases in which the owner does not want to breed from the dam again, ovarohysterectomy may be performed at the same time. This can be done following delivery via caesarean section although there is some increased risk of haemorrhage from a more vascular gravid uterus. Alternatively, the uterus can be removed and handed to assistants en bloc with subsequent delivery of the foetuses; this is potentially quicker but does rely on sufficient competent assistance. Ovarohysterectomy at the same time as caesarean section alleviates the need for repeat general anaesthesia and laparotomy in the future, and does not adversely affect milk production. In some cases ovarohysterectomy may be indicated to minimize maternal morbidity, for example if the uterus is grossly infected or necrotic.

Case example 1

PRESENTING SIGNS AND CASE HISTORY

A 22-month-old female Pug (7.8 kg) presented 6 hours after the onset of second stage labour. She had had 1 hour of strong nonproductive abdominal contractions initially but these had ceased.

The bitch had undergone planned mating with another Pug 64 days previously. Abdominal ultrasound had been performed 30 days after mating and had confirmed the presence of live foetuses and five foetal skeletons had been detected radiographically 45 days after mating. The bitch had been bright and appetent throughout gestation and had been maintained on a commercial dog food. She had suffered a previous episode of dystocia during her first pregnancy at 11 months of age for which oxytocin therapy had been required. There was no significant medical history and the bitch had received routine vaccinations.

Major body system examination

On presentation major body system examination was unremarkable. Abdominal palpation was comfortable and consistent with possible pregnancy. Good mammary development was present and milk that was grossly normal in appearance was readily expressed. Rectal temperature was 38.5°C and digital examination unremarkable. A clear vulval discharge with a small amount of green pigment was present and gentle digital examination per vaginam using aseptic technique and copious lubrication revealed a fully dilated cervix. Auscultation of the abdomen revealed several foetal heart rates of approximately 210 beats per minute; the dam's heart rate was 130 beats per minute.

CLINICAL TIP

- Normal foetal heart rate is approximately 170–250 bpm with the higher rates more common in cats than dogs. Rates lower than 160–170 bpm suggest foetal distress and should prompt a greater sense of urgency with respect to intervention.

Case management

An emergency database was performed and the dam was found to be normocalcaemic and normoglycaemic with a manual packed cell volume (PCV) of 35%. Conscious right lateral and dorsoventral abdominal radiographs were obtained that demonstrated five foetal skeletons all within the abdominal cavity with no obvious malposition. Obstruction of the pelvic canal was not suspected and a presumptive diagnosis of primary uterine inertia was made.

CLINICAL TIP

- Hypocalcaemia should be considered in any dystocic animal with neurological signs. However, it may also be present in nonneurological animals and can contribute to dystocia by reducing the strength of myometrial contractions. If facilities allow, serum ionized calcium concentration should be measured in preference to total calcium concentration.
- Calcium supplementation should definitely be provided if hypocalcaemia is documented and empirical supplementation may also be appropriate in animals in which oxytocin is ineffective (adequate calcium availability is required for oxytocin to be fully effective) or in which abdominal contractions appear to be weak (see Appendix 1).

CLINICAL TIP

- Mild normocytic normochromic anaemia may be detected in full-term bitches at parturition and is a normal finding.

CLINICAL TIP

- Abdominal radiography may be used to identify the number of foetuses present and to evaluate foetal presentation and size (Figure 37.1). Evidence of foetal death may also be detected in the form of intrafoetal gas shadows (can take 6 hours or more after death to appear) or overlapping of cranial bones and collapse of the spinal column (can take 48 hours or more to appear).
- A dorsoventral radiograph of the pelvis will allow the pelvic canal to be evaluated both for diameter and for the presence and presentation of a foetus. Radiographs of adequate quality are usually obtainable without the need for chemical restraint.

Oxytocin was administered (2 IU i.m.) and the bitch went on to deliver four puppies over the next 2 hours. Three were born alive but one was dead. A further dose of oxytocin (2 IU i.m.) was administered and the fifth puppy was also born alive. Five sets of placental and foetal membranes were expelled over the course of the whelping period. The bitch cleaned and nursed the puppies, all of which were suckling well and she was discharged shortly after.

The owners were advised to monitor the dam for any signs of a purulent malodorous vulval discharge, active vulval haemorrhage, evidence of mastitis or signs of

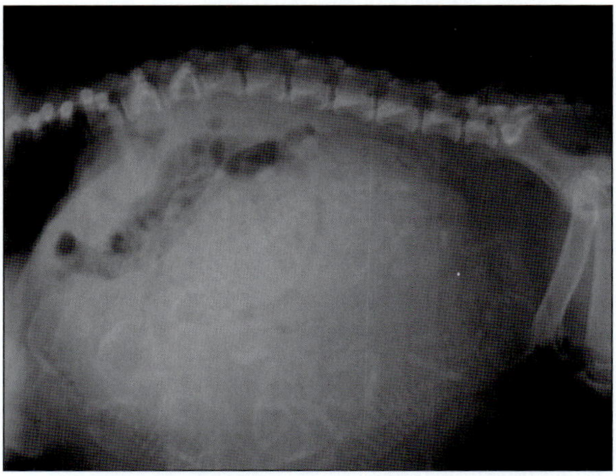

Figure 37.1 Right lateral abdominal radiograph of a pregnant dog; five foetal skulls are visible lying ventrally in the abdomen.

systemic illness, and to seek veterinary attention should they be concerned. In addition, they were asked to seek veterinary attention should the litter fail to thrive.

Case example 2

PRESENTING SIGNS AND CASE HISTORY

A 3-year-old female Yorkshire terrier (3.5 kg) presented 3 hours after the onset of abdominal contractions. A puppy had been noted protruding from the vulva in posterior presentation after approximately 2 hours but had not been delivered, thus prompting veterinary attention. The bitch had undergone accidental unwitnessed mating and the owner was unable to provide details regarding the sire or the timing. No imaging had been performed during gestation. The bitch had been bright and appetent throughout gestation and had been maintained on a commercial dog food. This was her first pregnancy and there was no significant medical history. The bitch had received routine vaccinations.

Major body system examination

On presentation the bitch was depressed but major body system examination was otherwise unremarkable. Abdominal palpation was comfortable and consistent with possible pregnancy. Good mammary development was present and milk that was grossly normal in appearance was readily expressed. Rectal temperature was 38.0°C but digital examination was not tolerated. A puppy was visible protruding in posterior presentation from the vulva. Auscultation of the abdomen failed to reveal foetal heart beats.

Case management

The protruding puppy was removed manually using sterile gloves and copious sterile lubrication. Gentle digital traction using a sterile gauze swab for increased grip was applied pulling slowly, steadily and without excessive force in a caudoventral direction. Unfortunately the puppy was found to have died.

An emergency database was performed and the dam was found to be normocalcaemic but mildly hypoglycaemic. An intravenous catheter was placed and glucose administered (0.25 g/kg diluted slow i.v. followed by a 2.5% glucose saline infusion at 4 ml/kg/hr).

CLINICAL TIP

- The use of copious sterile lubrication is essential during obstetric manoeuvres. It is possible to use instruments to manipulate and remove a foetus but this practice is discouraged due to increased risk of foetal and maternal injury. In addition, excessive traction should not be applied to a single extremity as severe injury is likely to occur.

CLINICAL TIP

- Periparturient hypoglycaemia in the dam is seen most commonly after prolonged labour, in toy breeds and with large litters.

Right lateral and dorsoventral abdominal radiographs were obtained that demonstrated three further foetal skeletons all within the abdominal cavity. The most caudal of the foetuses was malpresented, lying in transverse presentation. Abdominal ultrasound was able to detect at least two different foetal heart rates, both of which were approximately 170 beats per minute; maternal heart rate was 140 beats per minute. Given the malpresentation of the most caudal foetus caesarean section was recommended. Foetal heart rates were acceptable but borderline as an indication of foetal distress and immediate intervention was therefore recommended (see Box 37.2 for other indications for emergency caesarean section).

BOX 37.2 Indications for emergency caesarean section

Pelvic obstruction
Oversized (relative or absolute) foetus
Foetal malpresentation
Evidence of foetal distress (heart rate less than 170 beats per minute)
Failure of the medical approach
Meconium, excessive haemorrhage or purulent material in vulval discharge
Maternal systemic compromise

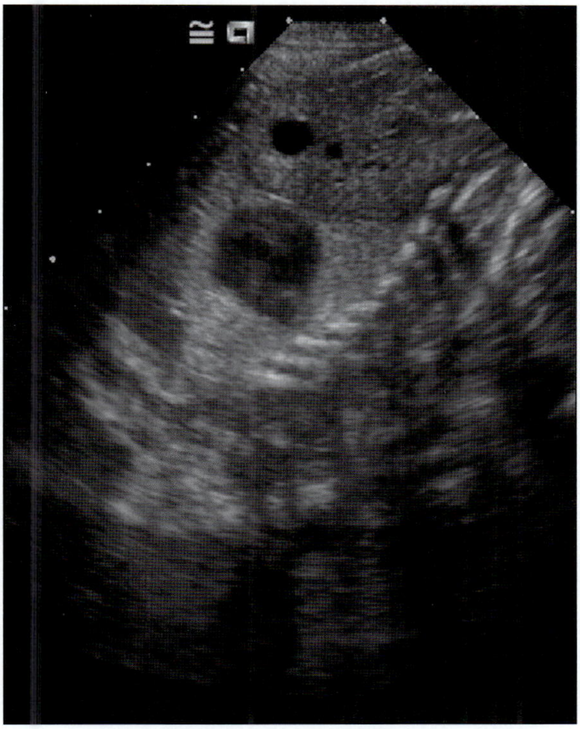

Figure 37.2 Ultrasound image of a canine foetus. The foetal heart is visible within the thoracic cavity (the left side of the rib cage is visible and associated with acoustic shadowing); the liver is visible (top of image) as well as the skull (bottom of image).

CLINICAL TIP

- Abdominal ultrasonography is relatively simple to perform for the purpose of detecting foetal heart beats and possibly foetal movements. The bitch may be in lateral recumbency or standing if preferred and the foetal rib cage should be identified. Within this it is usually possible to identify the heart and to count the heart rate if appropriate (Figure 37.2).
- If ultrasonography is not available and foetal heart beats cannot be heard on auscultation, it may be possible to identify them using an ultrasonic Doppler device for measuring blood pressure applied to the abdomen.

In addition to the glucose saline infusion the bitch was started on another isotonic crystalloid solution at 6 ml/kg/hr (making a total surgical infusion rate of 10 ml/kg/hr). Her ventral abdomen was clipped in preparation for surgery and an initial scrub performed. The bitch was then premedicated using low dose pethidine (2 mg/kg i.m.) and midazolam (0.1 mg/kg i.v.). After 5 minutes of preoxygenation, anaesthesia was induced in the operating theatre with intravenous propofol given slowly to effect (i.e. so that endotracheal intubation could be performed) and then maintained on isoflurane in oxygen. Prior to performing the final surgical scrub lidocaine (2 mg/kg diluted with 0.9% sodium chloride) was infiltrated subcutaneously around the laparotomy site. Caesarean section was performed and all puppies found to be alive. Carprofen (4 mg/kg i.v.) was administered following delivery and ovarohysterectomy was performed. A further dose of lidocaine was infiltrated into the midline during wound closure. Perioperative antibiosis was not administered.

CLINICAL TIP

- When calculating dosages for drugs to be administered to pregnant animals, it is important to dose to an estimate of the nongravid body weight of the dam as using full-term body weight will lead to relative overdosage.

The bitch recovered well from surgery and nursed her puppies well. Routine postpartum care was advised and the owners were also asked to monitor the surgical wound for evidence of infection, or seroma or haematoma formation. The bitch was discharged on a reduced dose of carprofen (2 mg/kg p.o. q 24 hr) for 5 days.

38 Heatstroke

THEORY REFRESHER

A spectrum of severity is seen in dogs suffering from heat-induced illness in terms of both pathophysiological derangements and clinical consequences. It may therefore be more accurate to employ a gradation of severity from heat stress to heat exhaustion to heatstroke. Nevertheless, the general term 'heatstroke' will be used here.

Heatstroke results from severe hyperthermia, although a specific threshold above which heatstroke occurs has not been defined in dogs. Cellular injury may occur above 41°C and permanent brain damage is reportedly possible. Enzyme dysfunction, protein denaturation and severe organ damage may occur above 43°C and are associated with a significant increase in mortality. Further information regarding the prognosis in dogs with heatstroke is provided in Box 38.1.

Pathogenesis

Heatstroke occurs when heat gain markedly exceeds heat loss and this is predominantly due to the cooling mechanisms stimulated by the hypothalamus becoming overwhelmed. These mechanisms include:

- Direct stimulation of panting to maximize evaporative heat loss – this is the predominant cooling mechanism in dogs
- Increased cardiac output and peripheral vasodilation to increase delivery of blood to the body surface – this increases heat loss via convection and radiation.

Heatstroke may occur more readily in dogs suffering from a lack of acclimatization to warmer weather. The acute phase response and heat shock proteins may also be involved in the pathogenesis of heatstroke.

Risk factors

A variety of predisposing factors exist that may be classified as endogenous or exogenous. Most of these factors impair heat loss and include:

- Exogenous
  - Confinement and/or poor ventilation
  - Increased humidity
  - Water deprivation
- Endogenous
  - Brachycephalic anatomy
  - Laryngeal dysfunction
  - Obesity
  - Darker and/or thicker coat.

Some factors affect heat gain, for example exercise, pyrexia, and especially external ambient temperature.

BOX 38.1 Prognostic considerations in dogs with heatstroke

The prognosis in heatstroke depends on a number of factors including:

- Duration of exposure
- Highest core body temperature reached
- Pre-existing medical conditions
- Development of secondary complications
- Speed and intensity of treatment

Unfavourable prognostic indicators include:

- Coma or hypothermia at presentation
- Progressive neurological deterioration
- Persistent/refractory hypoglycaemia
- Persistently unstable cardiovascular status
- Worsening azotaemia and oliguria despite appropriate fluid therapy
- Disseminated intravascular coagulation (DIC)

In fatal cases, death usually occurs within 24 hours. Death is unlikely to occur in patients surviving more than 48 hours.

BOX 38.2 Preventative measures for heatstroke in dogs

Heatstroke can be avoided in the majority of cases if appropriate preventative measures are employed. Preventative measures are especially important in dogs predisposed to heatstroke (e.g. brachycephalic breeds, dogs with laryngeal dysfunction, obese dogs) and include:

- Controlling exercise to allow acclimatization as summer approaches
- Avoiding exercise during the hottest times of the day
- Avoiding confinement in a car or other poorly ventilated space
- Ensuring shade is available if the dog is tied up outside
- Ensuring water is always available
- Keeping the coat short during warmer months

BOX 38.3 Potential pathophysiological derangements in heatstroke

- Increased metabolic demand
- Circulatory shock
- Hypoxia
- Excessive inflammation
- Coagulation abnormalities
- Endothelial injury and dysfunction

Measures designed to try to prevent heatstroke are summarized in Box 38.2.

Pathophysiology

Heatstroke may be divided into two types. Classic heatstroke occurs due to exposure to high environmental temperature, for example being locked in a car with shut windows on a warm day, or being tied up outside without shade/water. Exertional heatstroke is the result of strenuous exercise. Many pathophysiological derangements are possible in heatstroke due to both direct heat-induced cytotoxicity and acute physiological changes due to hyperthermia. These are summarized in Box 38.3. Multiple organ dysfunction syndrome (MODS) (Box 38.4) is the most serious potential sequela of heatstroke.

BOX 38.4 Potential components of multiple organ dysfunction syndrome (MODS)

- Circulatory collapse
- Brain dysfunction
- Disseminated intravascular coagulation (DIC)
- Acute renal failure
- Acute lung injury (ALI)/acute respiratory distress syndrome (ARDS)
- Acute hepatic failure
- Rhabdomyolysis
- Myocardial injury
- Intestinal injury (ischaemia, infarction)

NURSING ASPECT

On an emergency basis, nurses are often the first members of staff to speak to owners ringing about dogs with suspected heatstroke. While telephone diagnosis is generally to be avoided, the history in these cases is often very suggestive and early intervention can be crucial to a positive outcome. Advice includes:

- Check rectal temperature if possible
- Gently hose/soak the dog with cool (not cold) water; do not cover in wet towels
- Offer water if alert but withhold if vomiting
- Drive to the nearest clinic with the air conditioning on or windows open; do not dry the dog
- Do not administer antipyretic agents (e.g. paracetamol (acetaminophen), ibuprofen)

The possible effect of cooling measures implemented by the owner prior to presentation must be borne in mind as some dogs with heatstroke may be normothermic at presentation as a result.

Case example 1

PRESENTING SIGNS AND CASE HISTORY

A 2-year-old male neutered Newfoundland dog presented collapsed in the mid-afternoon on a warm summer's day. The dog had been out for a relatively long period of exercise in the middle of

Continued

PRESENTING SIGNS AND CASE HISTORY—cont'd

the day and had started to pant excessively on the way home. On returning home he had drunk a large volume of water, vomited a short while after, and then collapsed. Following a telephone conversation with the practice, the dog had been hosed down with cool water and then driven immediately to the practice with the air conditioning on maximum in the car. No other significant preceding history was reported.

Major body system examination

On presentation the dog was recumbent, markedly depressed and panting excessively. Cardiovascular examination revealed a heart rate of 160 beats per minute but it was very difficult to hear the heart sounds clearly due to the panting. Dorsal pedal pulses could not be palpated and femoral pulses were weak; pulse deficits were suspected. Mucous membranes were markedly hyperaemic with a rapid capillary refill time. Rectal temperature was 41.8°C and digital rectal examination revealed fresh blood. Pupillary light reflexes (direct and consensual) and menace responses were intact bilaterally.

CLINICAL TIP

The clinical findings in this case are relatively typical for dogs presenting with heatstroke. However, clinical findings depend on factors such as the severity and duration of hyperthermia, cooling measures performed prior to presentation, and the delay in presentation. As such a variety of clinical findings are possible.

Additional or alternative findings include:

- Normo- or hypothermia
- Hyper- or hypodynamic cardiovascular findings
- Ataxia
- Cortical blindness (usually transient)
- Tremors, seizures
- Petechiae/ecchymoses.

Assessment

The dog was assessed as suffering from severe hyperthermia due to heatstroke with evidence of cardiovascular, intestinal and possible neurological compromise. Given that cooling measures had already been started, it was suspected that rectal temperature would have been higher prior to presentation.

Emergency database

A short large bore intravenous catheter was placed in each cephalic vein and blood obtained via one of the catheters for an emergency database. This revealed haemoconcentration (manual packed cell volume 64%, reference range 37–55%; serum total solids 90 g/l, reference range 49–71 g/l), hypoglycaemia (blood glucose 2.0 mmol/l, reference range 3.3–6.1 mmol/l) and mildly raised blood urea nitrogen concentration (13.0 mmol/l, reference range 2.5–8.9 mmol/l). Blood smear examination at initial presentation was unremarkable.

Case management

Flow-by oxygen supplementation was provided and intravenous volume resuscitation was commenced using an isotonic replacement crystalloid solution. Hartmann's solution (buffered lactated Ringer's solution) was administered into each cephalic vein (total 40 ml/kg bolus) using pressure infusors (see Figure 4.1) and glucose supplementation (0.5 g/kg slow i.v. diluted) provided. The dog was soaked in cool water and multiple fans applied. Electrocardiography was performed and revealed predominantly sinus rhythm with intermittent ventricular premature complexes (VPCs) (see Figure 12.4).

The dog's cardiovascular status and mentation showed satisfactory improvement on this initial management. A further 15 ml/kg bolus of Hartmann's was administered and as the dog continued to pant excessively, butorphanol (0.2 mg/kg i.v.) was administered with good effect. Cooling measures were discontinued when the rectal temperature reached 39.5°C to avoid rebound hypothermia (see Ch. 16). The dog was maintained on intravenous fluid therapy with glucose supplementation (2.5% glucose/Hartmann's solution) and blood glucose monitored intermittently. Continuous electrocardiographic monitoring was performed but no antidysrhythmic therapy was indicated. Free catch urinalysis revealed moderate proteinuria, marked haemoglobinuria, no detectable glucosuria and an absence of urinary casts.

The dog remained clinically stable but developed widespread petechiation (see Ch. 21). Repeat peripheral blood smear examination performed several hours after presentation revealed marked thrombocytopenia, an increase in nucleated red blood cells and a mild subjective neutrophilia with some toxic change (see Ch. 3).

Table 38.1 Possible clinicopathological findings in dogs with heatstroke

Test	Possible findings
Packed cell volume (PCV)	Increased (haemoconcentration) or decreased (haemorrhage)
Serum total solids (TS)	Increased (haemoconcentration) or decreased (haemorrhage, leakage through inflamed vessel walls)
Blood glucose	Low, normal or high
Electrolytes	Hypernatraemia (dehydration); hyperkalaemia (muscle breakdown)
Venous acid–base status	Respiratory alkalosis, metabolic acidosis, hyperlactataemia
Arterial blood gas analysis	Hyper- or hypocapnia, hypoxaemia
Peripheral blood smear	Increased nucleated red blood cells, thrombocytopenia, neutrophilia or neutropenia
Biochemistry	Azotaemia (prerenal, renal), increased liver enzymes, hyperbilirubinaemia, increased creatine kinase (CK)
Urinalysis	Haematuria, haemoglobinuria, myoglobinuria, inappropriate glucosuria and casts (indicate renal damage)
Coagulation	Prolonged prothrombin time (PT), prolonged activated partial thromboplastin time (APTT)

Given the concerns regarding coagulopathy, and the lack of both a coagulation analyser and access to fresh frozen plasma (FFP), it was decided to refer the dog for more specialist management.

CLINICAL TIP

- The administration of antipyretic agents is contraindicated in dogs with heatstroke (see Ch. 16).

Follow-up

Follow-up information from the referral centre confirmed coagulopathy with marked prolongation of both prothrombin time (PT) and activated partial thromboplastin time (APTT). Multiple units of FFP were administered and intravenous glucose supplementation was required for a further 24 hours. A biochemistry profile revealed abnormalities consistent with muscle and hepatic parenchymal damage. No further complications were identified and the dog went on to make a complete recovery with intensive supportive care.

As demonstrated by this case, a variety of clinicopathological findings may be identified in dogs suffering from heatstroke. These are summarized in Table 38.1. In the author's experience petechiation is relatively common in dogs with heatstroke, not all of which are thrombocytopenic. This suggests probable vasculitis or platelet dysfunction as the cause of the petechiation.

SECTION 4

ADDITIONAL TOPICS

39 Notes on sedation and general anaesthesia

Shailen Jasani with Simon Ripoll

GENERAL CONSIDERATIONS

Successful management of the emergency patient frequently requires the use of sedative and anaesthetic drugs. However, it is in the emergency setting that the inherent risks and adverse effects of these drugs on patient physiology assume an increased significance and this should never be underestimated.

> **CLINICAL TIP**
>
> - Where the patient's condition allows, every effort should be made to delay anaesthesia until the patient is stabilized.
> - Cautious and extremely careful use of agents and techniques with which the clinician is personally familiar is more important than the choice of any particular agent.

Potential risks of sedation and anaesthesia

> **CLINICAL TIP**
>
> - Before commencing sedation or anaesthesia, the patient should be assessed in the context of how the major body systems are likely to cope with the adverse effects of the drugs employed, and also in turn how the course of anaesthesia is likely to be influenced by the patient's condition. Potential problems should be anticipated and prepared for in advance.

See Tables 39.1 and 39.2.

Hypothermia

Body temperature is likely to fall progressively in proportion to the duration of anaesthesia and may result in widespread detrimental effects, for example:

- Hypoventilation
- Hypoxaemia
- Cardiac dysrhythmias
- Central nervous system dysfunction
- Slowed drug metabolism, potentiating or prolonging sedative and anaesthetic effects.

Maximizing patient safety prior to sedation and anaesthesia

The fundamental goal is to ensure adequate oxygen delivery to the vital organs.

- By ensuring vital organ perfusion
  - Correct blood pressure
  - Correct hypovolaemia (± correct dehydration)
  - Normalize heart rate
  - Correct malignant or premalignant dysrhythmia
- By ensuring adequate blood oxygenation
  - Restore blood oxygen-carrying capacity (correct packed cell volume/haemoglobin content)
  - Improve ventilation (e.g. drain pleural fluid, relieve pneumothorax, treat pulmonary oedema)
- In addition
  - Reduce intracranial pressure if suspected to be elevated
  - Control seizures
  - Correct hypoglycaemia
  - Treat acute renal failure, improve urine output in oliguria/anuria, correct azotaemia
  - Correct any clinically significant electrolyte abnormality

Is general anaesthesia necessary?

Depending on the intended investigation or procedure, important questions to consider may be:

- Can general anaesthesia be avoided while still providing sufficient restraint and insensibility to pain to accomplish the task?

Table 39.1 Potential adverse effects of anaesthesia on body systems

Body system	Adverse effects
Cardiovascular	Hypotension Reversal of peripheral vasoconstriction which the patient may be relying on to maintain perfusion of vital organs Bradycardia or tachycardia Cardiac dysrhythmia
Respiratory	Reduced ventilation or apnoea Ventilation/perfusion mismatch Hypoxia Hypercapnia Respiratory acidosis
Nervous	Direct central nervous system suppression Raised intracranial pressure Reduced cerebral or spinal perfusion
Renal	Reduced renal perfusion
Hepatic	Reduced hepatic perfusion
Gastrointestinal	Increased risk of regurgitation and subsequent aspiration
Temperature	Hypothermia

Table 39.2 Potential effects of patient condition on the course of anaesthesia

Patient condition	Effect on anaesthesia
Cardiovascular compromise (e.g. hypovolaemia)	Risk of overdose (e.g. due to reduced volume of drug distribution, delayed response to intravenous injection) Reduced cardiac output increases rate of inhalation anaesthetic uptake resulting in more rapid inhalation induction Reduced hepatic and renal perfusion reduces metabolism and elimination of drugs
Respiratory compromise	Reduced ventilation results in slower onset of inhalation anaesthesia and a slowed response to altered inhalation anaesthetic concentration
Central nervous system disease	Reduced level of consciousness increases sensitivity to all sedatives and anaesthetic agents
Renal disease	Reduced renal elimination of drugs, prolonging duration of effect
Hepatic disease	Reduced hepatic metabolism of anaesthetic drugs, prolonging duration of effect
Hypoalbuminaemia	Increases nonprotein-bound, active concentration of many drugs, increasing sensitivity to these drugs

- Will appropriate analgesia, with or without additional sedation, be sufficiently effective?
- Could local anaesthesia be utilized in combination with sedation to perform a painful procedure?
- Or in fact, is general anaesthesia the safest option?

Maximizing patient safety during general anaesthesia

1. Select the most appropriate induction method.
2. Establish good venous access.
3. Do anything you can do without anaesthesia beforehand to minimize anaesthetic time (e.g. pre-clip surgical site).
4. Have all equipment and drugs well prepared (anticipate problems) (Table 39.3).
5. Preoxygenate via a facemask or flow-by oxygen until ready to intubate.
6. Adopt a calm, quiet approach – relaxing the patient minimizes the dose of anaesthetic required.
7. Take preinduction readings of vital parameters.
8. Attach the required monitoring equipment pre-induction if the patient allows it.
9. Intravenous fluids. Unless the patient's condition contraindicates it, run isotonic crystalloid fluids at surgical rates (typically 10 ml/kg/hr) as induction commences to offset any potential drop in blood pressure. The type and rate of fluids employed subsequently under anaesthesia in general will be based on that already instituted for stabilization (see Ch. 4). To what extent these rates are modified for anaesthesia depends on:
   (a) Cardiovascular status at induction
   (b) Packed cell volume, albumin and electrolyte levels

Table 39.3 Being prepared for anaesthesia of critical patients

Anaesthetic aspect	Equipment
Intubation	Laryngoscope Range of ET tubes – include several much smaller tubes where potential for unexpectedly narrow airway exists (e.g. upper airway obstruction) Tube tie Local anaesthetic spray for cats
Complications of intubation	Face mask Alternative narrow endotracheal oxygen delivery device: long narrow bore tube such as urinary catheter which can be adapted to connect to oxygen supply ET tube stylets/wire to act as guide and thread tube over in event of partial obstruction of nasopharynx Suction apparatus Emergency tracheotomy kit
Oxygen administration and ventilation	Appropriate breathing circuit: if continuous IPPV anticipated, use T-piece for <10 kg, use Bain or Circle for >10 kg
Monitoring	Pulse oximeter, ECG, blood pressure monitor, capnograph, thermometer or temperature probe, glucometer
Intravenous fluids	Include those that might be required later or in event of patient deterioration: crystalloids, colloids, Oxyglobin®, appropriate blood products as indicated and as available Fluid administration equipment, preferably including infusion pumps
Temperature control	Preventing heat loss: blanket, bubble wrap, heat and moisture exchanger on circuit (Thermovent®), warm ambient temperature of room Heat sources if appropriate: warm air blanket, warm water bed, 'hot hands'
Emergency drugs	Atropine, adrenaline (epinephrine), lidocaine (only indicated if there is continuous ECG monitoring to characterize nature of cardiac dysrhythmia)

ECG, electrocardiograph; ET, endotracheal; IPPV, intermittent positive pressure ventilation.

   (c) Expected on-going pathological fluid losses (bleeding, body cavity effusions or gut sequestration)
   (d) Intraoperative blood loss.
10. Calculate the approximate expected dose of anaesthetic agent required – be conservative. Consider using an intravenous sedative pre-induction to minimize the intravenous anaesthetic dose (e.g. diazepam). Dose in increments until the desired effect is reached (usually to allow smooth intubation), allowing plenty of time between doses if the patient is cardiovascularly unstable. More rapid administration may be justified if patent airway or intermittent positive pressure ventilation (IPPV) is a priority.
11. Ensure smooth intubation. Use local anaesthetic spray in cats in a timely fashion and allow it time to work.
12. Perform an airway, breathing, circulation (ABC) check immediately on intubation and be prepared to implement IPPV:
    (a) Airway = check correct intubation and secure the tube in place
    (b) Breathing = confirm breathing through tube (chest movement produces bag movement) or give a breath if no breath observed (bag movement produces chest movement)
    (c) Circulation = check pulse.
13. Use a balanced anaesthetic technique for the maintenance of anaesthesia: use nitrous oxide in the gas mixture if it is safe to do so, timely opioid analgesia bolus or constant rate infusion (local anaesthetic techniques, muscle relaxants if familiar with their use). Minimize anaesthetic concentrations at all times.

CLINICAL TIP

- Because anaesthetic drugs cause cardiorespiratory depression in a dose-dependent manner, it is important to try to minimize the dose used. Anaesthetic administration can be minimized by the rational use of additional drugs which contribute to the anaesthetic state, without producing significant cardiorespiratory effects of their own.
- The anaesthetic state consists of unconsciousness, analgesia and muscle relaxation. The provision of effective analgesia using opioids and, where possible, local anaesthesia in particular can go a long way to reducing anaesthetic dosage.

14. Control temperature (see Table 39.3). Rebreathing circuits (circle systems) recycle exhaled breath (minus carbon dioxide) and so help to retain warmth and moisture.
15. Monitor appropriately (see below).
16. Ensure that intensive patient monitoring and support continue through the recovery as well.

Patient monitoring during general anaesthesia

Under anaesthesia, the following questions should constantly be asked:

- Is there adequate circulation and perfusion?
- Is the patient adequately oxygenated?
- Is there adequate ventilation to get rid of carbon dioxide from the body?
- Is there adequate kidney function to ensure other waste products are removed from the body?

The emphasis should be on continuous monitoring of physical examination parameters, ideally by a member of staff dedicated to this purpose:

- Pulse rate and quality – ideally access to a central (femoral) and peripheral (distal limb, tongue) pulse. This should be supplemented by heart auscultation by stethoscope or oesophageal stethoscope
- Respiratory rate and quality – observation of chest and reservoir bag movement
- Capillary refill time and mucous membrane colour
- Core temperature and the temperature of the extremities
- Eye position, palpebral reflex, pupil size, jaw tone.

CLINICAL TIP

- Recording of measurements every 5 minutes is to be encouraged, primarily to focus the mind and alert the recorder to important trends in vital parameters over time.

CLINICAL TIP

Monitoring such as pulse oximetry, blood pressure measurement, capnography and electrocardiography should be used as available. There are two golden rules with monitoring:

1. When in doubt, always look at the patient and rely on your own senses.
2. Do not rely on what just one monitor is telling you; always consider it in the context of all the other information you have available – from the patient, from other monitors, and from what is being done to the patient (surgery, drugs, fluids, anaesthetic, etc.).

SEDATIVE AND ANAESTHETIC DRUGS

Benzodiazepines

These are especially useful for sedation or calming in emergency patients when combined with an opioid; if possible, give the opioid first and allow time for it to take effect.

- Minimal cardiovascular or respiratory effects at standard doses.
- Can be given i.v., showing an obvious effect within less than 1 minute.
- Diazepam is poorly absorbed following i.m. administration; use midazolam.
- Either drug can be combined with a low dose of ketamine to provide more profound sedation without undue cardiovascular compromise.

CLINICAL TIP

- A combination of benzodiazepine, opioid and low dose ketamine may provide particularly effective sedation without needing to use a high dose of any of the individual drugs.

Opioids

CLINICAL TIP

- Opioids have an important role to play in the anaesthetic management of the emergency patient, and as a general rule they should be utilized whenever possible.
- It should be remembered, however, that what is an acceptable dose for analgesia in the conscious patient may sometimes represent overdose if given in the anaesthetized patient.

See Chapter 5.

Medetomidine and dexmedetomidine

- Potent agonists at alpha$_2$-adrenoceptors in the brain and spinal cord.
- Cause profound and predictable sedation as well as good analgesia.
- Use with caution in the emergency patient because of marked physiological effects.
- Cause widespread peripheral vasoconstriction and significant bradycardia; also cause a reduction in cardiac output, although perfusion of vital organs is considered to be well preserved.
- Very low doses of medetomidine (1–2 μg/kg) have very much reduced side effects, while still contributing to effective sedation in combination with other drugs:
  - Combines well with opioids
  - Higher doses of opioids or addition of small doses of benzodiazepine can improve sedation whilst allowing the medetomidine dose to remain low
  - Combination with low dose ketamine can provide good sedation whilst offsetting bradycardia to some extent.

Contraindications for use

Absolute contraindications

- Any form of shock
- Severe hypotensive state
- Bradycardia or pathophysiological tachycardia
- Cardiac dysrhythmia
- Significant respiratory compromise.

Relative contraindications

- Potential to seizure
- Raised intracranial pressure (bradycardia)
- Unstable diabetic patients (hyperglycaemic effects)

Acepromazine

- Anxiolytic agent.
- Combines effectively with opioids to produce good sedation.
- Arterial hypotensive effects unhelpful in many emergency patients and cannot be pharmacologically reversed.
- Lacks significant direct respiratory depressant effects; can be useful in calming certain patients in respiratory distress (e.g. upper respiratory tract obstruction, rib injury).
- History of seizures is not a contraindication for judicious use.

Ketamine

- Minimal cardiovascular and respiratory effects at lower doses.
- Can contribute to sedation or general anaesthesia, and is also an effective analgesic (see Ch. 5).
- Should almost always be combined with another agent (benzodiazepine, medetomidine or acepromazine); addition of an opioid helps to produce smooth sedation whilst adding to analgesia.

Contraindications

- May increase heart rate which is unhelpful in certain patients, e.g. cats with hypertrophic cardiomyopathy; any patient with cardiac disease where increased myocardial oxygen demand would be detrimental.
- May increase intracranial pressure and is potentially pro-convulsant, therefore avoid in head trauma and seizuring patients.
- Ketamine is excreted primarily unchanged by the kidneys in cats, therefore use judiciously if there is severe renal dysfunction; primary hepatic metabolism in dogs.

Propofol

- Rapid-acting; can be used as both a sedative and anaesthetic.
- Causes dose-related hypotension and respiratory depression so use judiciously.
- Can be titrated to effect and slow, incremental dosing should always be employed:
  - Failure to do this in the shocked or severely hypotensive patient can easily prove fatal
  - Cardiovascular-sparing sedative agents should be used whenever possible to minimize the dose of propofol in animals with cardiovascular

compromise; combination of opioid and benzodiazepine often ideal
  - If sedation only is required, small sub-anaesthetic doses of propofol can be used to 'top up' a diazepam/opioid combination.
- Tendency to cause apnoea at induction (particularly in dogs); easily rectified by IPPV following intubation but allowance must be made for the possibility of delayed or difficult intubation:
  - Preoxygenate
  - Administer propofol slowly
  - Use good premedication to minimize propofol dose.

Alfaxalone

- Good alternative to propofol in many situations; can also be used as both a sedative and general anaesthetic.
- Also produces dose-dependent hypotension and respiratory depression at higher doses.
- Use of cardiovascular-sparing premedication is recommended to minimize the total dose of alfaxalone used.
- Best administered in increments allowing 15–20 s between boluses; given in this way, it appears to be less likely to produce apnoea than propofol:
  - May be the intravenous agent of choice in respiratory compromised patients
  - Low doses of alfaxalone, titrated to effect, are useful in head trauma where apnoea and consequent hypercapnia is particularly undesirable.

See Tables 39.4 and 39.5 for information on drugs used for sedation and anaesthesia; see Table 5.1 for information regarding opioids.

Sedative combinations

These may allow a reduced dose of each drug to be used, thus reducing the potential for side-effects (Box 39.1).

INHALATION ANAESTHESIA

Induction

- Induction with inhalant agents is generally less desirable in critical patients.
- Especially avoid it where it is important to establish a secure airway rapidly, e.g. respiratory compromise, risk of airway obstruction, high risk of regurgitation and aspiration of stomach contents.
- May be the induction technique of choice in paediatric, especially neonatal and juvenile, animals.

Maintenance

- Drugs of choice in most critical patients.
- Depth of anaesthesia readily controlled; cardiorespiratory depressant effects readily reversible because the anaesthetic can be rapidly removed from the body via the lungs.
- Greatest clinical familiarity.
- Dose-related arterial hypotension and respiratory depression can be minimized by supplemental sedation and analgesia using cardiovascular-sparing drugs, in particular opioids.
- Sevoflurane is the most rapidly responsive form of anaesthesia of the commonly available agents and is the author's preferred agent in the emergency patient.
- Nitrous oxide can be used to reduce the concentration of inhalant and so help to reduce the cardiorespiratory depressant effects of these agents:
  - Avoid if arterial saturation of haemoglobin with oxygen (SpO_2) less than 95%
  - Will rapidly diffuse into any abnormal air-filled spaces in the body; avoid in pneumothorax, gastric dilation and gastrointestinal obstruction in particular.

CONSIDERATIONS IN SPECIFIC DISORDERS

Caesarean section

Anaesthetic considerations for dam

- Increased risk of regurgitation/vomiting due to pressure from gravid uterus and not being starved.
- Anaesthetic doses must be calculated according to estimated non-pregnant weight.
- Inhalation induction more rapid but overdose more likely.
- Displacement of diaphragm by gravid uterus interferes with ventilation.
- Positioning in dorsal recumbency may cause hypotension due to compression of the caudal vena cava by the gravid uterus.
- Intraoperative and postoperative pain.

Anaesthetic considerations for neonates

- Periods of hypotension or vasoconstriction may reduce placental blood flow.
- Anaesthetics cross the placenta and cause neonatal depression.
- Potential for hypothermia.
- Smooth, rapid recovery of dam required for optimum nursing of neonates.

Table 39.4 Information for drugs used for sedation and general anaesthesia

Drug	DOSE RANGE AND DURATION OF ACTION		Notes
	Dog	Cat	
Diazepam	0.1–0.5 mg/kg Up to 1 hr	0.1–0.5 mg/kg Up to 1 hr	Slow i.v. or rectal Cannot mix in syringe with other agents, do not use in drip lines
Midazolam	0.1–0.4 mg/kg Up to 90 min	0.1–0.4 mg/kg Up to 90 min	Slow i.v. or i.m.
Medetomidine	1–5 μg/kg i.v. 5–20 μg/kg i.m. 2–3 hr	2–10 μg/kg i.v 10–40 μg/kg i.m. 2–3 hr	Avoid if cardiovascular instability, shock, severe head trauma, renal failure, diabetes Easily reversible
Dexmedetomicine	Half medetomidine dose	Half medetomicine dose	Avoid if cardiovascular instability, shock, severe head trauma, renal failure, diabetes Easily reversible
Acepromazine	0.005–0.05 mg/kg 4–6 hr	0.005–0.05 mg/kg 4–6 hr	Avoid if cardiovascular instability, shock, head trauma, severe renal or hepatic disease Cannot reverse
Ketamine	*Sedation*: 1–2 mg/kg i.v. 1–5 mg/kg i.m. 30–45 min *GA (with premed)*: 2–5 mg/kg i.v. 5–10 mg/kg i.m.	*Sedation*: 1–5 mg/kg i.v. 2–10 mg/kg i.m. 30–45 min *GA (with premed)*: 3–10 mg/kg i.v. 10–20 mg/kg i.m.	Only anaesthetic which is also good analgesic Good preservation of protective airway reflexes Must combine with sedative – poor muscle relaxation when used alone Avoid in hyperdynamic cardiac disease states, head trauma/seizures Dose conservatively in severe renal disease
Propofol	*Sedation*: Up to 2 mg/kg i.v. *GA (with premed)*: Up to 4 mg/kg i.v. CRI: 3–36 mg/kg/hr	*Sedation*: Up to 3 mg/kg i.v. *GA (with premed)*: Up to 6 mg/kg i.v. CRI: 3–10 mg/kg/hr	Always give carefully to effect – no prescribed dose Bolus effect lasts 5–10 minutes Higher doses may be required for anaesthesia if used alone No analgesia For CRI without syringe driver, add 50 ml propofol to 450 ml 0.9% sodium chloride to give 1 mg/ml propofol Limit prolonged infusion/repeat dosing in cats (Heinz body anaemia)
Alfaxalone	*Sedation*: Up to 1 mg/kg i.v. *GA (with premed)*: Up to 2 mg/kg i.v. but typically 1–1.5 mg/kg	*Sedation*: Up to 2 mg/kg i.v. *GA (with premed)*: Up to 5 mg/kg i.v. but typically 3–4 mg/kg	Always give to effect – no prescribed dose Bolus effect lasts 5–10 minutes No analgesia

CRI , constant rate infusion; i.m., intramuscular; i.v., intravenous; GA, general anaesthetic.

Example anaesthetic protocol

Premedication: Pethidine (1–2 mg/kg i.m.)
Pre-clip ventral abdomen and perform initial surgical scrub
Preoxygenate

Induction: Propofol

Maintenance: Isoflurane in oxygen/nitrous oxide mixture (discontinue nitrous oxide prior to removal of foetuses to avoid potential diffusional hypoxia when they start to breathe)

Table 39.5 Reversal agents for sedatives

Drug	Reversing agent	Dose and route
Medetomidine, dexmedetomidine	Atipamezole	5× dose in mg/kg of medetomidine (same volume) in dogs Usually given at 2.5× dose in mg/kg of medetomidine (half volume) in cats, but repeat the dose if sedation poorly reversed Licensed for i.m. use, but use i.v. in an emanergency
Full (pure) opioid	Naloxone	0.01–0.1 mg/kg slow i.v. to effect, i.m. Short duration of action (20–60 minutes) due to rapid metabolism therefore repeat doses may be required
Diazepam, midazolam	Flumazenil	0.01 mg/kg rapid i.v Onset of action 1–2 minutes Short duration of action (60 minutes)

BOX 39.1 Sedative combinations for emergency patients

Very unstable patient, low pain

Butorphanol 0.2–0.3 mg/kg i.v. followed 5–10 minutes later by diazepam/midazolam 0.2 mg/kg i.v.

Unstable patient, high pain

Substitute butorphanol with morphine/methadone 0.1–1.0 mg/kg (dogs) or 0.1–0.5 mg/kg (cats) i.v. or i.m.; use buprenorphine 0.02 mg/kg i.v. or i.m. if no full opioid

Critical but stable, and not sedated enough or likely to be sedated enough with above combinations

ADD acepromazine 0.005–0.01 mg/kg i.v.
OR medetomidine 1–2 µg/kg i.v.
OR ketamine 2–3 mg/kg i.v.
Choice depending on patient condition, temperament

Critical but stable, and temperament suggests more predictable sedation required

Leave out diazepam/midazolam, go straight for a triple combination of opioid (as above) + ketamine + acepromazine OR medetomidine – choice depending on patient condition. Medetomidine combinations will usually give the most profound sedation and should be used with care

Lively or aggressive patient with potential critical illness or unpredictable response to sedatives

Go for medetomidine 3–5 µg/kg + appropriate opioid at above doses i.v. or i.m. Medetomidine can always be topped up if there is not enough sedation

Primary clinical problem is respiratory compromise

Acepromazine 0.01 mg/kg i.v. + butorphanol 0.1 mg/kg i.v.
Acepromazine 0.01 mg/kg i.v. + ketamine 2–3 mg/kg i.v.
Diazepam/midazolam 0.2 mg/kg i.v. + ketamine 2–3 mg/kg i.v.
Acepromazine + diazepam/midazolam + ketamine at same doses if smoother sedation required

Additional notes

- Medetomidine doses may need to be up to two times higher in cats
- All combinations can be mixed in one syringe, except diazepam which must be given separately
- These doses are a guide only, based on personal experience. They are deliberately intended to be for the emergency patient with critical illness, and so are deliberately conservative 'starter' doses, on the grounds that it is better to top up poor sedation as required, rather than to risk destabilization of a patient
- In patients with the potential for severe respiratory compromise, general anaesthesia and intubation may be safer than any of these sedative combinations

Intravenous fluids:	Isotonic crystalloid at 10 ml/kg/hr
Analgesia:	Lidocaine (diluted with saline) infiltrated into abdominal midline prior to final scrub and at time of laparotomy closure
	Carprofen or meloxicam i.v. following delivery

Intractable blood loss: surgery for ruptured splenic haemangiosarcoma

- Anaesthesia may interfere with compensatory mechanisms for hypovolaemia and cause hypoperfusion of vital organs (brain, heart, lungs).
- Appropriate fluid resuscitation and possible abdominal counterpressure are essential preoperatively (see Ch. 29) and increase the margin of safety for anaesthesia.
- Packed red blood cell transfusion if indicated; Oxyglobin® may be used but small bag size so may not be practical for big dogs.

Example anaesthetic protocol

Premedication:	Full opioid (e.g. morphine 0.3 mg/kg slow i.v.)
	Pre-clip ventral abdomen and perform initial surgical scrub
Induction:	Preoxygenate
	Diazepam 0.2 mg/kg i.v.
	Propofol or alfaxalone i.v.
Maintenance:	Inhalant anaesthesia in 100% oxygen
Intravenous fluids:	Isotonic crystalloid at 10–20 ml/kg/hr ± synthetic colloid (5 ml/kg boluses or appropriate infusion) as necessary
Analgesia:	Full opioid premedication, intra- and postoperatively
	Carprofen or meloxicam only when cardiovascular status is completely stable

Diaphragmatic rupture

Anaesthesia only indicated following adequate and sustained patient stabilization (see Ch. 28).

Example anaesthetic protocol

Premedication:	Midazolam 0.2 mg/kg, ketamine 2 mg/kg and acepromazine 0.01 mg/kg i.v.
Induction:	Preoxygenate
	Attach pulse oximeter if available
	Propofol i.v.
	Lidocaine spray on larynx (cats)
	Commence IPPV as quickly as possible
	Maintain initially in sternal recumbency with chest raised above abdomen while the anaesthesia is stabilized and good oxygenation confirmed
	Clip in lateral and dorsolateral recumbency with the chest raised above the abdomen
Breathing circuit:	Must allow manual IPPV (e.g. modified Ayres T-piece for smaller patients)
Maintenance:	Inhalant anaesthesia in 100% oxygen
	Continuous manual IPPV throughout surgery until the diaphragm is repaired and air drained from thoracic cavity
Intravenous fluids:	Isotonic crystalloid at 10 ml/kg/hr
Analgesia:	Full opioid immediately after induction i.v. or i.m.; topped up as necessary
	Carprofen or meloxicam after induction if the cardiovascular status is stable

Gastric dilatation and volvulus syndrome

Anaesthesia is only indicated following adequate patient stabilization with fluid therapy and gastric decompression (see Ch. 29).

Anaesthetic considerations

- Compression of the caudal vena cava is likely to be worse in dorsal recumbency exacerbating reduced venous return to the heart and depressing cardiac output; gastric decompression is essential before induction.
- Aggressive fluid therapy must be continued during anaesthesia.
- Cardiac dysrhythmia may exist before induction and exacerbate hypoperfusion; anaesthetic agents may sensitize the myocardium to dysrhythmogenic molecules with a risk of deterioration into malignant and potentially fatal rhythm disturbances. Minimize risk by using high inspired oxygen concentrations, preventing

hypoventilation with IPPV, and minimizing anaesthetic doses. Monitor and treat if indicated (see Ch. 12).

Example anaesthetic protocol

Premedication:	Methadone 0.3 mg/kg slow i.v. (avoid morphine as more emetic)
Induction:	Preoxygenate
	Aggressive intravenous crystalloids as indicated (10–40 ml/kg/hr)
	Attach ECG electrodes prior to induction
	Diazepam 0.2 mg/kg i.v.
	Alfaxalone or propofol i.v. 30 seconds later
Maintenance:	Isoflurane in 100% oxygen
Analgesia:	Methadone continued regularly
	Carprofen or meloxicam only when the cardiovascular status is completely stable; also delay administration depending on the severity of gastrointestinal compromise

Traumatic brain injury

- Only anaesthetize in exceptional circumstances.
- Anaesthetics directly suppress central nervous system activity, therefore there is a particular risk in any patient with significant, symptomatic brain pathology.
- Avoid ketamine.
- Inhalant anaesthetics tend to elevate intracranial pressure; use with extreme caution; consider propofol infusion instead.
- Try to avoid the patient being in a relatively head-down position or continuous pressure over the jugular veins as this may worsen intracranial hypertension.

40 Notes on transfusion medicine

There is an increasing availability to nonreferral practices of products for transfusion through commercial and charitable pet blood banks, and a good understanding of the basic principles of transfusion medicine is essential. This is to ensure that the recipient is treated in the safest and most appropriate way, that the owner's resources are put to greatest use, and that the product which was donated by another animal, sometimes requiring sedation, is in fact used in the most beneficial manner. In the author's opinion, the latter is sometimes readily overlooked and ultimately it must be remembered that animal blood donors do not volunteer for the task!

BLOOD COMPONENTS

Use only the blood product indicated to minimize risk of a transfusion reaction and reduce the total volume to be administered (Table 40.1).

Anaemia – normovolaemic versus hypovolaemic

Normovolaemic anaemia

- e.g. chronic nonregenerative anaemia, acute haemolytic anaemia.
- These patients require oxygen-carrying capacity and therefore ideally packed red blood cells (pRBC) only.
- Separation of feline whole blood into components is not commonplace, so cats typically receive fresh whole blood (FWB) transfusion.
- It is often less wasteful to use FWB for small dogs (although smaller or half-units of pRBC may be satisfactory).
- Recipients should be monitored for volume overload.

Hypovolaemic anaemia

- Due to blood loss.
- These patients require both intravascular volume expansion and oxygen-carrying capacity.
- Typically use aggressive isotonic crystalloid or synthetic colloid therapy to correct the hypovolaemia (see Ch. 4), and lower rate FWB or pRBC transfusion for the anaemia.
- Haemoglobin-based oxygen-carrying solutions may have a role in the treatment of hypovolaemic anaemia (see Ch. 4).

BLOOD TYPES

These are determined by species-specific inherited antigens on the red blood cell surface.

Canine blood types

- Dog erythrocyte antigen (DEA) 1.1, 1.2, 3, 4, 5, 6, 7 and 8 (plus others); positive or negative for each DEA type.
- DEA 1.1 is extremely antigenic.
- Blood typing is typically restricted to determining DEA 1.1-positive or -negative status.

CLINICAL TIP

- If blood typing cannot be performed, DEA 1.1-negative blood should ideally be given if available. However, dogs are not believed to have clinically significant, naturally occurring antibodies against foreign red blood cell surface antigens (alloantibodies) and therefore the first blood transfusion between two dogs of opposite blood types is unlikely to cause an acute transfusion reaction. Therefore DEA 1.1-positive blood can be used for the first transfusion if necessary. However, it will induce alloantibody production that may then shorten the lifespan of the transfused red blood cells.

Continued

Table 40.1 Summary of main blood components in veterinary use

Blood component	Relevant functional constituents	Indications for use	Other comments
Fresh whole blood	RBC Platelets Coagulation factors (labile and stable) Plasma proteins	Anaemia with haemostatic abnormalities Hypovolaemic anaemia	pRBC preferred in normovolaemic anaemia (e.g. IMHA) FWB is typically used instead of pRBC in cats and small dogs but must be monitored for volume overload Must be type-specific in cats; preferred but not necessary for first transfusion in dogs Typically give 10–20 ml/kg Requires transfusion within 6–8 hours of collection (platelets and some clotting factors are rapidly inactivated by storage)
Packed red blood cells	RBC	Normovolaemic anaemia Used for nonregenerative (typically chronic) anaemia and haemolysis	Transfuse when clinical signs attributable to anaemia (e.g. weakness, collapse, tachycardia, tachypnoea, bounding pulses) are present as opposed to PCV threshold Typically used for medium-to-large size dogs; type-specific blood preferred but this is not necessary for the first transfusion Typically give 10 ml/kg at low rate over 4–6 hours to avoid volume overload Intravascular volume expansion should be provided by intravenous fluid therapy in hypovolaemic animals (e.g. following haemorrhage) Shelf life of 35–37 days with added preservative
Fresh frozen plasma	Coagulation factors (including vWF) Plasma proteins	Coagulation factor deficiency, both acquired (e.g. vitamin K deficiency, severe liver disease) and hereditary	Typically frozen within 6–8 hours of collection Theoretically type-specific product is preferred in dogs but clinically this is not necessary; currently not available for cats Typically give 10–20 ml/kg Not suitable for albumin replacement as large volumes and repeated transfusions are required for any clinically significant effect. The priority is to treat the underlying disorder and provide nutritional and synthetic colloid support After 1 year this material is reclassified as stored frozen plasma
Stored frozen plasma	Labile coagulation factors (V, VIII) are lost Does contain vitamin K-dependent factors (II, VII, IX, X)	Vitamin K deficiency	Describes plasma frozen more than 6–8 hours following collection, plasma stored frozen for more than 1 year, or FFP that was thawed and then refrozen

FFP, fresh frozen plasma; FWB, fresh whole blood; IMHA, immune-mediated haemolytic anaemia; PCV, packed cell volume; pRBC, packed red blood cells; RBC, red blood cells; vWF, von Willebrand factor; WBC, white blood cells.

CLINICAL TIP—cont'd

- Once a dog has received a blood transfusion, regardless of whether this was type specific or not, sensitization may occur. It is probably only safe to repeat the transfusion within 4 days before crossmatching becomes essential.

Feline blood types

Routine testing is carried out for blood types A, B and AB.

Type B

- More common among exotic and pure breeds – e.g. British short hair, Devon Rex, Cornish Rex, Abyssinian, Persian, Himalayan, Somali and Maine Coon.
- Most type B cats have high levels of strong, naturally occurring anti-type A alloantibodies (from 2 months of age).
- Severe and potentially fatal transfusion reaction is a very real possibility if a type B cat is given type A blood.

Type A

- The majority are type A.
- A small percentage of type A cats have weak, naturally occurring anti-type B alloantibodies (from 2 months of age).
- A type A cat receiving type B blood is at risk of a transfusion reaction but this should be relatively mild and certainly not fatal.

Type AB

- Relatively rare.
- These cats do not possess naturally occurring antibodies to type A or B red cell antigens.
- They could therefore receive type A or type B (or type AB) red blood cells; however, because cats typically receive fresh whole blood, a type A donor is preferred as anti-type A alloantibodies in the plasma of a type B donor cat could result in a transfusion reaction.

CLINICAL TIP

- Ideally cats must be blood typed prior to even the first transfusion and receive type-specific blood; crossmatching must be performed for any subsequent transfusion. If blood typing is

CLINICAL TIP—cont'd

not possible, use of a haemoglobin-based oxygen-carrying solution (see Ch. 4) should be considered as a readily available and often invaluable substitute that does not carry risks with respect to transfusion reactions. If this is not available, immediate referral of the case should be considered, although some severely anaemic cats are too unstable to travel.
- In the exceptional circumstance when an untyped blood transfusion must be given, it is essential to try to minimize the associated risks by using a donor cat that is likely to have the same blood type as the recipient (e.g. domestic short hair donor for a domestic short hair recipient as both are likely to be type A; exotic breed donor for an exotic breed recipient to at least try to increase the likelihood that both are type B). This situation is far from ideal, especially if the recipient is potentially type B, and the owner must be warned of the significant risks.

In-house blood typing

All practices likely to perform regular transfusions should invest in this facility. Most methods involve visualization of an agglutination reaction between a red cell surface antigen if present and antibodies specific for that antigen.

- Blood-typing cards (RapidVet-H Canine DEA 1.1® and RapidVet-H Feline A, B, AB®, DMS Laboratories, New Jersey, USA) are currently used most widely
- Other systems are increasingly available and may offer advantages, especially easier interpretation (e.g. DME VET DEA 1.1® and DME VET DEA A+B®, Alvedia, Lyon, France; DiaMed ID-Card Anti-DEA 1.1 (Dog)® and DiaMed ID-Card Anti A+B (Cat)®, Bio-Rad Laboratories, Inc., California, USA).

CROSSMATCHING

This is used to detect existing antibodies to red cell antigens, but does not test for antibodies against white blood cell or platelet antigens that may cause non-haemolytic transfusion reactions. Compatible crossmatches do not guarantee normal red blood cell survival as delayed transfusion reactions may occur.

In-house testing (e.g. RapidVet-H Crossmatch®, DMS Laboratories, New Jersey, USA) is becoming increasingly available.

Major crossmatch

This tests for alloantibodies in the recipient's plasma to donor red cell antigens. This type of incompatibility has the potential to be associated with the most severe transfusion reactions as the recipient plasma volume, and therefore alloantibody concentration, is large (hence major).

Minor crossmatch

This tests for alloantibodies in the donor's plasma to recipient red cell antigens. Transfusion reactions are likely to be less severe as the donor plasma volume, and therefore alloantibody concentration, is smaller (hence minor).

Controls

A donor and a recipient control test is usually also performed that checks for any reaction between each individual's serum and its own red blood cells.

TRANSFUSION REACTIONS

CLINICAL TIP

- All animals receiving a blood component transfusion should be monitored closely for an acute transfusion reaction, ideally using a dedicated transfusion monitoring chart.
- A number of parameters, including heart and pulse rate, respiratory rate and effort, mucous membrane colour and capillary refill time, rectal temperature, and mentation are monitored before, regularly during and for a period after the transfusion. Plasma and urine colour should also be monitored if possible.
- The reader is referred to other sources for more information on transfusion monitoring.

Transfusion reactions are typically classified as acute or delayed and then further classified as immunological (haemolytic or nonhaemolytic) or nonimmunological.

Acute haemolytic transfusion reaction

This is a type of immunological reaction (immunoglobulin (Ig) M (or IgG)-mediated type II hypersensitivity reaction). It occurs when the recipient has pre-existing alloantibodies to donor red blood cell surface antigens, and is the most concerning type of transfusion reaction.

Canine acute haemolytic transfusion reaction

- The normal lifespan of canine red blood cells is 100–120 days.
- The half-life of transfused canine red blood cells in the recipient is approximately 21 days.
- It can be as little as 30 minutes with acute haemolysis.

Clinical findings

- Tachycardia, tachypnoea or dyspnoea, weakness, collapse, salivation, vomiting and pyrexia.
- Evidence of haemolysis:
  - Intravascular: haemoglobinaemia and haemoglobinuria; may become apparent within minutes of starting the transfusion
  - Extravascular: hyperbilirubinaemia and bilirubinuria are usually associated with less severe signs.

Intervention

- Stop transfusion immediately.
- Start appropriate fluid therapy to treat hypoperfusion if it is present.
- Other symptomatic treatment.
- Corticosteroids are not used in human medicine.

Feline acute haemolytic transfusion reaction

- The normal lifespan of feline red blood cells is 70–80 days.
- The half-life following appropriately matched allogenic transfusion is 29–39 days.

Type B blood given to a type A cat

- A minor transfusion reaction is possible, reducing red cell half-life to approximately 2 days.
- Clinical signs may occur within minutes but should be mild – lethargy, restlessness, tachycardia and tachypnoea.
- Possible evidence of intravascular haemolysis, i.e. haemoglobinaemia, haemoglobinuria.

Type A blood to be given to a type B cat

- This is likely to cause a severe and potentially fatal transfusion reaction, with red cell half-life reduced to several hours or less.
- Clinical signs include gastrointestinal signs, salivation, vocalization and marked cardiorespiratory abnormalities.

- There may be evidence of intravascular haemolysis, i.e. haemoglobinaemia, haemoglobinuria.
- Systemic inflammatory response syndrome (SIRS), maldistributive shock, disseminated intravascular coagulation (DIC) and multiple organ dysfunction syndrome (MODS) are all possible.
- The severity of the reaction is usually proportional to the amount of blood transfused but even 1 ml may be enough to trigger a reaction.

Intervention

- Stop transfusion immediately.
- Give appropriate fluid therapy to treat hypoperfusion if it is present.
- Other symptomatic treatment.
- Corticosteroids are not used in human medicine.

Acute allergic transfusion reaction

- This is a nonhaemolytic immunological reaction (type I hypersensitivity reaction, usually IgE or mast-cell mediated).
- It occurs within seconds to minutes of the transfusion being started.
- An allergic reaction to plasma proteins is a potential cause of transfusion reactions when only plasma is transfused (i.e. despite absence of red blood cells).

Clinical signs

- These are usually mild, self-limiting or readily amenable to treatment and include erythema, pruritus, urticaria and oedema.
- Occasionally there are more severe anaphylactic reactions with cardiovascular, respiratory or gastrointestinal signs.

CLINICAL TIP

- An acute haemolytic transfusion reaction may be clinically indistinguishable from an allergic reaction and it is therefore important to check for evidence of intravascular (haemoglobinaemia, haemoglobinuria) and extravascular (hyperbilirubinaemia, bilirubinuria) haemolysis.

Intervention

- Discontinuing the transfusion may be all that is needed.
- Restart at a slower rate (e.g. half of the original rate) if the reaction subsides and monitor closely.
- Intravenous fluid therapy, corticosteroid or antihistamine may be required – judge on the individual case basis. Anaphylactic shock requires aggressive management (see Ch. 26).

41 Notes on paediatric medicine

The term paediatric refers to animals under 6 months of age that can be further subdivided into neonates, infants, weanlings and juvenile animals. Changes in physiology and haemodynamics occur as animals progress through these stages. In particular, there are important pharmacological considerations with respect to neonates (up to 2 weeks old) and infants (2–6 weeks old).

Neonatal and infant medicine is one area with which veterinary surgeons and nurses are often least familiar. In the author's experience, many owners are unwilling to commit substantial resources for veterinary care of the sickest neonates and infants and this lack of familiarity and experience is therefore not surprising.

THE HEALTHY NEONATE

- Spends almost all its time nursing or sleeping until 2–3 weeks old.
- Inadequate milk intake usually results in constant crying, failure to gain weight, and reluctance to nurse; supplemental feeding or a healthy vaccinated foster dam may be required.

Physical examination

Approximate normal physiological parameters are shown in Table 41.1. Healthy neonates are lively and plump. An estimation of general health and physical condition can be made by assessing the following:

- Suckling reflex
- Rooting reflex (opening and closing of the lips, moving the head in search for milk)
- Righting reflex when placed in dorsal recumbency: present at birth and strengthens over the first 4 weeks
- Adequate weight gain (see below)
- Coat condition: should be shiny
- Bowel sounds: usually auscultable.

Specific problems to examine neonates for include:

- Cleft palate
- Umbilical hernia
- Umbilical infection: the umbilical cord usually falls off by 3 days of age and the umbilicus should be dry. A soft erythematous umbilicus, possibly with a discharge, is suggestive of bacterial omphalitis
- Open fontanelle: may be associated with fading or future neurological signs. Many toy canine breeds have open fontanelles and small open fontanelles may be normal in kittens
- Cardiac murmur: may be innocent or pathological
- Protruding eyelids: ophthalmia neonatorum may cause protrusion of the eyelids before they are fully open, with or without a purulent discharge; due to infection with *Staphylococcus sp* or other normal flora
- Nonpatent urogenital or anal opening.

Body weight

Birth weight

Canine

- 100–200 g for toy breeds
- 400–500 g for large breeds
- More than 700 g for giant breeds

Feline

Average birth weight 90–110 g.

Weight gain

Approximate guidelines for daily weight gain:

- Puppies should gain 2.2–2.7 g for every kg of anticipated adult weight each day, or have a daily weight gain of 5–10% of their birth weight. Healthy puppies usually will have doubled their birth weight by 10 days of age.

Table 41.1 Approximate guidelines for physiological parameters in neonatal puppies and kittens

Physiological parameter	Normal values or findings
Heart rate	Puppies: 180–200 beats per minute; kittens: 250 beats per minute; decreases from 4 weeks old
Respiratory rate	20–30 breaths per minute
Rectal temperature	Average 36.0°C at birth; adult values by 4 weeks old
Mean arterial blood pressure	Considerably lower than adults; may not normalize until several months of age
Opening of eyes	Usually by 14 days old (5–14 days)
Vision	Usually normal by 3–4 weeks old
Menace response	May take 2–3 months to develop but can be sooner
Pupillary light reflexes	Present when eyes first open; normal by 3 weeks old
Opening of ear canals	Usually 6–14 days old
Hearing	Mature by 3–4 weeks old
Olfaction	Well developed at birth
Pain sensation	Present at birth
Withdrawal reflex	Usually develops by 1 week old
Ambulation	Usually develops by 2–3 weeks old
Gag reflex	Usually not present until after 10 days old

- Kittens should gain a minimum of 7–10 g per day (can be as much as 15–30 g) and healthy kittens usually will have doubled their birth weight by 14 days of age.

CLINICAL TIP

- Weight is a very useful parameter to assess in neonates and failure to gain weight is a consistent early sign of illness.
- Neonates should ideally be weighed daily, and in order to maximize the reliability of these data, weighing should be done at the same time of the day and at the same time with respect to feeding.

Urination and defecation

- Unable to urinate voluntarily for the first 2–3 weeks of life; urination stimulated by maternal licking of the genital region.
- Can only defecate when stimulated by maternal licking of anal region:
  - Meconium (soft, yellow-brown, relatively odour-free) passed for the first 2 days of life
  - Faeces then become light to medium brown in colour and pasty in consistency; typically they do not become solid until after weaning
  - Overfeeding by owners is a common cause of diarrhoea.

CLINICAL TIP

- Neonates require maternal licking of the genital and anal regions in order to urinate and defecate, and this is potentially readily overlooked if neonates are hospitalized away from the dam. In such cases the genital and anal regions can be stimulated by gentle stroking for example with a warm moist cotton wool ball.

CLINICAL PATHOLOGY

CLINICAL TIP

- Venepuncture in neonates is usually performed using a jugular vein and the author would strongly encourage the prior application of EMLA® cream 5% (AstraZeneca) (see Ch. 5). Both the difficulties in obtaining samples and especially the small blood volume of these animals mean that it is absolutely crucial to plan tests carefully so as to coordinate interventions, to take the minimum volume of blood required, and to run only tests that are essential. Maximum use should be made of any blood taken and chemistry analysers that only require low volume samples should be used as much as possible. In addition, peripheral blood smear examination is usually more than adequate and uses much less blood than performing a full haematology profile.
- At least in the context of clinical pathology that requires blood sampling, it is an unavoidable reality that neonates are unlikely to receive as intensive investigation or monitoring as an older animal. This needs to be accepted and embraced from the outset and does not preclude these patients from nevertheless receiving excellent care. Common sense is very much needed so that for example empirical glucose supplementation may be provided to sick neonates as they are prone to hypoglycaemia rather than performing frequent venepuncture for blood glucose measurement.

See Table 41.2. Reference ranges used for adult animals are not always appropriate for neonates and this is essential to remember in order to avoid misdiagnosis. In addition, there is limited information available in the veterinary literature and what is available is regrettably typically based on studies performed on laboratory or experimental animals.

GENERAL TREATMENT CONCEPTS

NURSING ASPECT

Very young animals are much less able to cope with illness than older animals and require much

NURSING ASPECT—cont'd

more attentive nursing and monitoring. The role of the nurse is never more important than in the care of neonates and infants. Although most of the treatment measures implemented are nonspecific and supportive in nature, these animals are almost entirely dependent on their caretakers in the absence of their dams.

Treatment of neonates typically consists of:
- Temperature control
- Fluid therapy and glucose supplementation
- Nutritional support
- Stimulation of urination and defecation
- Infection control.

Hypothermia

- Neonates are highly susceptible, e.g.
  - Relatively large body surface area
  - Reduced subcutaneous fat
  - Immature thermoregulatory system (e.g. poor peripheral vasoconstriction, inability to shiver until after 1 week of age).
- Causes significant additional energy demand.
- May manifest as unresponsiveness, bradycardia and respiratory depression; may also promote ileus and cause gastro-oesophageal reflux.
- Common sign of sepsis.

CLINICAL TIP

- Hypothermic neonates should only be warmed once hypovolaemia, if present, has been addressed. They should not, however, be fed until warmed.
- Warming should be performed slowly and the animal must be able to move away from the heat source to avoid thermal injury. In addition, it must be remembered that neonates have a lower normal rectal temperature than older animals and are also unable to pant; they are therefore readily at risk of being overheated.

Warming

- Ambient temperature of 29–32°C recommended.
- Guidelines for target rectal temperatures at which the intensity of warming can be reduced:

Table 41.2 Guidelines for interpretation of clinicopathological findings in puppies and kittens

Parameter	Puppies	Kittens
Haematocrit, packed cell volume (PCV)	Within adult range at birth Decreases thereafter Nadir usually at about 4 weeks old (coincides with weaning) Normalizes by 3–6 months old	Within adult range at birth Decreases thereafter (usually decreases proportionally less than in puppies) Nadir usually at about 4–6 weeks old (coincides with weaning) Normalizes by 3–6 months old
Leucogram, platelet count	Typically as for adult dogs Possible mild lymphocytosis based on adult range by 3 weeks old	Typically as for adult cats Possible leucocytosis based on adult range by 8–9 weeks old
Glucose	Similar to adult range	Similar to adult range
Albumin	Lower than adult range at birth Increases thereafter and usually normalizes by 2–4 months old	Lower than adult range at birth Increases thereafter and usually normalizes by 2–4 months old
Globulin	Lower than adult range at birth Increases thereafter and usually normalizes by 6 months old	Lower than adult range at birth Increases thereafter and usually normalizes by 6 months old
Bilirubin	May be greater than adult range (perhaps 2–3 times maximum) Usually normalizes by 6 weeks old	May be greater than adult range (perhaps 5 times maximum) Usually normalizes by 6 weeks old
Alkaline phosphatase (ALP)	Greater than adult range (perhaps 40–80 times maximum)	Greater than adult range (perhaps 3–6 times maximum)
Gamma glutamyl transferase (GGT)	Greater than adult range (perhaps 150–500 times maximum)	Similar to adult range
Blood urea nitrogen (BUN)	May be lower than adult range	May be lower than adult range
Creatinine	May be lower than adult range	May be lower than adult range
Calcium, phosphorus	Increased due to bone growth	Increased due to bone growth
Urine specific gravity	Isosthenuric (1.007–1.015) for a few days after birth Increases with age to reach normal concentrating ability by 8–10 weeks old (can take up to 6 months)	Isosthenuric (1.007–1.015) for a few days after birth Increases with age to reach normal concentrating ability by 8–10 weeks old (can be delayed but less so than puppies)
Glucosuria, proteinuria	May be normal in puppies (usually less than 8 weeks old)	May be normal in kittens (usually less than 8 weeks old)

  - 1–3 days old: 36.5–37°C
  - 4–7 days old: 37–37.5°C
  - >7 days old: 37.5–38.0°C.
- Warmed (but not hot!) fluids should be administered: warm the fluid line in relatively close proximity to the patient so that the fluid is still warm when it enters the body. This is best achieved using an in-line fluid warmer (e.g. Tempcare® Veterinary Fluid Warmer) but wrapping the line around several hot hands or a hot water bottle may be satisfactory. You must ensure that the patient is not at risk of thermal injury.

- Warming of fluid bags is far less effective, as cooling occurs within a matter of minutes. Even if the fluid bag can be kept warm, cooling is likely en route to the patient.

Hypoglycaemia

- Neonates are highly susceptible, e.g.
  - Immature glucose feedback mechanisms
  - Inefficient hepatic gluconeogenesis
  - Decreased glycogen stores
  - Brain (and heart) are highly dependent on glucose as the energy substrate
  - Increased loss of glucose in urine.
- Causes of hypoglycaemia include:
  - Vomiting and diarrhoea due to primary gastrointestinal disease or another cause
  - Inadequate food and fluid intake
  - Infection.
- Hypoglycaemia may manifest as lethargy, depression, poor feeding, crying, and a limp body.

Treatment

- Enteral supplementation
- Parenteral supplementation:
  - Intravenous or intraosseous but not subcutaneous or intraperitoneal route
  - Glucose solutions (1.25–5%) made up in 0.9% sodium chloride (normal, physiological saline) or Hartmann's solution (buffered lactated Ringer's solution) should be used
  - A 4% glucose solution in 0.18% sodium chloride is commercially available but should not be used. This solution is markedly hypotonic compared to plasma and can cause potentially very serious electrolyte derangements (see Ch. 4).

CLINICAL TIP

- It can be both difficult and potentially undesirable to check blood glucose regularly in neonates. The author tends to take an empirical approach to hypoglycaemic neonates, providing a conservative basal level of supplementation with additional treatments being guided by deterioration in the clinical status more than blood glucose measurements.
- The route of administration depends on whether parenteral access is available. Intravenous administration is generally preferred, but the author has used oral glucose solutions (e.g. Glucogel©, BBI Healthcare, Swansea, UK) applied topically to the oral mucosa with good success in a number of cases. As always the level and route of supplementation must be guided by the individual requirements of the patient.
- It is also noteworthy that while hypoglycaemia is clearly undesirable, excessive glucose supplementation may be more problematic in neonates than it is in older animals.

Fluid therapy

Fluid requirements of very young animals are much higher than for adults, for example due to:

- Higher percentage of total body water
- Greater surface area to body weight ratio
- Higher metabolic rate.

Maintenance rates as high as 10 ml/kg/hr may be required for replacement isotonic crystalloid solutions. However, it is noteworthy that excessive fluid administration may have more serious consequences than in older animals as immature animals have a reduced ability to dilute their urine and thereby excrete the surplus fluid. Close monitoring is therefore indicated, although in practical terms this may be difficult to achieve (e.g. monitoring of packed cell volume and total solids is very difficult). Monitoring weight may be helpful, especially if weight loss occurs as these animals should be gaining weight daily and weight loss may be due to dehydration. Monitoring for an increase in respiratory rate and effort may be the most practical evidence of fluid overload.

Route and rate of fluid therapy depend on the individual patient's requirements but may also be affected by patient size and compliance, and the expertise of the personnel.

- Enteral feeding if the patient is normothermic and still nursing; warmed subcutaneous or intraperitoneal isotonic crystalloid fluid therapy may also be appropriate for these cases depending on the suspected degree of dehydration and the success of enteral feeding; glucose should not be included in fluids given by these parenteral routes.
- Intravenous or intraosseous fluid therapy for moderate to severe dehydration or hypovolaemia.

Hypovolaemia can be very difficult to detect as changes in perfusion parameters may be due to immature compensatory mechanisms; a conservative approach to fluid resuscitation is recommended. Severe dehydration is the most common cause of hypovolaemia in the very young.

Drug therapy

- Altered drug absorption, distribution, metabolism, efficacy and elimination are likely when compared to adults, for example due to:
  - Greater surface area to body weight ratio
  - Reduced body fat and greater water composition (may affect distribution)
  - Lower serum concentration of total protein and especially albumin (to which most drugs preferentially bind)
  - Reduced renal clearance
  - Immature hepatic enzyme systems for oxidation and glucuronidation
  - Greater permeability of the neonatal blood–brain barrier
  - Immature autonomic nervous system.
- Factors change as animal gets older.
- Neonates are dependent on a high respiratory rate to prevent hypoxia and on a relatively fast heart rate to maintain cardiac output; use drugs causing cardiorespiratory depression very judiciously.
- Try opioids first for sedation; additional drugs should only be added if still required.

CLINICAL TIP

- Although perhaps not applicable to all drugs, in general dose reduction is appropriate for animals up to 12 weeks of age, and older in some cases. The reader is encouraged to consult datasheets and authoritative drug formularies for more information about specific drugs prior to their use.
- Dose reduction often involves reducing the recommended adult dose by up to 50% and/or increasing the recommended adult dosing interval by up to 50%.

Antimicrobial therapy

- The intestinal flora is more susceptible to disruption by antimicrobial therapy and will cope less well with any subsequent diarrhoea.
- Only use antimicrobial treatment if there is a good clinical indication.
- Beta-lactam antibiotics (e.g. amoxicillin/clavulanic acid, cephalosporins) are usually the first choice and require an increased dosing interval due to the prolonged half-life.
- Metronidazole is recommended for giardiasis and anaerobic infections; dose reduction is required.

Analgesia

Analgesia is highly important in young animals and many of the same principles apply as for adults (see Ch. 5).

Opioids

- Can be used very safely.
- Full (pure) opioids are preferred as they can be readily titrated.
- Avoid preconceptions about the required dose, i.e. whether you should use more or less compared to adults; start at bottom end of the adult dose range and titrate upwards according to the response.
- Naloxone can be used to reverse the effects.

Nonsteroidal anti-inflammatory agents

Avoid at least until the animal is more than 12 weeks of age due to the immaturity of hepatic and renal systems, and inherent difficulties in assessing volume and hydration status.

Local anaesthesia

Use lidocaine at reduced doses (due to immaturity of the peripheral nerves).

CLINICAL TIP

- EMLA® cream 5% (AstraZeneca) (see Ch. 5) is safe in young animals and the author would strongly encourage its use as extensively as possible.

APPENDICES

APPENDIX
MCQs

1. **Which of the following is most correct? The major body systems are:**
   (a) The cardiovascular and respiratory systems
   (b) The cardiovascular and neurological systems
   (c) The cardiovascular, respiratory and neurological systems
   (d) The cardiovascular, neurological and musculoskeletal systems

2. **Which is the most common type of shock in dogs and cats?**
   (a) Hypovolaemic
   (b) Maldistributive
   (c) Cardiogenic
   (d) Obstructive

3. **Which of the following is most correct? The main physical examination parameters for assessing perfusion are:**
   (a) Heart rate, mucous membrane colour and capillary refill time
   (b) Heart rate, peripheral pulse quality and mucous membrane colour
   (c) Heart rate, peripheral pulse quality, mucous membrane colour and capillary refill time
   (d) Heart rate, peripheral pulse quality, mucous membrane colour, capillary refill time and skin turgor

4. **Which of the following is most true about prerenal azotaemia?**
   (a) The azotaemia is severe and associated with increased packed cell volume, plasma total solids and urine specific gravity
   (b) The azotaemia is severe and associated with decreased packed cell volume, plasma total solids and urine specific gravity
   (c) The azotaemia is mild and associated with decreased packed cell volume, plasma total solids and urine specific gravity
   (d) The azotaemia is mild and associated with increased packed cell volume, plasma total solids and urine specific gravity

5. **Which of the following is correct? In uncomplicated severe hypovolaemia the size of the initial isotonic crystalloid bolus should be:**
   (a) 20–40 ml/kg for both dogs and cats
   (b) 60–90 ml/kg for dogs, 40–60 ml/kg for cats
   (c) 60–90 ml/kg for dogs, 10–20 ml/kg for cats
   (d) 20–40 ml/kg for dogs, 40–60 ml/kg for cats

6. **Which of the following opioids has the slowest onset of action?**
   (a) Morphine
   (b) Methadone
   (c) Butorphanol
   (d) Buprenorphine

7. **Which of the following causes of acute abdomen is not a surgical emergency?**
   (a) Perforated gastric ulcer
   (b) Nonperforated gastric ulcer
   (c) Uterine rupture
   (d) Intestinal obstruction

8. **Which of the following is not an indication to treat ventricular tachycardia with lidocaine?**
   (a) Associated with haemodynamic compromise
   (b) Recurrent R-on-T phenomenon
   (c) Multiform complexes
   (d) Sustained rate of 140 beats per minute

9. Which of the following statements about hyperthermia is not true?
- **(a)** Hyperthermia should be treated with an antipyretic agent
- **(b)** Hyperthermia should be treated by active cooling
- **(c)** Active cooling should cease when temperature reaches 39.5°C
- **(d)** Hyperthermia may be caused by heat stress or severe seizure activity

10. Which of the following statements about hypothermia is not true?
- **(a)** Hypovolaemic hypothermic animals should be treated with appropriate fluid therapy before warming
- **(b)** Animals that present with hypothermia as a result of cardiac dysfunction should be warmed aggressively
- **(c)** Hypothermic animals should not be fed until temperature has improved
- **(d)** Hypothermia can have adverse effects on many body systems

11. Which of the following is not associated with hepatic jaundice in cats?
- **(a)** Feline cholangitis/cholangiohepatitis complex
- **(b)** Hepatic lipidosis
- **(c)** *Mycoplasma haemofelis* infection
- **(d)** Hepatic lymphoma

12. The lag phase for red blood cell regeneration (preregenerative anaemia) following significant blood loss is:
- **(a)** Up to 3 days
- **(b)** Up to 7 days
- **(c)** Up to 14 days
- **(d)** Up to 21 days

13. Which of the following statements is not true about regurgitation?
- **(a)** Regurgitation is most commonly due to small intestinal disease
- **(b)** Regurgitation is a passive event
- **(c)** Regurgitation is associated with an increased risk of aspiration pneumonia
- **(d)** Regurgitation shows no consistent relationship with feeding

14. Which of the following statements is not true about lung sounds?
- **(a)** Pulmonary oedema is associated with loud harsh lung sounds and possible crackles
- **(b)** Pulmonary contusions are associated with loud harsh lung sounds and possible crackles
- **(c)** Pleural effusion is associated with dull lung sounds
- **(d)** Pneumothorax is associated with loud harsh lung sounds dorsally

15. Idiopathic epilepsy is most likely to be diagnosed in which of the following?
- **(a)** A 2-year-old German shepherd
- **(b)** A 10-year-old Boxer
- **(c)** A 6-year-old Pug
- **(d)** A 6-month-old Yorkshire terrier

16. Following a motor vehicle accident, a cat presents with evidence of multiple traumatic injuries including to the head. The cat is found to be hypertensive and bradycardic. This is most likely due to:
- **(a)** Pain
- **(b)** Myocardial injury
- **(c)** Raised intracranial pressure
- **(d)** Ruptured urinary bladder

17. Which of the following statements is true following blunt thoracic trauma?
- **(a)** Pulmonary contusions and pneumothorax are the most common injuries
- **(b)** Diaphragmatic rupture is the most common injury
- **(c)** Flail segments usually occur without other injuries
- **(d)** Haemothorax requiring drainage is common

18. Which of the following is the most common cause of haemoabdomen in dogs?
- **(a)** Gastric dilatation/volvulus syndrome (GDV)
- **(b)** Coagulopathy
- **(c)** Rupture of an intra-abdominal neoplasm
- **(d)** Trauma

19. Which of the following statements is not true about abdominal counterpressure bandages?
- **(a)** They should be placed as tightly as possible
- **(b)** They should be placed starting caudally and moving cranially

(c) They should be removed starting cranially and moving caudally
(d) They should not be used in animals with respiratory compromise

20. Which of the following statements is not true about uroabdomen?
(a) Trauma is the most common cause
(b) Azotaemia is typically mild at the time of diagnosis
(c) Urea, creatinine and potassium concentrations in the peritoneal fluid are typically higher than concomitant plasma concentrations
(d) The presence of a palpable bladder does not rule out leakage of urine from the bladder

21. Which of the following is not considered a risk factor for gastric dilatation and volvulus?
(a) Large/giant breed
(b) Narrow and deep chest
(c) Feeding multiple small meals daily
(d) Fearful/agitated demeanour

22. Which of the following is not a contraindication for induction of emesis following oral toxin exposure?
(a) Significantly altered mentation
(b) Respiratory distress
(c) Ingestion of a caustic or corrosive agent
(d) More than 1 hour since ingestion

23. Intoxication with which of the following is not potentially associated with acute renal failure in dogs?
(a) Metaldehyde
(b) Grapes/raisins
(c) Ethylene glycol
(d) Nonsteroidal anti-inflammatory agents

24. Which of the following is not a vitamin-K dependent coagulation factor?
(a) II
(b) VIII
(c) IX
(d) X

25. Which of the following contains the lowest concentration of theobromine?
(a) White chocolate
(b) Milk chocolate
(c) Dark chocolate
(d) Cocoa powder

26. Which of the following has not been reported to occur following xylitol poisoning in dogs?
(a) Hypoglycaemia
(b) Acute renal failure
(c) Acute liver failure
(d) Coagulopathy

27. Which of the following is not a compensatory mechanism in heart disease?
(a) Tachycardia
(b) Increased inotropy
(c) Peripheral vasodilation
(d) Sodium and water retention

28. Which of the following is not indicated in all animals with acute decompensated congestive heart failure?
(a) Oxygen supplementation
(b) Digoxin
(c) Furosemide
(d) Low dose morphine

29. Which of the following is the most commonly diagnosed feline cardiomyopathy?
(a) Hypertrophic cardiomyopathy
(b) Dilated cardiomyopathy
(c) Restrictive cardiomyopathy
(d) Unclassified cardiomyopathy

30. Clinical signs in cats with aortic thromboembolism correlate least with which of the following?
(a) Whether complete or only partial obstruction occurs
(b) The duration of obstruction
(c) The extent and diameter of any collateral circulation
(d) The severity of the underlying heart disease

31. Which of the following tumours is most commonly identified in dogs with malignant pericardial effusion?
(a) Lymphoma
(b) Haemangiosarcoma
(c) Chemodectoma
(d) Mesothelioma

32. Which of the following is the least common cause of pleural effusion in cats?
- (a) Neoplasia
- (b) Congestive heart failure
- (c) Haemothorax
- (d) Pyothorax

33. Which of the following statements is not true about feline bronchial disease?
- (a) Siamese cats are over represented
- (b) Antibiotics are indicated in the treatment of all affected cats
- (c) Allergens or nonspecific airway irritants are likely to be involved in the pathogenesis
- (d) Clinical signs are the result of lower airway obstruction

34. Which of the following statements is not true about canine laryngeal paralysis?
- (a) It is usually bilateral
- (b) In most cases laryngeal paralysis is an acquired condition
- (c) There is a high incidence of megaoesophagus in affected dogs
- (d) Emergency tracheostomy is frequently required in dogs suffering an acute respiratory crisis

35. Which of the following is not considered a component of brachycephalic airway obstruction syndrome?
- (a) Tracheal hypoplasia
- (b) Elongated soft palate
- (c) Stenotic nares
- (d) Everted laryngeal saccules

36. Which of the following is not consistent with immune-mediated haemolytic anaemia?
- (a) Nonregenerative anaemia
- (b) Positive in-saline agglutination test
- (c) Spherocytosis
- (d) Positive Coombs' test

37. How many platelets do animals with primary (idiopathic) immune-mediated thrombocytopenia (ITP) typically have per high power field (×100) on peripheral blood smear examination?
- (a) 3–4
- (b) 2–3
- (c) 1–2
- (d) 0–1

38. Which of the following is least consistent with primary hypoadrenocorticism (Addison's disease)?
- (a) Hyponatraemia
- (b) Hyperkalaemia
- (c) Hyperglycaemia
- (d) Mild azotaemia

39. Which of the following statements is not true about diabetic ketoacidosis?
- (a) It occurs most commonly in animals without a prior diagnosis of diabetes mellitus
- (b) Most animals have another concurrent precipitating disorder
- (c) There is no risk of recurrence following one episode of ketoacidosis
- (d) It is diagnosed most often in middle-aged to older male cats and female dogs

40. Iatrogenic hypocalcaemia following bilateral thyroidectomy usually occurs how many days after surgery?
- (a) 1–5
- (b) 6–10
- (c) 11–15
- (d) 16–20

41. Which of the following does not distinguish acute anterior uveitis from acute glaucoma?
- (a) Miotic pupil
- (b) Painful red eye
- (c) Abnormal iris
- (d) Low intraocular pressure

42. Which of the following statements is not true about feline urethral obstruction?
- (a) Mechanical urethral obstruction is much more common in male cats
- (b) Urethral plugs are the most common cause in male cats
- (c) Struvite urolithiasis in cats is typically associated with a urease-producing bacterial infection
- (d) Prolonged urethral obstruction results in hypovolaemia and profound electrolyte and acid–base disturbances

43. Which of the following is the most common cause of acute renal failure in dogs and cats?
(a) Infection
(b) Trauma
(c) Disseminated intravascular coagulation (DIC)
(d) Toxins

44. Which of the following is not a recognized electrocardiogram abnormality in hyperkalaemia?
(a) Sinoventricular rhythm
(b) Sinus tachycardia
(c) Atrial standstill
(d) Peaked T waves

45. Which of the following is the most common cause of dystocia in dogs and cats?
(a) Mechanical obstruction
(b) Foetal malpresentation
(c) Primary uterine inertia
(d) Maternal anxiety

46. Which of the following is not considered to be an indication for immediate veterinary attention during parturition?
(a) Weak irregular nonproductive straining for more than 30 minutes
(b) A green (bitch) or brown (queen) vulval discharge without a foetus being born in the subsequent 2 hours
(c) Flank biting or other signs suggesting severe abdominal discomfort in the dam
(d) The presence of a foetus or foetal membranes protruding from the vulva for more than 15 minutes

47. Which of the following is not good advice to a client ringing about a dog with heatstroke before bringing the dog down to the clinic?
(a) Gently hose/soak the dog with cool (not cold) water
(b) Cover the dog in wet towels
(c) Offer water if alert but withhold if vomiting
(d) Drive to the nearest clinic with the air conditioning on or windows open

48. When considering general anaesthesia in a pregnant animal, which of the following is incorrect?
(a) There is an increased risk of regurgitation/vomiting due to pressure from the gravid uterus and not being starved
(b) Anaesthetic doses must be calculated according to the estimated nonpregnant weight
(c) Positioning in dorsal recumbency may cause hypotension due to compression of the caudal vena cava by the gravid uterus
(d) Inhalation induction occurs more slowly and overdose is less likely

49. Which of the following statements is not true with respect to feline blood transfusion?
(a) Most cats are blood type A
(b) Blood type B is more common among exotic and pure breeds
(c) A severe and potentially fatal transfusion reaction is a very real possibility if a type A cat is given type B blood
(d) Type AB cats do not possess naturally occurring antibodies to type A or B red cell antigens

50. Which of the following statements is incorrect about a 4-week-old kitten?
(a) Total protein concentration is within the adult reference range
(b) Haematocrit is lower than the adult reference range
(c) Blood glucose concentration is within the adult reference range
(d) Vision should be normal

APPENDIX MCQs – Answers

1. **(c)** Severe abnormalities in these three systems have the potential to be rapidly fatal.
2. **(a)** Hypovolaemia is a reduction in the effective circulating intravascular volume and is the most common cause of shock in companion animals.
3. **(c)** Answers (a) and (b) do not include all the perfusion parameters; skin turgor included in answer (d) is an indicator of hydration, not perfusion.
4. **(d)** Severe azotaemia is usually postrenal or renal in origin; prerenal azotaemia is usually due to dehydration which causes increased PCV and TS, and fluid conservation (hence high urine specific gravity).
5. **(b)**
6. **(d)** Onset may be up to 45 minutes therefore typically not appropriate as first line analgesic.
7. **(b)**
8. **(d)** Sustained (more than 30 seconds) ventricular tachycardia at a rate above 180 beats per minute is an indication to treat.
9. **(a)** In hyperthermia the thermoregulatory set point is unchanged and the hypothalamus attempts to return core temperature to normal limits. Clinically significant consequences occur when physiological attempts to cool the body become overwhelmed and active cooling is therefore appropriate. Antipyretic agents reset the thermoregulatory set point and should not be used.
10. **(b)** Warming will lead to cutaneous vasodilation that may exacerbate hypotension; these animals should therefore not be warmed. An increase in temperature in these cases may be supportive of a positive response to appropriate treatment of the heart disease.
11. **(c)** *Mycoplasma haemofelis* causes haemolytic anaemia that results in prehepatic jaundice if it occurs.
12. **(b)**
13. **(a)** Regurgitation is most commonly due to oesophageal disease, especially megaoesophagus and oesophageal foreign bodies.
14. **(d)** Pneumothorax is associated with quiet lung sounds dorsally (and possibly diffusely).
15. **(a)**
16. **(c)** The Cushing response constitutes raised intracranial pressure giving rise to systemic hypertension and a reflex bradycardia.
17. **(a)**
18. **(c)**
19. **(a)** Realistically intra-abdominal pressure is only likely to be increased sufficiently to exceed venous pressure and reduce venous haemorrhage. Therefore excessively tight bandages do not offer any greater advantage and are likely to be associated with greater complications.
20. **(b)** Azotaemia is typically severe at the time of diagnosis.
21. **(c)** Feeding a single large meal daily is considered a risk factor.
22. **(d)** Induction of emesis is appropriate for several hours following oral exposure.
23. **(a)** Metaldehyde is associated with central nervous system signs (and occasionally temporary blindness or liver failure).
24. **(b)** Factor VII is the missing vitamin K-dependent factor.
25. **(a)**
26. **(b)** Hypoglycaemia and acute liver failure reported; coagulopathy secondary to liver failure.
27. **(c)** Peripheral vasoconstriction occurs to counter the tendency towards arterial hypotension in heart disease.

28. **(b)** Digoxin is now only considered appropriate in a specific population of cases.

29. **(a)** Hypertrophic cardiomyopathy (HCM) is the most commonly diagnosed feline heart disease and is inherited in some breeds (e.g. the Maine coon).

30. **(d)** There is no reported correlation between the severity of heart disease and the clinical signs of obstruction.

31. **(b)** Haemangiosarcoma is the most commonly diagnosed canine cardiac tumour and arises most often from the wall of the right atrium or auricle. It is the most common cause of canine pericardial effusion and is assumed to have metastasized in virtually all cases at the time of diagnosis.

32. **(c)**

33. **(b)** The relationship between respiratory infection and feline bronchial disease remains to be clarified. Antibiotics should only be used if infection is documented.

34. **(d)** Emergency tracheostomy is rarely required.

35. **(a)** Tracheal hypoplasia of variable severity may or may not be present in dogs with BAOS.

36. **(a)** IMHA is typically associated with a (strongly) regenerative anaemia.

37. **(d)** The diagnosis of immune-mediated thrombocytopenia is routinely made on the basis of identifying a thrombocytopenia of this severity in an animal with compatible clinical signs. Thereafter, investigations are performed to identify a primary cause and if one cannot be found, a presumptive diagnosis of ITP is made.

38. **(c)** Mild hypoglycaemia is a relatively common finding in Addison's disease.

39. **(c)** There is a constant risk of recurrence in these animals, especially cats.

40. **(a)**

41. **(b)** Acute glaucoma is also associated with a painful red eye but characterized by mydriasis, raised intraocular pressure and a normal iris.

42. **(c)** This is true in dogs but not in cats; antibiotics should not be used without documenting infection.

43. **(d)**

44. **(b)** Sinus bradycardia is recognized.

45. **(c)**

46. **(a)** Weak irregular nonproductive straining for more than 2 hours is an indication for veterinary attention, as is strong active but nonproductive abdominal contractions for more than 30 minutes.

47. **(b)** Covering the dog in wet towels is a significant impediment to heat loss and should be avoided.

48. **(d)** Inhalation induction occurs more rapidly but overdose is more likely

49. **(c)** The answer is the wrong way round; in fact a severe and potentially fatal transfusion reaction is a very real possibility if a type B cat is given type A blood (as most type B cats have high levels of strong, naturally occurring anti-type A alloantibodies).

50. **(a)** Total protein (both albumin and globulin) is lower than the adult reference range.

1 APPENDIX
Drug formulary

Agent	Dose/routes of administration	Indication(s) in emergency patients	Adverse effects/other comments
Acepromazine	D, C: 0.005–0.05 mg/kg slow i.v., i.m., s.c. q 4–6 hr	Sedation and anxiolysis, including for upper respiratory tract obstruction	Phenothiazine Allow adequate time for full clinical effect (15 min) before administering further doses Causes peripheral vasodilation and potentially hypotension; also bradycardia Avoid if there is cardiovascular instability, shock, head trauma or severe renal or hepatic disease Cannot reverse No analgesic effect Some antidysrhythmic effects
Activated charcoal	D, C: 1–5 g/kg p.o. Repeat q 4–6 hr until faeces are black	Adsorbent for treatment of oral poisoning	Not absorbed or metabolized in the gut Potential adverse effects are vomiting and constipation after multiple doses; diarrhoea possible Black faeces
Adrenaline (epinephrine)	D, C: low dose 0.01–0.02 mg/kg i.v., i.o.; 0.02–0.04 mg/kg via endotracheal tube; q 3–5 min D, C: high dose 0.1–0.2 mg/kg i.v., i.o.; 0.2–0.4 mg/kg via endotracheal tube; q 3–5 min	Cardiopulmonary cerebral resuscitation	Endotracheal administration should be performed using a urinary catheter to administer at the level of the carina Try low dose first; then high dose if no response
	D, C: 0.01 mg/kg slow i.v. (or i.m., s.c. in less severe cases); 0.01 mg/kg into tongue vein or parenchyma; 0.02 mg/kg via endotracheal tube	Anaphylaxis/ anaphylactic shock	Endotracheal administration should be performed using a urinary catheter to administer at the level of the carina Repeat after 20–30 min (or sooner if necessary) if the response is inadequate Appropriate fluid therapy and adrenaline administration should cause clinical improvement within minutes
Alfaxalone	D: up to 1 mg/kg slowly i.v. C: up to 2 mg/kg slowly i.v.	Sedation	Always give to effect – no prescribed dose Bolus effect lasts 5–10 min No analgesia
	D: up to 2 mg/kg slowly i.v. but typically 1–1.5 mg/kg C: up to 5 mg/kg slowly i.v. but typically 3–4 mg/kg	General anaesthesia with premedication	As above

Agent	Dose/routes of administration	Indication(s) in emergency patients	Adverse effects/other comments
Aminophylline (theophylline + ethylenediamine)	D: 9–11 mg/kg slowly i.v. (diluted), (i.m.) C: 2–5 mg/kg slowly i.v. (diluted), (i.m.)	Emergency bronchodilation	i.m. administration is locally painful; avoid if at all possible Theophyllines relax smooth muscle in the bronchi and pulmonary vasculature Weak chronotropic and inotropic action Mild diuretic action
Amlodipine	C: 0.625–1.25 mg/cat p.o. q 12–24 hr D: 0.05–0.2 mg/kg p.o. q 12–24 hr	Hypertension, especially in cats	Calcium channel blocker; causes peripheral arteriolar vasodilation Relatively slow onset of action (maximum effect within 7 days)
Amoxicillin/clavulanic acid	D, C: 20 mg/kg i.v. q 8 hr; 12.5–25 mg/kg p.o. q 8–12 hr	Bacterial infections	Amoxicillin is bactericidal; clavulanic acid is a beta-lactamase inhibitor that increases the spectrum of activity Broad spectrum activity against some Gram-positive and Gram-negative aerobes; many obligate anaerobes Time-dependent activity so avoid missing doses Hypersensitivity reactions are occasionally reported
Apomorphine	D: 0.04–0.1 mg/kg s.c., i.m., ocular (i.v.) C: 0.02 mg/kg s.c., i.m.	Induction of emesis following oral poisoning	Stimulates dopamine receptors in the chemoreceptor trigger zone causing emesis Highly reliable emesis in dogs, usually within 5–15 min Ocular route: apply to conjunctival sac; lavage thoroughly following emesis to minimize drug absorption; highly dependent on compliance. Centrally acting Sedation, respiratory depression, ataxia, protracted vomiting Use in cats not recommended by some
Ascorbic acid (vitamin C)	D, C: 30 mg/kg p.o. q 6 hr for 6 doses	Reduction of methaemoglobinaemia associated with paracetamol (acetaminophen) poisoning	Preparations for i.v. use may be available; treatment regimen as for oral preparations
Aspirin (acetylsalicylic acid)	C: 22–25 mg/kg p.o. q 48–72 hr; 75 mg p.o. q 48–72 hr (high dose) C: 5 mg/cat p.o. q 72 hr (low dose)	Antithrombotic in feline cardiomyopathy; prophylaxis of arterial thromboembolism	Reduces platelet aggregation Beneficial effect of high dose regimen has not been proven Further clarification required regarding efficacy of low dose regimen Do not use in dehydrated or hypovolaemic animals or those with gastrointestinal disease; use cautiously in renal disease Gastrointestinal side effect is the most common Care needed as cats have reduced ability to metabolize and excrete salicylates

Continued

Agent	Dose/routes of administration	Indication(s) in emergency patients	Adverse effects/other comments
	D: 0.5 mg/kg p.o. q 24 hr	Antithrombotic in immune-mediated haemolytic anaemia (IMHA)	Ultralow dose therapy Discontinued at the same time as prednisolone administration ceases
Atipamezole	D: 5× dose in mg/kg of medetomidine (same volume) i.m., s.c. C: 2.5× dose in mg/kg of medetomidine (half volume) i.m., s.c.	Selective $alpha_2$-adrenergic antagonist – reversal agent for medetomidine, dexmedetomidine	Can give half the quoted dose and repeat if poor reversal of sedation Avoid i.v. administration unless in emergency due to possible hypotension and/or aggression Reverses analgesic effect, so ensure alternative analgesia is provided
	C: 50 µg/kg i.m.	Medetomidine (20 µg/kg) reversal following induction of emesis	
Atropine sulphate	D, C: 0.02–0.04 mg/kg i.v., i.m., s.c.	Vagally mediated clinically significant bradydysrhythmia	Antimuscarinic agent (vagolytic) Dose-related pharmacological effects; multisystemic adverse effects possible at high doses Peak effects within 2–4 min following i.v. administration (up to 10 min with i.m. administration); wait for full effect before repeating dose due to an apparently poor response
Atropine sulphate ophthalmic preparation	D, C: 1 drop or small amount of ointment q 8–12 hr until pupil dilated then q 24–72 hr as necessary to maintain mydriasis	Miosis in anterior uveitis	Causes pupillary dilation and cycloplegia
Azathioprine	D: 2 mg/kg p.o. q 24 hr for up to 7–10 days, then q 48 hr long-term	Immune-mediated haemolytic anaemia (IMHA) Immune-mediated thrombocytopenia	Typically used with corticosteroid Delayed onset of action (may be up to 6 weeks, generally 10–14 days) therefore not useful in initial stabilization; however, provides a long-term corticosteroid-sparing effect and allows a quicker dose reduction Monitor for bone marrow suppression and hepatotoxicity; gastrointestinal signs and acute pancreatitis are also reported Do not administer to cats due to a marked bone marrow toxicity
Benazepril	D: 0.25–0.5 mg/kg p.o. q 12–24 hr C: 0.25–1.0 mg/kg p.o. q 12–24 hr	Heart failure Hypertension Chronic renal failure Protein-losing glomerulonephropathy	Angiotensin converting enzyme (ACE) inhibitor; causes vasodilation and decreased salt and water retention (decreased aldosterone production) Requires hydrolysis in the liver to benazeprilat for pharmacological activity Amlodipine is more effective for hypertension in cats Monitor for hypotension, hyperkalaemia and renal impairment

Agent	Dose/routes of administration	Indication(s) in emergency patients	Adverse effects/other comments
Buprenorphine	D: 0.01–0.02 mg/kg i.v., i.m. or s.c. q 6–8 hr C: 0.01–0.02 mg/kg i.v., i.m., . s.c. or o.t.m. q 6–8 hr	Analgesia for mild to moderate pain	Partial μ (OP3) agonist, also has antagonistic actions Typically not appropriate as the first line analgesic due to its slow onset of action (usually up to 45 min) Especially effective in cats
Butorphanol	D, C: 0.1–0.6 mg/kg i.v., i.m. or s.c. q 1–4 hr, prn; 0.05–0.4 mg/kg/h CRI	Sedation (analgesia) Antitussive effect	μ (OP3) antagonist, κ (OP2) agonist, Onset of action 15–20 min Not appropriate as the sole analgesic
Calcium gluconate (10%)	D, C: 0.5–1.5 ml/kg i.v. bolus over 5–20 min (equivalent to 50–150 mg calcium gluconate/kg, or 4.5–13.4 mg elemental calcium/kg) Then 0.3–0.6 ml/kg/hr CRI (equivalent to 30–60 mg calcium gluconate/kg/hr, or 2.7–5.4 mg elemental calcium/kg/hr)	Clinically significant hypocalcaemia	Repeat boluses until signs have resolved Dilute with 0.9% sodium chloride for CRI; using buffered lactated Ringer's solution for dilution may result in calcium precipitation Monitor for bradycardia ECG monitoring recommended during administration
Calcium gluconate (10%)	D, C: 0.5–1.5 ml/kg i.v. bolus over 30–60 s (equivalent to 50–150 mg calcium gluconate/kg, or 4.5–13.4 mg elemental calcium/kg)	Clinically significant hyperkalaemia	Given more quickly than for treatment of hypocalcaemia as it is a potentially life-saving treatment for cardiotoxicity Rapid onset of action (can be a few seconds) and first line choice in a crisis Short duration of action (often 10–15 min) Monitor ECG during administration Does not lower serum potassium concentration but restores normal cell membrane excitability Will also address any possible ionized hypocalcaemia Bolus can be repeated while other measures are used to improve hyperkalaemia directly
Calcium	D, C: 15–100 mg elemental calcium/kg/day (typically divided into 2–4 equal doses)	Chronic therapy for hypocalcaemia	1 mg elemental calcium is equivalent to 11.2 mg calcium gluconate, 7.7 mg calcium lactate, and 2.5 mg calcium carbonate Typically used together with vitamin D therapy but tapered earlier while continuing with long-term vitamin D Calcium carbonate preferred as it contains the highest concentration of elemental calcium, so reducing the number of tablets to be administered

Continued

Agent	Dose/routes of administration	Indication(s) in emergency patients	Adverse effects/other comments
Carprofen	D: ≤4 mg/kg i.v., s.c. (i.m.) q 24 hr (or divided into 2 equal doses q 12 hr); reduce to 2 mg/kg/day single dose after 7 days C: 1–2 mg/kg s.c., i.v. single dose perioperatively	Analgesia Antiinflammatory effect Antipyretic activity	Nonsteroidal antiinflammatory agent; preferential COX-2 inhibitor Do not administer if the patient has dehydration or hypovolaemia/ hypoperfusion Contraindicated with gastrointestinal and bleeding disorders Gastrointestinal, renal, hepatic and coagulopathic adverse effects have been reported Do not administer to animals less than 12 weeks old
Chlorambucil	C: 2 mg (total dose) p.o. q 24–72 hr	Immunosuppressive therapy in cats	Less toxic than azathioprine and cyclophosphamide in cats 2 mg tablets not readily dividable hence total dose recommendation; use longer dosing intervals in smaller cats Myelosuppression and gastrointestinal toxicity are the predominant adverse effects (generally 7–14 days after starting treatment)
Chlorpheniramine	D: 2–12 mg (maximum 0.5 mg/ kg) p.o. q 8–12 hr; 2.5–10 mg i.m. q 8–12 hr C: 2(–4) mg/cat p.o. q 8–12 hr	Hypersensitivity (allergic) disease	Antihistamine (H_1-receptor antagonist) Central nervous system depression and gastrointestinal adverse effects reported (likely to be mild)
Ciclosporin	D: 5–10 mg/kg p.o. q 12–24 hr	Long-term therapy for immune-mediated haemolytic anaemia (IMHA)	Monitor trough blood concentrations intermittently to achieve effective but safe levels Primarily adverse gastrointestinal effects but these are uncommon
Cimetidine	D, C: 5–10 mg/kg p.o., slow i.v. q 6–8 hr	Gastric mucosal injury/ ulceration Gastritis Oesophagitis secondary to gastric reflux	Histamine (H_2) receptor antagonist, increasing gastric acid pH by reducing acid production Inhibits hepatic microsomal enzymes and may alter the metabolic rates of other drugs (e.g. benzodiazepines, beta-blockers) Newer agents (e.g. ranitidine, famotidine) are more effective, have fewer drug interactions and longer dosing interval Other agents (e.g. omeprazole) are more effective
	D, C: 5 mg/kg slow i.v. q 8 hr	Paracetamol (acetaminophen) poisoning	Administer as early as possible for greatest efficacy

Agent	Dose/routes of administration	Indication(s) in emergency patients	Adverse effects/other comments
Dexamethasone (2 mg/ml)	D, C: 0.3–0.6 mg/kg i.v., s.c. q 24 hr	Immune-mediated haemolytic anaemia (IMHA) Immune-mediated thrombocytopenia	Corticosteroid with high glucocorticoid but low mineralocorticoid activity Use initially in animals that are vomiting or anorexic
	D, C: 0.25–1 mg/kg i.v., i.m. q 24 hr	Feline bronchial disease Upper respiratory tract dyspnoea	Initial dose may need to be given i.m. in animals with respiratory distress Typically start lower and then repeat dose if there is an inadequate response
	D, C: 0.1–1 mg/kg i.v. bolus	Urticaria, angioedema, anaphylaxis	Choose dose based on the severity of the signs Adrenaline administration and aggressive fluid therapy are the priority in anaphylaxis
	D: 0.5 mg/kg i.v. q 2–6 hr initially; then 0.05–0.1 mg/kg i.v. q 8–12 hr until oral medication is possible	Acute hypoadrenocorticism (Addisonian crisis)	Can be administered prior to or during an ACTH stimulation test
	D: 0.1 mg/kg i.v. q 24 hr for 3–7 days	*Angiostrongylus vasorum* infection	Administer in conjunction with antiparasitic treatment Intended to reduce inflammatory reaction associated with dying larvae Typically used in dogs with (marked) respiratory, neurological or ocular signs, or those with heavy worm burdens
Dexmedetomidine	Use half of medetomidine dose	Sedation Premedication for anaesthesia	As for medetomidine Use atipamezole for reversal
Diazepam	D, C: 0.1–0.5 mg/kg slow i.v.; 1–2 mg/kg p.r.; 0.1–1.0 mg/kg/hr CRI	First line management of seizures and muscle tremors	Benzodiazepine Rapid onset of action; duration of action likely to be 15–60 min Cannot mix in syringe with other agents May adsorb to plastic so do not store drawn up in syringes; consider midazolam for infusions Higher rectal dose used in animals receiving concurrent phenobarbital therapy Acute hepatic failure has been reported in cats as an idiosyncratic adverse drug reaction several days after starting oral therapy
	D, C: 0.1–0.5 mg/kg slowly i.v	Sedation in combination with an opioid and/or ketamine	As above May cause excitement if used alone Cannot give i.m.

Continued

Agent	Dose/routes of administration	Indication(s) in emergency patients	Adverse effects/other comments
Diltiazem	D: 0.1–0.25 mg/kg slow i.v. (over 2–3 min); can repeat q 5–15 min up to maximum total dose of 0.75 mg/kg; 0.5–2 mg/kg p.o. q 8 hr C: 0.05–0.2 mg/kg slow i.v. (over 3 min); 1.5–2.5 mg/kg p.o. q 8 hr	Clinically significant supraventricular tachycardia	Calcium channel blocker; slows atrioventricular node conduction and prolongs refractory times Treatment of congestive heart failure if present is the first step Attempt vagal manoeuvres before giving diltiazem Minimal negative inotropic effect
Diphenhydramine	D: 2–4 mg/kg p.o. q 8–12 hr; 1–2 mg/kg i.m., s.c., i.v. q 8–12 hr C: 0.5–4 mg/kg p.o. q 8–12 hr; 1–2 mg/kg i.m., s.c., i.v. q 8–12 hr	Hypersensitivity (allergic) disease	Antihistamine (H_1-receptor antagonist) Antipruritic, antitussive and antiemetic effects Central nervous system depression and anticholinergic effects (dry mouth, urinary retention) are the most common adverse effects
Doxycycline	C: 5–10 mg/kg p.o. q 24 hr for 10–21 days	*Mycoplasma haemofelis* (previously *Haemobartonella felis*) infection	Tetracycline antibiotic Direct oral administration must be followed by syringing a small amount (5 ml) of water to prevent lodging in the oesophagus and possible severe oesophagitis Use with caution in pregnant and young animals (bone and teeth abnormalities)
EMLA® cream 5% (2.5% lidocaine, 2.5% prilocaine)	D,C: topical application of empirical volume	Skin desensitization for venepuncture	Recommended especially for use in young animals and cats Usually covered with an occlusive dressing Onset of action may be less than the 30–60 min reported Minimal if any systemic drug absorption is likely
Enrofloxacin	C: 5 mg/kg slow i.v. diluted, s.c., p.o. q 24 hr	*Mycoplasma haemofelis* (previously *Haemobartonella felis*) infection	Fluoroquinolone antibiotic; concentration-dependent bactericidal (Gram negative, Gram positive, not anaerobes) Minimize use due to increasing resistance Especially useful for mycoplasmosis when enteral doxycycline is not possible or too stressful Has been associated with permanent blindness due to retinal toxicity in cats at higher doses than recommended here
Ethanol (20%)	D: 5.5 mL/kg i.v. q 4 hr for 5 doses then q 6 hr for 4 doses C: 5.0 mL/kg i.v. q 6 hr for 5 doses then q 8 hr for 4 doses D, C: give the same total dose as above over the same time period as a CRI	Ethylene glycol poisoning	Dilute in normal saline (0.9% sodium chloride) Central nervous system depression; intensive and supportive care may be required Fomepizole is the treatment of choice

Agent	Dose/routes of administration	Indication(s) in emergency patients	Adverse effects/other comments
Ethanol (40% as alcoholic beverage)	D: 4.4–6.6 mL/kg p.o. q 4 hr for 5 doses then q 6 hr for 4 doses C: 4.4 mL/kg p.o. q 6 hr for 5 doses then q 8 hr for 4 doses	Ethylene glycol poisoning	Central nervous system depression; intensive and supportive care may be required May cause gastric irritation and vomiting Do not use other ethanol-containing fluids (e.g. surgical spirit) Fomepizole is the treatment of choice
Famotidine	D: 0.5–1 mg/kg p.o., s.c., i.v. q 12–24 hr C: 0.5–1 mg/kg p.o., s.c. q 12–24 hr	Gastric mucosal injury/ulceration Gastritis Oesophagitis secondary to gastric reflux	Histamine (H_2) receptor antagonist, increasing gastric acid pH by reducing acid production Longer duration of action and fewer drug interactions than cimetidine There have been anecdotal reports of intravascular haemolysis following i.v. administration in cats
Fenbendazole	D: 50 mg/kg p.o. q 24 hr for 7–28 days	*Angiostrongylus vasorum* infection	Benzimidazole antiparasitic with very high safety index Not licensed for canine *A. vasorum* infection in the UK
Fludrocortisone	D: 0.01–0.02 mg/kg p.o. daily (single dose or divided into 2 equal doses) C: 0.05–0.1 mg/cat p.o. q 12–24 hr	Maintenance therapy for primary hypoadrenocorticism (Addison's disease)	Mainly mineralocorticoid but also has glucocorticoid activity that may produce clinically significant side effects Usually start at 0.01 mg/kg p.o. daily; monitor sodium and potassium levels q 1–2 weeks, and adjust daily dose by 0.05–0.1 mg as appropriate
Flumazenil	D, C: 0.01 mg/kg rapid i.v.	Benzodiazepine reversal agent	Competitive antagonist at benzodiazepine receptors in the central nervous system Onset of action 1–2 min Short duration of action (60 min)
Fomepizole	D: 20 mg/kg i.v. for first dose, followed by 15 mg/kg i.v. at 12 and 24 hr, and 5 mg/kg i.v. at 36 hr C: 125 mg/kg i.v. for first dose, followed by 31.25 mg/kg i.v. at 12, 24 and 36 hr	Ethylene glycol poisoning	Treatment of choice for ethylene glycol poisoning Mild dose-related central nervous system depression may be seen, especially in cats
Furosemide	D: 2–6 mg/kg i.v., i.m. q 1–2 hr until clinical improvement; then q 6–12 hr C: 1–4 mg/kg i.v., i.m. q 1–2 hr until clinical improvement; then q 12 hr	Acute decompensated congestive heart failure	Initial dose may need to be given i.m. depending on patient stability Loop diuretic; inhibits sodium and chloride reabsorption in thick ascending limb of loop of Henle – promotes natriuresis and reduces water resorption Response usually noted within 1 hr (e.g. urination) Ensure ad lib water available Excessive administration can cause severe dehydration, electrolyte abnormalities and renal failure

Continued

Agent	Dose/routes of administration	Indication(s) in emergency patients	Adverse effects/other comments
	D, C: give 2 mg/kg i.v.; if no significant diuresis after 1 hr, give 4 mg/kg i.v.; if no significant diuresis after 1 hr, give 6 mg/kg; if diuresis established, give 2–6 mg/kg i.v. q 6–8 hr or 0.1–1.0 mg/kg/hr CRI	Oliguric acute renal failure	Ensure adequate fluid replacement first Contraindicated if there is complete anuria If there is a poor initial response, try mannitol with the additional furosemide boluses If the patient remains anuric or is severely oliguric, needs dialysis
	D, C: 2–4 mg/kg i.v., s.c., p.o. q 8–12 hr	Hypercalcaemia	Only administer following volume expansion with normal saline (0.9% sodium chloride)
Glucose/dextrose (50%)	D, C: 0.25–0.5 g/kg diluted slow i.v. (0.5–1.0 ml/kg)	Treatment of clinically significant hypoglycaemia	Frequently needs to be followed by infusion (see p. 289)
Glyceryl trinitrate (2% topical preparation)	D: ½–2 inch q 6–8 hr C: ¼ inch q 6–8 hr	Acute decompensated congestive heart failure	Systemic venodilator reducing preload and potentially helping with pulmonary oedema Apply to clipped or hairless skin; rotate site of application (inner pinna, groin, axilla) Can be absorbed through human skin – wear gloves to apply; mark kennel and kennel sheet clearly to alert other personnel to its use and include the site of application
Heparin – low molecular weight (fractionated)	C: 100–300 IU/kg s.c. q 6–12 hr	Prevention of further thrombus formation following systemic thromboembolism	Beneficial effect not proven Much debate regarding dosage ranges and overall approach Beware of bleeding (and hypersensitivity reactions)
Hydrocortisone	D: 0.5–0.625 mg/kg/hr CRI; 2–4 mg/kg i.v. q 3–6 hr	Acute hypoadrenocorticism (Addisonian) crisis	Perform ACTH stimulation test prior to commencing treatment Mainly glucocorticoid but has some mineralocorticoid activity
Hydrogen peroxide (3%)	D, C: 1–3 ml/kg p.o.	Induction of emesis at home following oral poisoning	Ensure no contraindications to induction of emesis (see p. 153) Take care during administration to avoid aspiration Emesis usually within 10 min May be repeated once
Imidacloprid + moxidectin	D: 10 mg/kg imidacloprid + 2.5 mg/kg moxidectin topically (equivalent to 0.1 ml/kg)	*Angiostrongylus vasorum* infection	Advocate Spot-on solution® (Bayer plc, Newbury, UK) licensed
Insulin, neutral (regular, soluble)	D, C: 0.1–0.5 IU/kg i.v.	Clinically significant hyperkalaemia	Administer together with glucose (0.25–0.5 g/kg i.v.) Onset of action can be more than 15 min Lowers serum potassium concentration by moving potassium into cells Intravenous glucose supplementation is typically required for several hours subsequently (monitor and adjust accordingly)

Agent	Dose/routes of administration	Indication(s) in emergency patients	Adverse effects/other comments
Ketamine	D, C: 0.1–1 mg/kg i.v. prn (often q 30 min) or followed by 0.1–1.0 mg/kg/hr CRI	Analgesia for moderate to severe pain without profound sedation, typically in combination with an opioid	An *N*-methyl-*D*-aspartate (NMDA) receptor antagonist Variable cardiovascular effects; increase in heart rate, cardiac output and blood pressure may occur (centrally mediated sympathetic response and endogenous catecholamine release) Avoid if hyperdynamic cardiac disease is present Primarily excreted unchanged by the kidneys in cats, therefore use judiciously if there is renal dysfunction Cleared by primary hepatic metabolism in dogs Should not be used alone, especially in dogs
	D: 1–2 mg/kg i.v.; 1–5 mg/kg i.m; q 30–45 min C: 1–5 mg/kg i.v.; 2–10 mg/kg i.m.; q 30–45 min	Sedation	As above Typically combined with a benzodiazepine and often an opioid
	D: 2–5 mg/kg i.v.; 5–10 mg/kg i.m. C: 3–10 mg/kg i.v.; 10–20 mg/kg i.m.	General anaesthesia with premedication	As above Dissociative anaesthetic The only anaesthetic which is also a good analgesic Good preservation of protective airway reflexes Must combine with sedative – poor muscle relaxation when used alone Cats' eyes remain open after ketamine administration so lubricate
Lidocaine (2%)	D: 2 mg/kg i.v. bolus; 50–80 μg/kg/min CRI following successful bolus administration C: 0.25–0.75 mg/kg i.v. bolus; repeat in 0.25–0.5 mg/kg increments; 10–40 μg/kg/min CRI following successful bolus administration	Clinically significant ventricular dysrhythmia	Class 1b antidysrhythmic actions Alternative therapy is usually attempted if a satisfactory improvement is not noted after the maximum dose of 8 mg/kg in dogs, 4 mg/kg in cats Effective bolus administration is usually followed by CRI; cats more susceptible to adverse effects with infusion Signs of toxicity include vomiting, depression, hypersalivation and neurological signs It may be less effective with hypokalaemia
	D: 2 mg/kg topical application or infiltration; max dose 12 mg/kg C: 2 mg/kg topical application or infiltration; max dose 6 mg/kg	Local anaesthesia during surgical intervention	Causes reversible blockade of sodium channels Rapid onset of action (may be as short as 3–5 min) Short duration of action (1–2 hr) Especially recommended as an abdominal midline block during caesarean section

Continued

Agent	Dose/routes of administration	Indication(s) in emergency patients	Adverse effects/other comments
	D: 1–2 mg/kg i.v. loading dose followed by 50–80 μg/kg/min CRI	Analgesia	Infusion for analgesia is not recommended in cats due to the risk of significant cardiovascular depression
Mannitol	D, C: 0.5–1.5 g/kg i.v. over 10–20 min	Raised intracranial pressure	Osmotic diuretic; onset of osmotic effect 15–30 min Can be repeated every 2–8 hr but no more than three doses in a 24-hr period Discontinue therapy if there is no positive response Contraindicated in hypovolaemia, dehydration, congestive heart failure, pulmonary oedema and anuric renal failure Follow administration with isotonic crystalloid to prevent dehydration or hypovolaemia Dissolve crystals before use; in-line filter also recommended
	D, C: 0.5–1.5 g/kg i.v. over 10–20 min If diuresis occurs, can repeat q 4–6 hr for first 12–24 hr of treatment	Oliguric acute renal failure	As above Ensure adequate fluid replacement first Contraindicated in anuric renal failure (may worsen fluid overload and pulmonary oedema) Discontinue administration if there is no positive response to the first dose
Maropitant	D: 1 mg/kg s.c. q 24 hr for up to 5 consecutive days C: 0.5 mg/kg s.c. q 24 hr for up to 5 consecutive days	Antiemetic therapy	Neurokinin (NK_1) receptor antagonist in medullary vomiting centre Suppresses peripheral and centrally mediated emesis Injection may be painful; drug refrigeration may alleviate some associated discomfort If longer than 5 days treatment needed, allow 48 hr washout period between courses (due to drug accumulation) Use in cats is extra-label at the time of writing
Medetomidine	D: 1–5 μg/kg slow i.v.; 5–20 μg/kg i.m. C: 2–10 μg/kg i.v; 10–40 μg/kg i.m.	Sedation in combination with opioid	Profound changes in cardiac output and blood pressure Bradycardia and peripheral vasoconstriction (pale to white mucous membranes) Respiratory depression Avoid use if cardiovascular instability, shock, severe head trauma, renal failure or diabetes is present Easily reversible
	D, C: 2–5 μg/kg slow i.v. or i.m. prn (often q 30–90 min); 1–3 μg/kg/hr CRI	Analgesia	Especially useful in animals requiring some degree of concurrent sedation (e.g. due to anxiety or distress) Cardiovascular and respiratory effects likely to be minimal at these microdoses Dosing interval is significantly increased with concurrent opioid use

Agent	Dose/routes of administration	Indication(s) in emergency patients	Adverse effects/other comments
	C: 20 μg/kg i.m., i.v.; single dose only	Induction of emesis following oral poisoning	May sedate animal without causing emesis Conservative dosing is highly recommended
Meloxicam	D: ≤0.2 mg/kg i.v., s.c. or p.o. once; then ≤0.1 mg/kg i.v., s.c. or p.o. q 24 hr C: ≤0.3 mg/kg i.v., s.c. or p.o. once; then ≤0.1 mg/kg i.v., s.c. or p.o. q 24 hr	Analgesia Antiinflammatory effect Antipyretic activity	Nonsteroidal antiinflammatory agent; preferential COX-2 inhibitor Do not administer in cases with dehydration or hypovolaemia/hypoperfusion Use cautiously in cases with hepatic or renal dysfunction and bleeding disorders Gastrointestinal, renal and hepatic adverse effects are reported Do not administer to animals less than 12 weeks old
Methadone	D: 0.1–1.0 mg/kg slow i.v., i.m. or s.c. q 4 hr, prn C: 0.1–0.5 mg/kg slow i.v., i.m. or s.c. q 6 hr, prn	Analgesia Premedication Anxiolysis	Full μ (OP3) agonist The analgesia is equipotent with morphine Emesis rarely occurs following administration Panting commonly occurs in dogs
Methocarbamol	D, C: 44–220 mg/kg i.v.; ideally no more than 330 mg/kg/24 hr	Intoxication with tremorogenic toxins	Centrally acting skeletal muscle relaxant It may cause salivation, emesis; sedation, lethargy, weakness and ataxia
Methylprednisolone	D, C: 1–2 mg/kg i.v. over 15–20 min	Urticaria, angioedema, anaphylaxis	Adrenaline administration and aggressive fluid therapy are the priority in anaphylaxis
	D: 1–2 mg/kg i.v. q 2–6 hr	Acute hypoadrenocorticism (Addisonian crisis)	Negligible mineralocorticoid activity Perform ACTH stimulation test prior to starting treatment
Metoclopramide	D, C: 1–2 mg/kg i.v. over 24 hr as CRI; 0.2–0.5 mg/kg s.c. q 6–8 hr	Antiemetic therapy Upper gastrointestinal prokinetic	The antiemetic effect is mainly due to dopamine receptor antagonism in the chemoreceptor trigger zone Not licensed for antiemetic therapy (maropitant is licensed) Contraindicated in gastrointestinal obstruction Neurological signs and behavioural changes may occur as adverse effects; especially in cats
Metronidazole	D, C: 10 mg/kg slow i.v. q 12 hr; 15–25 mg/kg p.o. q 12 hr	Appropriate bacterial and protozoal infections	Bactericidal, especially for anaerobes; it also has antiprotozoal activity (especially giardiasis) Neurological toxicity is reported after high acute doses or chronic moderate-to-high doses; mydriasis, nystagmus, ataxia, head tilt, tremors, seizures; also anorexia, lethargy, vomiting
	D, C: 10–15 mg/kg p.o. q 12 hr	Large intestinal diarrhoea	Postulated to have some immunomodulatory effects (on cell-mediated immune responses)

Continued

Agent	Dose/routes of administration	Indication(s) in emergency patients	Adverse effects/other comments
Mexiletine	D: 4–8 mg/kg p.o. q 8–12 hr	Clinically significant ventricular tachycardia Supraventricular tachycardia in some dogs	Class 1b antidysrhythmic agent; similar to lidocaine Usually effective in lidocaine-responsive dysrhythmias Adverse effects include nausea, vomiting, depression and neurological signs Use in cats is not recommended
Midazolam	D, C: 0.1–0.5 mg/kg i.v., i.m., s.c.; 0.1–0.8 mg/kg/hr CRI	Sedation/premedication in combination with an opioid or ketamine (cats) Seizures Muscle tremors	Benzodiazepine Rapid onset of action Duration up to 90 min Unlike diazepam, it can be given i.m. Preferred over diazepam in cats because of the potential for idiosyncratic acute hepatic failure in this species Lactated Ringer's solution should not be used for CRI preparation
Milbemycin oxime + praziquantel	D: 0.5 mg/kg milbemycin oxime + 5 mg/kg praziquantel p.o. weekly for 4 weeks	*Angiostrongylus vasorum* infection	Milbemax® (Novartis Animal Health, Frimley, UK) licensed
Misoprostol	D: 2–5 µg/kg p.o. q 8–12 hr	Nonsteroidal antiinflammatory agent (NSAIA) intoxication Gastric ulcer prophylaxis and treatment	Prostaglandin E_1 analogue; cytoprotective for gastric mucosa Most useful for prevention rather than treatment of NSAIA-associated gastrointestinal ulceration Most prevalent adverse effects involve the gastrointestinal system Contraindicated in pregnant animals due to the risk of abortion Not recommended for cats Gloves should be worn when handling and stricter safety precautions taken in women of childbearing age
Morphine	D: 0.1–1.0 mg/kg slow i.v., i.m. or s.c. q 4 hr, prn; 0.1–0.5 mg/kg/hr CRI C: 0.1–0.5 mg/kg slow i.v., i.m. or s.c. q 6 hr, prn; 0.05–0.2 mg/kg/hr CRI	Analgesia for moderate to severe pain Premedication	Full µ (OP3) agonist Gold standard analgesic for severe pain Onset of action 10–15 min following i.v. administration Vomiting is more likely than with other opioids, therefore avoid use in cases with raised intracranial or intraocular pressure and gastric dilatation and volvulus syndrome Rapid i.v. administration may be associated with histamine release (transient vasodilation and hypotension)
	D, C: 0.1 mg/kg slow i.v., s.c., q 6 hr	Dyspnoea, especially acute congestive heart failure	Anxiolysis Vasodilation Must give slowly if using the i.v. route to avoid vomiting and vagally mediated bradycardia

Agent	Dose/routes of administration	Indication(s) in emergency patients	Adverse effects/other comments
Mycophenolate mofetil	D: 10–15 mg/kg p.o. q 12–24 hr	Long-term therapy for immune-mediated haemolytic anaemia (IMHA)	Limited veterinary experience at the time of writing No information for cats
N-acetylcysteine	D, C: initial loading dose of 140 mg/kg i.v.; further 5–7 doses of 70 mg/kg i.v. q 6 hr	Paracetamol (acetaminophen) poisoning	Rapidly hydrolysed to cysteine in vivo that is required for intracellular glutathione synthesis; glutathione conjugates NAPQI Administer intravenously undiluted or diluted in a 5% glucose solution Oral administration is possible if there is no vomiting but this is not particularly patient friendly
Naloxone	D, C: 0.01–0.1 mg/kg slow i.v. to effect, i.m. or s.c., prn	Opiate antagonist	Reverses the majority of opiate effects including respiratory and central nervous system depression Does not reverse emetic effect of apomorphine but reverses other effects Short duration of action (20–60 min) due to rapid metabolism, therefore repeat doses may be required
Omeprazole	D, C: 0.5–1 mg/kg slow i.v., p.o. q 24 hr	Gastric and duodenal ulceration Gastritis Oesophagitis secondary to gastric reflux	Proton pump inhibitor, reduces gastric acid secretion and raises gastric pH Intravenous use for more than 3 days is not recommended Reduce dose in patients with severe hepatic or renal disease
Ondansetron	D, C: 0.1–0.2 mg/kg slow i.v. q 6–12 hr	Antiemetic and antinausea therapy	Serotonin type 3 receptor antagonist Expensive; try if response to other drugs (e.g. maropitant) is inadequate
Oxytocin	D: 1–2 IU/kg i.m. (or s.c.), maximum dose 20 IU C: 2–4 IU total dose i.m. (or s.c.)	Dystocia due to primary uterine inertia	Lower doses may be equally effective Contraindicated in cases with pelvic obstruction, inadequate cervical dilation, vaginal masses or strictures, and in those with inguinal hernias Repeated doses may be given every 20–30 min Failure to respond to 2–3 doses is considered an indication for surgical intervention Check serum calcium concentration; perhaps supplement empirically if oxytocin ineffective
Paracetamol (acetaminophen)	D: 10–15 mg/kg p.o. q 8–12 hr	Analgesia Antipyretic activity	Should never be administered to cats Poor antiinflammatory activity Minimal gastrointestinal side effects May be used in conjunction with conventional nonsteroidal antiinflammatory agents Hepatotoxicity is possible

Continued

Agent	Dose/routes of administration	Indication(s) in emergency patients	Adverse effects/other comments
Pentobarbital	D, C: 5–20 mg/kg slowly i.v. to effect (e.g. 3 mg/kg aliquots q 90 s); may need to repeat q 4–8 hr	Seizures and muscle tremors refractory to diazepam if propofol cannot be used or afforded	Barbiturate Aim for deep sedation rather than a surgical plane of anaesthesia Monitor closely for excessive respiratory depression The sterile preparation is no longer clinically available in the UK
Pethidine	D: 2–10 mg/kg i.m., 5–15 mg/kg s.c. q 1–2 hr, prn C: 5–10 mg/kg i.m., 8–15 mg/kg s.c. q 2 hr, prn	Analgesia for moderate pain Premedication	Full μ (OP3) agonist Rapid onset of action Not suitable for maintenance analgesia as it cannot be given intravenously (carries significant risk of severe histamine reaction) May provide useful sedation
Phenobarbital	D, C: 3 mg/kg slow i.v. q 30–60 min, up to total dose of 18–24 mg/kg in 24 hr; then 3–5 mg/kg slow i.v. q 12 hr for 24–48 hr before enteral therapy	Rapid loading in management of status epilepticus or severe tremorogenic intoxication	Barbiturate Onset of action likely to be 15–30 min Sedation occurs commonly Other (long-term) side effects include polyuria/polydipsia, liver injury and (rarely) cytopenias
Pimobendan	D: 0.1–0.3 mg/kg p.o. q 12 hr, give 1 hr before feeding	Congestive heart failure secondary to dilated cardiomyopathy or mitral valve insufficiency	Positive inotrope and vasodilatory properties Contraindicated in hypertrophic cardiomyopathy and where cardiac output cannot be enhanced by increased contractility (e.g. aortic stenosis) Bioavailability is significantly reduced in the presence of food A variety of nonspecific adverse effects are reported
Prednisolone	D: 2 mg/kg p.o. q 12 hr initially then tapered gradually C: 2–4 mg/kg p.o. q 12 hr initially then tapered gradually	Immunosuppression	Common adverse effects include polyuria/polydipsia, increased appetite, panting (dogs), muscle wastage Adverse effects are often worse in larger dogs necessitating lower doses
	C: 1–2 mg/kg p.o. q 12 hr	Oral treatment for feline bronchial disease following initial stabilization	Can start to taper (over 2–3 months) after 7–10 days if there is a satisfactory response
	D: 2–5 mg/kg i.v. q 3–6 hr initially; then 0.1–0.2 mg/kg p.o. q 12–24 hr	Acute hypoadrenocorticism (Addisonian) crisis	Perform ACTH stimulation test prior to starting treatment Mainly glucocorticoid but has some mineralocorticoid activity
	D: 0.7 mg/kg p.o. q 24 hr for 3–7 days	*Angiostrongylus vasorum* infection	Administer in conjunction with antiparasitic treatment Intended to reduce the inflammatory reaction associated with dying larvae Typically used in dogs with (marked) respiratory, neurological or ocular signs, or those with a heavy worm burden

Agent	Dose/routes of administration	Indication(s) in emergency patients	Adverse effects/other comments
Procainamide	D: 6–10 mg/kg slow i.v.; 25–50 µg/kg/min CRI; 8–20 mg/kg p.o. q 6 hr C: 1–2 mg/kg slow i.v.; 10–20 µg/kg/min CRI; 3–8 mg/kg p.o. q 6–8 hr	Ventricular tachycardia inadequately responsive to maximal lidocaine therapy	Class 1a antidysrhythmic agent Use with caution in cases with significant hepatic or renal disease or with congestive heart failure Adverse effects are generally related to blood drug concentration and are mainly gastrointestinal or cardiovascular
Propofol	D: up to 2 mg/kg i.v. C: up to 3 mg/kg i.v.	Sedation	Always give carefully to effect – not a prescribed dose Bolus effect lasts 5–10 min Causes peripheral vasodilation and myocardial depression, so use cautiously if there is cardiovascular instability Significant respiratory depression is possible No analgesia
	D: up to 4 mg/kg i.v.; 3–36 mg/kg/hr CRI C: up to 6 mg/kg i.v.; 3–10 mg/kg/hr CRI	General anaesthesia with premedication	As above For CRI without syringe driver, add 50 ml propofol to 450 ml normal saline (0.9% sodium chloride) to give 1 mg/ml propofol Limit prolonged infusion/repeat dosing in cats (Heinz body anaemia)
	D, C: 2 mg/kg aliquots slow i.v. to effect; CRI starting at 3 mg/kg/hr and titrating upwards as necessary	Seizures and muscle tremors refractory to diazepam	As above
Ranitidine	D: 0.5–2 mg/kg slow i.v. q 8–12 hr; 1–2 mg/kg p.o. q 12 hr C: 2.5 mg/kg slow i.v. q 12 hr; 3.5 mg/kg p.o. q 12 hr	Gastric and duodenal ulcers Gastritis Oesophagitis secondary to gastric reflux Prokinetic activity	Histamine (H_2) receptor antagonist, increasing gastric acid pH by reducing acid production Preferred over cimetidine as it has fewer drug interactions and less frequent dosing
S-Adenosylmethionine (SAMe)	D: initial dose of 40 mg/kg p.o.; then 20 mg/kg p.o. q 24 hr for 9 days C: 180 mg (total dose) p.o. q 12 hr for 3 days; then 90 mg p.o. q 12 hr for 14 days	Paracetamol (acetaminophen) poisoning	The feline protocol has only been reported experimentally
Soda crystals (washing soda)	D, C: one crystal on tongue at back of mouth May be repeated	Induction of emesis following oral poisoning	It is extremely important to make sure that caustic soda (sodium hydroxide) is not used by accident Emesis usually within 10 min
Sodium bicarbonate	D, C: 1–2 mmol/kg slow i.v.	Clinically significant hyperkalaemia	Can repeat dose if necessary Lowers serum potassium concentration by moving potassium into cells Effect can persist for several hours Access to on-site acid–base analyser is much preferred

Continued

Agent	Dose/routes of administration	Indication(s) in emergency patients	Adverse effects/other comments
Sotalol	D: 1–2 mg/kg slow i.v. (over 5 min); 1–2.5 mg/kg p.o. q 12 hr C: 1 mg/kg slow i.v. (over 5 min)	Ventricular tachycardia inadequately responsive to maximal lidocaine therapy	Nonselective beta-blocker and Class III antidysrhythmic The main concerns are its potential for negative inotropy and prodysrhythmic effects
Sucralfate	D: 0.5–2 g/dog p.o. q 8–12 hr C: 0.25–0.5 g/cat p.o. q 8–12 hr	Oral, oesophageal, gastric and duodenal ulcer treatment Gastric ulcer prophylaxis in high risk cases Oesophagitis	Tablets can be crushed and mixed with water Administration 30–60 min before food is recommended Coats ulcerated/exposed mucosa and promotes reepithelialization; possible cytoprotective effects
Syrup of ipecacuanha (7%)	D: 1–2 ml/kg p.o. C: 3.3 ml/kg p.o. May be repeated once	Induction of emesis at home following oral poisoning	If emesis is induced, it usually occurs within 30 min Bitter taste therefore potential problems with compliance
Terbutaline	C: 0.01 mg/kg slow i.v., s.c. q 4 hr; 0.312–1.25 mg/cat p.o. q 8–12 hr	Feline bronchial disease	Beta-adrenergic agonist; bronchodilator Parenteral administration is essential in an emergency patient Adverse effects are dose related and are usually mild and transient
	D: 0.005–0.01 mg/kg i.m., s.c. q 4–6 hr; 1.25–5 mg/dog p.o. q 8–12 hr C: 0.005–0.015 mg/kg i.m., s.c. q 4–6 hr; 0.625–1.25 mg/cat p.o. q 8–12 hr	Clinically significant sinus bradydysrhythmia	Due to stimulation of cardiac beta-receptors Improvement is usually only partial and short lived
Tramadol	D, C: 1–5 mg/kg p.o., i.v. q 6–12 hr	Analgesia (antitussive activity)	Synthetic mu-receptor opiate agonist; also inhibits serotonin and noradrenaline (norepinephrine) uptake The main clinical adverse effects are sedation and nausea Naloxone will partially antagonize its effects Start at upper end of dose range and upper end of dosing intervals in cats Avoid oral preparations containing paracetamol (acetaminophen) in cats
Vitamin D	Dihydrotachysterol: 0.01–0.03 mg/kg p.o. q 24–48 hr Alfacalcidol: 0.01–0.05 µg/kg p.o. q 24 hr Calcitriol: 0.01–0.03 µg/kg p.o. q 24 hr	Chronic therapy for hypocalcaemia	The daily dose is usually divided into 2 equal doses administered initially together with oral calcium supplementation but the latter is usually tapered while vitamin D is continued

Agent	Dose/routes of administration	Indication(s) in emergency patients	Adverse effects/other comments
Vitamin K_1 (phytomenadione)	D, C: 2–5 mg/kg s.c. in multiple sites, p.o. q 24 hr (divide into 2–3 administrations)	Treatment of anticoagulant rodenticide poisoning Treatment of coagulopathy secondary to acute hepatic failure (e.g. xylitol poisoning)	Some preparations are licensed for i.v. administration; anaphylaxis has been associated with the i.v. administration of some preparations i.m. administration is not recommended in coagulopathic animals as this may induce painful and potentially severe haemorrhage Full haemostatic benefit likely within 12 hr Bioavailability of oral vitamin K_1 is increased when given with fatty (e.g. canned) food
Xylazine	C: 0.4–0.5 mg/kg i.m., s.c.	Induction of emesis following oral poisoning	Sedation, respiratory depression

ACTH, adrenocorticotrophic hormone; C, cats; COX-2, cyclooxygenase-2; CRI, constant rate infusion; D, dogs; ECG, electrocardiogram; i.m., intramuscular; i.o., intraosseous; IU, international units; i.v., intravenous; NAPQI, N-acetyl-para-benzoquinoneimine; o.t.m., oral transmucosal; p.o., per os; p.r., per rectum; prn, pro re nata (as needed); s.c., subcutaneously.

ADDITIONAL USEFUL INFORMATION

Intravenous glucose supplementation

Glucose solution required	SIZE OF ISOTONIC CRYSTALLOID FLUID BAG	
	500 ml	***1000 ml***
	Volume to be removed and added	
1.25% (12.5 mg/ml)	12.5 ml	25 ml
2.5% (25 mg/ml)	25 ml	50 ml
5% (50 mg/ml)	50 ml	100 ml
7.5% (75 mg/ml)	75 ml	150 ml
10% (100 mg/ml)	100 ml	200 ml

This table presumes the use of a 50% (500 mg/ml) glucose (dextrose) solution and either 0.9% sodium chloride (normal saline) or buffered lactated Ringer's solution (Hartmann's solution, compound sodium lactate).

The volumes listed are the amount of fluid that should be removed from the isotonic crystalloid bag, and then replaced by an equal volume of 50% glucose solution in order to make a glucose solution of the desired concentration.

For example, to make a 5% glucose saline solution, remove 50 ml from a 500 ml bag of 0.9% sodium chloride and then add 50 ml of 50% glucose solution to the bag.

Intravenous potassium chloride supplementation

Serum potassium concentration (mmol/l)	AMOUNT OF POTASSIUM CHLORIDE REQUIRED (mEq)	
	Per 500 ml fluid	**Per 1000 ml fluid**
3.5–5.5	10	20
3.0–3.5	15	30
2.5–3.0	20	40
2.0–2.5	30	60
< 2.0	40	80

Note: 1 mEq of potassium is equivalent to 1 mmol of potassium.

This table is one example of a number of similar tables presenting comparable guidelines. These guidelines are very much empirically derived and clearly the amount of potassium delivered to the patient depends on the fluid rate as much as the potassium concentration. If a satisfactory response to empirical supplementation is not achieved, the actual rate of potassium administration should be calculated and used to guide subsequent therapy.

Potassium supplementation should not exceed a rate of 0.5 mEq/kg/h and the use of enteral supplementation should not be overlooked. In the exceptional circumstance where it is necessary to exceed this rate, continuous electrocardiogram monitoring should be used if available, and great care must be taken to alert all staff to the use of such a high potassium supplementation in order to avoid inadvertent bolus administration that could well be fatal. This rate of potassium supplementation must only be administered using an infusion pump or syringe driver, and the fluid bag and infusion device must be clearly labelled, e.g. 'high potassium concentration, do not bolus!'.

Conversion factors

1% solution = 10 mg/ml = 1 g/100 ml

1 mmol = 1 mEq divided by the valence of the ion (e.g. 1+, 2+)

- e.g. valence of sodium is 1 (i.e. Na^{1+}) so 1 mmol of sodium = 1 mEq divided by 1 = 1 mEq of sodium
- e.g. valence of calcium is 2 (i.e. Ca^{2+}) so 1 mmol of calcium = 1 mEq divided by 2 = 0.5 mEq of calcium

1 standard teaspoon = 5 ml; 1 standard tablespoon = 15 ml

1 fluid ounce (oz) = 29.6 ml; 1 ml = 0.034 oz

1 lb = 0.454 kg; 1 kg = 2.2 lb

1 part per million (ppm) = 1 mg/kg for solid substances, 1 mg/l for liquid substances

Weight conversion factors:

- 1 kg = 1000 g
- 1 g = 1000 mg
- 1 mg = 1000 μg

2 APPENDIX Procedures – equipment and techniques

IN-DWELLING NASAL OXYGEN CATHETER PLACEMENT

Equipment required

- Topical local anaesthetic solution (e.g. proxymetacaine drops)
- Appropriately sized red rubber catheter or soft flexible paediatric feeding tube (8-French for most dogs, 5-French for small dogs) or veterinary nasal oxygen catheter if available
- Some means of marking the tube (e.g. piece of tape, appropriate pen)
- Lubricant gel, preferably containing local anaesthetic
- Butterfly tape and suture material, skin stapler or skin glue
- (Elizabethan collar)

Procedure

- Elevate the patient's nose and drip a small amount of local anaesthetic solution into the nostril.
- Allow enough time for the local anaesthetic to take effect (e.g. 10 min).
- Measure the catheter from the tip of the nose to the medial canthus and mark it.
- Lubricate the tip of the tube.
- Hold the animal's head with the nose pointing upwards and insert the catheter along the ventromedial aspect of the nasal cavity until the mark is reached; being too forceful here can cause epistaxis.
- Fix the catheter in place, first to the lateral aspect of the nose and then to the skin, either between the eyes or to the side of the face. It is important to ensure that the catheter is out of the animal's visual field. The catheter may be fixed using tape tags that are sutured, using skin staples or with skin glue.
- Loop the catheter along the animal's neck (dorsally or laterally depending on how it has been fixed) and bandage over it with a light dressing. This will help to minimize traction on the fixation. An intravenous fluid line or some other form of tubing may be used to extend the catheter if it is too short to reach the neck.
- Connect the catheter to the oxygen supply using appropriate tubing (see Figure 6.3).
- Repeat the procedure on the other side if two indwelling catheters are required; a commercial or improvised Y-connector can be used to connect both catheters to the same oxygen tubing.
- Use of an Elizabethan collar may be indicated in some patients.
- Commence humidified oxygen supplementation at 50–150 ml/kg/min.
- Local anaesthetic drops may be reapplied as necessary.

Additional notes

A nasopharyngeal oxygen catheter is placed in the same way but the catheter is premeasured to the ramus of the mandible.

THORACOCENTESIS

Equipment required

- Clippers
- Surgical scrub equipment
- Sterile gloves
- Appropriately sized butterfly needle (typically 21 or 23 gauge for an adult cat or small dog), or intravenous catheter (14–20 gauge depending on the size of the patient) and extension tubing. The size of the needle or catheter is guided both by patient size and the nature of the material to be aspirated
- Sterile three-way tap
- Appropriately sized syringe (typically 20 ml for cats and small dogs, 60 ml for bigger dogs)
- Sample containers (sterile EDTA, serum and additive-free containers)
- Jug, bowl or other collection vessel
- Ideally a total of three people

Procedure

- The animal is allowed to stand or to sit in sternal recumbency as preferred and gently restrained by one individual; minimal restraint often works best. Lateral recumbency may be acceptable for pneumothorax.
- Flow-by oxygen supplementation is provided (if tolerated).
- A patch of fur is clipped in the 7th, 8th or 9th intercostal space on both sides of the chest and the area is aseptically prepared on one side (the side that is chosen initially may be guided by auscultation, ultrasonography or a dorsoventral radiograph if one has been obtained). If pleural fluid is suspected, an area in the ventral third of the thorax is chosen for aspiration; if pneumothorax is suspected, an area in the dorsal third of the thorax is chosen; if pleural space disease has yet to be confirmed, an area half-way up the thorax is chosen.
- The location for needle insertion should lie just cranial to the rib to avoid the neurovascular bundle that lies caudal to each rib. In smaller animals, this essentially involves inserting the needle in the middle of the intercostal space.
- Depending on the animal in question, and wearing sterile gloves, a suitable butterfly needle, or an intravenous catheter attached to extension tubing, is attached to a three-way tap and then to a 20 ml or 60 ml syringe (Figure App2.1). Note that the three-way tap is therefore located away from the patient.
- The needle is inserted by a second person gently but briskly into the pleural space at a right angle to the chest wall with the bevel facing dorsally – lingering on the skin is undesirable as this is often a highly sensitive area.
- Gentle suction is applied to the syringe by a third person as the needle is inserted into the pleural space. Once in the pleural space the needle can be angled caudally or ventrally to lie flat against the chest wall to reduce the risk of lung trauma.
- Aspiration is continued until negative pressure is reached or it feels like the lung is being scratched by the needle.
- It may be necessary to reposition the needle (and sometimes the patient) gently either initially or during the procedure to maximize the amount of material removed.
- Samples of pleural fluid are collected in sterile EDTA, serum and additive-free containers for cytology, haematocrit measurement, culture and sensitivity or other analyses as appropriate.
- The total volume of material removed is recorded.

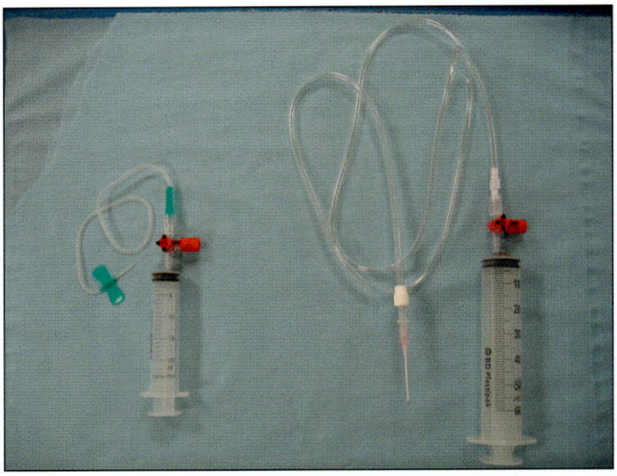

Figure App2.1 Equipment for thoracocentesis. Butterfly needle attached to 20 ml syringe for cats and small dogs (left); intravenous catheter; extension tubing and 60 ml syringe for larger dogs.

- The procedure may need to be performed on both sides of the thorax – this is decided based on the results of the procedure on the first side and the individual patient's circumstances. For example:
  - Is residual pleural space material likely to be reabsorbed?
  - Is additional material likely to accumulate?
  - Are there concurrent intrathoracic abnormalities that make the animal less tolerant of residual material?
  - How compliant was the patient for thoracocentesis on the first side?

Additional notes

Clinically significant respiratory compromise is generally associated with approximately 20 ml/kg or more of pleural air or fluid. Removal of a smaller volume than this is therefore unlikely to cause significant clinical improvement although smaller volumes may be of greater significance in the presence of concurrent injuries (e.g. pulmonary contusions). If clinical signs do not improve following aspiration of an appropriate volume of pleural air or fluid it suggests that another abnormality exists and is predominantly responsible for the dyspnoea.

This may be the case for example in an animal that has suffered blunt thoracic injury resulting in both pneumothorax and pulmonary contusions. Aspiration of 20 ml/kg of air may only cause partial improvement in clinical signs if pulmonary contusions are significantly involved in the dyspnoea noted. Nevertheless, therapeutic thoracocentesis is still appropriate as it will be of some benefit in improving expansion of the already compromised lungs.

PERICARDIOCENTESIS

Equipment required

- Sedative agents (e.g. butorphanol ± midazolam) – not required in many cases
- Lidocaine 2% solution (without adrenaline), 2 ml syringe, 23 gauge needle – for local anaesthesia
- Lidocaine 2% solution (without adrenaline), 10 ml syringe, needle in case of significant ventricular dysrhythmia
- Clippers
- Surgical scrub equipment
- Sterile gloves
- Sterile no. 11 blade
- Over-the-needle BD Angiocath™ 14 or 16 gauge, 3¼ or 5 inch (a variety of other instruments including central venous catheters and small chest drains may be used for pericardiocentesis; the latter may be left in situ in the pericardial sac for repeat drainage short-term)
- Three-way tap
- Extension tubing
- 60 ml syringe
- Sample containers (sterile EDTA and additive-free containers)
- Jug, bowl or other collection vessel

Procedure

- Place and secure a peripheral intravenous catheter.
- Restrain the dog in left lateral recumbency so that aspiration is performed from the right side. If lateral recumbency is not tolerated, sternal recumbency may be used. If available, ensure electrocardiogram (ECG) monitoring is in place.
- Clip an area ventrally (from sternum to mid-thoracic level) extending from the 3rd to 8th intercostal space.
- Identify the site at which the Angiocath™ will be inserted: this is usually cranial to the rib (to avoid the intercostal artery in particular that lies caudal to the rib) at the level of the costochondral junction in the 4th, 5th or 6th intercostal space. Ultrasonography can be used to help identify the best site.
- Infiltrate lidocaine (1 ml of 2% solution) at the chosen site subcutaneously and down to the parietal pleura.
- Perform a surgical scrub of the clipped area.
- Wearing sterile gloves, make a stab incision in the skin and then insert the Angiocath™ at the chosen site pointing towards the heart – the catheter is usually inserted approximately perpendicular to the thoracic wall pointing slightly dorsally. Ultrasonography may be used to guide catheter positioning but is usually not required.
- Advance the Angiocath™ until the pericardial sac is penetrated – it may be possible to feel a 'pop' as the catheter goes through the pericardium. Pericardial effusion, which is usually sanguineous or port-wine coloured, is not under negative pressure within the pericardial sac and is therefore expelled forcefully once the pericardium has been penetrated. Pericardial effusion may be mistaken for pleural effusion that can have a very similar appearance. However, the latter should not be expelled forcefully through the catheter.
- Advance the catheter over the stylet slightly further and then remove the stylet.
- Attach one end of the extension tubing to the catheter and hand the other end to an assistant who should then connect the three-way tap and the 60 ml syringe.
- Pericardial fluid is then aspirated until no further fluid is returned or the patient is no longer compliant.
- Fluid samples should be transferred using sterile technique into the sterile sample containers.
- The catheter is then removed and there is usually no need to cover the insertion site.

Additional notes

The ECG should be monitored for significant ventricular dysrhythmia (see Ch. 12) throughout – if this is noted, it may be that the catheter is making contact with the myocardium and it should be withdrawn slightly. If the dysrhythmia is very severe or if it does not improve when the catheter is withdrawn slightly, the catheter should be removed completely. Lidocaine (start with 2mg/kg bolus) should be administered intravenously if a ventricular dysrhythmia is haemodynamiacally significant and fails to improve with catheter withdrawal.

A sample of pericardial effusion withdrawn at the start of the procedure should be checked frequently for clotting while the procedure progresses. Pericardial effusion is devoid of platelets and clotting factors and will not clot unless it is from active or very recent haemorrhage. If the catheter has inadvertently punctured a cardiac chamber or there is rupture of a sizeable vessel, blood will be aspirated and will clot. The haematocrit of pericardial fluid is usually less than that of the patient. In addition drainage of pericardial fluid is typically associated with a rapid improvement in patient status.

ABDOMINOCENTESIS

Equipment required

- Clippers
- Surgical scrub equipment

- Sterile gloves
- Appropriately sized hypodermic needle (20, 21 or 23 gauge; ½ or 1 inch long) and syringe (2 or 5 ml)
- Sample containers (sterile EDTA, serum and additive-free containers)

Procedure

- Restrain the animal in right lateral recumbency (or standing).
- Clip and scrub the ventral abdomen around the umbilicus – the site chosen is typically just caudal to the umbilicus and lateral to the midline; alternatively ultrasonography may be used to guide the site of aspiration.
- Wearing sterile gloves attach the needle to the syringe.
- Advance the needle perpendicular to the abdominal wall into the abdomen in one gentle but purposeful motion.
- Aspirate intermittently as the needle is advanced further.
- Transfer any fluid removed into the sample containers using aseptic technique.

Additional notes

- Lateral recumbency is preferred as it reduces the likelihood of splenic injury.
- If aspirated fluid is grossly suggestive of blood, it should be observed for clotting. In contrast to blood accidentally aspirated from the spleen or a vessel, sanguineous effusion is devoid of platelets and clotting factors and will not clot unless it is from active or very recent haemorrhage.
- An over-the-needle catheter may be used instead of a hypodermic needle.
- An open system using one or more needles inserted into the abdomen without syringes attached may be used to retrieve peritoneal fluid and may be more rewarding in some cases (reduces likelihood of omentum or viscera occluding the needle). However, this technique allows air to leak into the abdominal cavity which may confuse subsequent diagnostic imaging.
- If single quadrant abdominocentesis is unrewarding, the technique is repeated in the three other abdominal quadrants (four quadrant abdominocentesis). If free peritoneal fluid is still not obtained, diagnostic peritoneal lavage should be considered (see below).
- Abdominocentesis is not recommended in coagulopathic patients.

DIAGNOSTIC PERITONEAL LAVAGE

Equipment required

- Clippers
- Surgical scrub equipment
- Sterile gloves
- Sterile no. 15 blade
- Appropriately sized long over-the-needle intravenous catheter (16, 18 or 20 gauge)
- Closed fluid administration system – the precise system will depend on the patient in question (e.g. a single 60 ml syringe may be adequate for a small cat; a fluid bag, infusion set and three-way tap may be needed for a big dog)
- 10–20 ml/kg of warmed sterile normal saline (0.9% sodium chloride solution)
- Standard abdominocentesis equipment (see above)

Procedure

- Restrain the animal in lateral recumbency (or standing).
- Clip and scrub the ventral abdomen around the umbilicus – the site chosen is typically just caudal to the umbilicus and lateral to the midline.
- Wearing sterile gloves cut two or three additional (side) holes into an appropriately sized over-the-needle intravenous catheter using a scalpel blade. In order not to weaken the catheter, the holes should not be longer than 50% of the circumference of the catheter and should not be made opposite each other.
- Insert the catheter in a caudodorsal direction into the abdomen in one gentle but purposeful motion.
- Once the abdominal wall has been penetrated, advance the catheter over the stylet and then remove the stylet. Connect the fluid administration system.
- Infuse 10–20 ml/kg of warmed sterile saline into the abdomen under gravity or via gentle injection pressure.
- Allow a dwell time of several minutes (20–30 min if possible) and gently agitate the patient's abdomen intermittently in the interim to aid dispersal.
- Retrieve as much fluid as possible using standard abdominocentesis technique (see above).

Additional notes

It is common to retrieve only a small proportion of the lavage fluid originally infused (the remainder will be absorbed via the peritoneum or removed at surgery).

Due to dilution, fluid obtained via diagnostic peritoneal lavage cannot reliably be subjected to biochemical quantitative analysis; the main uses are cytology and microbiology.

GASTRIC DECOMPRESSION – OROGASTRIC INTUBATION

Equipment required

- Roll of tape or mouth gag
- Appropriately sized stomach tube, preferably with multiple fenestrations

- Lubricant for stomach tube
- Means of marking the stomach tube (e.g. piece of tape, suitable marker pen)
- Bucket (or similar) for collecting gastric effluent and lavage fluid
- Funnel and jug for performing lavage

Procedure

- Ideally have the patient in sternal recumbency but allow to adopt his/her preferred position.
- Place a roll of tape (or gag) in the mouth to prevent chewing of the tube.
- Premeasure the stomach tube from the tip of the nose to the last rib and mark it.
- Lubricate the tube well and pass it through the roll of tape down the oesophagus; the oesophagus starts dorsal to, and to the (patient's) left of, the larynx. Some resistance is usually encountered as the tube is passed through the distal oesophageal sphincter. Excessive force is to be avoided to reduce the risk of gastric perforation.
- Collect the effluent and examine it grossly for evidence of haemorrhage or gastric mucosal sloughing suggestive of more severe ischaemia.
- Lavage the stomach several times with warm water (20–50 ml/kg/lavage).

Additional notes

In addition to the opioid that should already have been administered, sedation with an agent that is cardiovascular sparing may be needed for orogastric intubation to be performed (e.g. diazepam to effect).

It must be remembered that the ability to pass a stomach tube does not exclude the presence of some degree of gastric volvulus in gastric dilatation/volvulus syndrome.

GASTRIC DECOMPRESSION – PERCUTANEOUS NEEDLE DECOMPRESSION

Equipment required

- Clippers
- Surgical scrub equipment
- Sterile gloves
- 16 or 18 gauge over-the-needle intravenous catheter (or similar sized hypodermic needle)

Procedure

- Restrain the patient in sternal (or left lateral) recumbency.
- Identify the point of maximal abdominal distension on the right side of the abdomen and percuss the area for tympany to ensure the stomach and not the spleen lies beneath.
- Clip and aseptically prepare the chosen site.
- Insert the intravenous catheter percutaneously into the stomach at the chosen site and remove the stylet. Gas with a characteristic smell is released immediately through the catheter.

Additional notes

Needle decompression is a quick and easy procedure that is effective in relieving gaseous distension. However, it does involve blindly placing a needle through a gastric wall that may already be severely compromised. It should perhaps therefore be reserved for the following types of cases:

- Animals that are intolerant of orogastric intubation despite appropriate sedation
- Animals that are intolerant of orogastric intubation and that are deemed too unstable to sedate
- Animals in which a stomach tube cannot be passed.

NASOOESOPHAGEAL FEEDING TUBE PLACEMENT

Equipment required

- Topical local anaesthetic solution (e.g. proxymetacaine drops)
- Appropriately sized soft flexible paediatric feeding tube (8-French for most dogs, 3.5 to 5-French for most cats and small dogs)
- Some means of marking the tube (e.g. piece of tape, appropriate pen)
- Lubricant gel, preferably containing local anaesthetic
- Appropriately sized syringe (2.5–10 ml) filled with sterile saline or water for injection
- Butterfly tape and suture material, skin stapler or skin glue
- (Elizabethan collar)

Procedure

- Elevate the patient's nose and drip a small amount of local anaesthetic solution into the nostril.
- Allow enough time for the local anaesthetic to take effect (e.g. 10 min).
- Measure the feeding tube from the tip of the nose to the 9th intercostal space and mark it.
- Lubricate the tip of the tube.
- Hold the animal's head with the nose pointing upwards and insert the tube along the ventromedial aspect of the nasal cavity. The tube should be inserted in short controlled steps allowing the animal to adjust between

each step if necessary. An increase in resistance is likely to be encountered in the mid-nasal region.

- Once the tube has passed through the nose, lower the head and continue to advance the tube until the mark is reached. If the animal coughs during placement, the tube is potentially in the trachea and should be withdrawn and the procedure recommenced; no tube placement is contraindicated in patients unable to cough (e.g. due to reduced mentation).
- Inject 2.5–10 ml of saline/water down the tube followed by an equal amount of air – if the animal coughs, the tube is potentially in the trachea.
- Fix the tube in place, first to the lateral aspect of the nose and then to the skin, either between the eyes or to the side of the face. It is important to ensure that the tube is out of the animal's visual field. The tube may be fixed using tape tags that are sutured, using skin staples or with skin glue.
- Confirm correct tube placement radiographically; the end should lie in the distal oesophagus.
- Loop the feeding tube along the animal's neck (dorsally or laterally depending on how it has been fixed) and bandage over it with a light dressing. This will help to minimize traction on the fixation. An intravenous fluid line or some other form of tubing may be used to extend the feeding tube if it is too short to reach the neck.

Additional notes

Correct tube placement can also be checked by connecting the feeding tube to a capnograph. If the tube is in the oesophagus, end-tidal carbon dioxide should be approximately 0 mmHg with no waveform. Tracheal placement results in a higher $ETCO_2$ and a capnograph waveform.

- Use of an Elizabethan collar may be indicated in some patients (typically young animals and cats).
- The small diameter of feeding tubes mandates the use of liquid diets.

GASTRIC LAVAGE

Equipment required

- Appropriate set-up for general anaesthesia, including cuffed endotracheal tube
- Roll of tape or mouth gag
- Large bore stomach tube with terminal fenestrations
- Means of marking the tube (e.g. piece of tape, suitable marker pen)
- Lubricant
- Bucket (or similar) for collecting gastric effluent and lavage fluid
- Funnel and jug for performing lavage

Procedure

- General anaesthesia is mandatory (unless the patient is unconscious).
- The use of a cuffed endotracheal tube is mandatory.
- Position the animal in sternal (or right lateral) recumbency with the head lower than the thorax.
- Insert the roll of tape (or gag) into the mouth to facilitate stomach tube passage.
- Premeasure the stomach tube from the tip of the nose to the last rib and mark it.
- Lubricate the tube well and then pass it down the oesophagus up to the mark – the opening of the oesophagus lies dorsally and to the (patient's) left of the trachea.
- Some resistance is usually encountered as the tube is passed through the distal oesophageal sphincter; excessive force should be avoided to reduce the risk of iatrogenic damage.
- Lavage the stomach with warm water (or normal saline) until the returning effluent is clear (20–50 ml/kg lavage).
- If appropriate, administer activated charcoal via the stomach tube.

Additional notes

- Great care must be taken throughout and especially during stomach tube removal to prevent aspiration.
- The majority of commercial stomach tubes are likely to be too big for use in cats. However, a tube for gastric lavage may be improvised for example by using the tubing from an oesophageal stethoscope into which terminal fenestrations are cut.

URETHRAL CATHETERIZATION OF MALE CATS WITH URETHRAL OBSTRUCTION

Equipment required

- Minimum of two individuals usually required
- Clippers
- Surgical scrub equipment
- Sterile gloves
- Sterile lubricant
- Lidocaine 2% solution (without adrenaline)
- Feline urethral catheter – typically 3- to 5-French
- Lacrimal irrigation cannula (Figure App2.3) or over-the-needle intravenous catheter with needle withdrawn

- Warmed 500 ml bag of 0.9% sodium chloride (normal, physiological saline)
- Fluid administration set
- Three-way tap
- 20 ml syringe
- Sterile additive-free containers
- Jug, bowl or other collection vessel
- Urine collection system

Procedure

- Generously clip around the preputial opening.
- Position the cat in lateral or dorsal recumbency.
- Set up the fluid bag, administration set, three-way tap and 20 ml syringe.
- Perform a surgical scrub of the clipped area.
- Mix 2 mg/kg of lidocaine thoroughly with a small amount of sterile lubricant; use this to coat both the irrigation cannula and the urethral catheter.
- Extrude the penis with the nondominant hand and evaluate its appearance; gently palpate the distal urethra for evidence of obstruction. If the obstruction is very distal, the tip of the penis may have a blue appearance and it may be possible gently to massage the obstructing material out.
- Gently insert the irrigation cannula or over-the-needle intravenous catheter (with the needle withdrawn to act as a stylet) into the urethra. If the cannula passes, it can be withdrawn and the urethral catheter inserted. Otherwise flushing should commence.
- It is usually necessary to flush the urethra in order to facilitate catheter placement. Inject the warmed saline in short sharp bursts with the catheter being simultaneously gently advanced in a twisting motion. In addition, once the catheter has passed a short distance from the external orifice, it is essential to release the penis back into the prepuce and straighten the normal bend in the feline urethra in order for the catheter to pass further. This is achieved by pulling the prepuce caudally (and dorsally).
- Once the catheter has been fully inserted, the bladder should be thoroughly lavaged with warmed saline using the fluid administration set, three-way tap and 20 ml syringe. The urine can be markedly haematuric and lavage is ideally continued until the fluid returning from the bladder is clear. However, this is dependent on the patient's compliance and a risk–benefit assessment of the level of chemical restraint required. The first urine sample obtained via the catheter prior to bladder lavage can be kept for analysis as required.
- Connect the urethral catheter to a urine drainage bag in a closed collection system (Figure App2.5). Tape the collection tubing both to the cat's tail and to the kennel subsequently in order to minimize pull on the urethral catheter.
- Apply an Elizabethan collar to the cat to prevent interference with the urinary catheter

Additional notes

Great care must be taken throughout catheterization to minimize trauma to the already inflamed and friable urethra and avoid rupture. Although it can take copious flushing and much patience to achieve catheterization in some cases, in the author's experience it is almost always achievable.

A number of different types of feline urethral catheters are available (Figures App2.2 and App2.3). It is

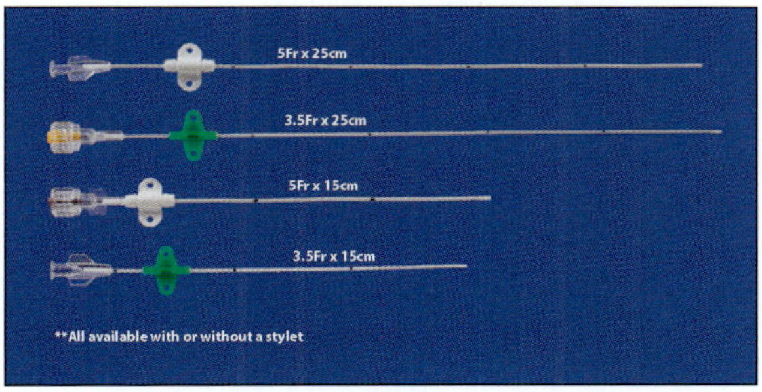

Figure App2.2 MILA International, Inc. Tomcat Urethral Catheters.

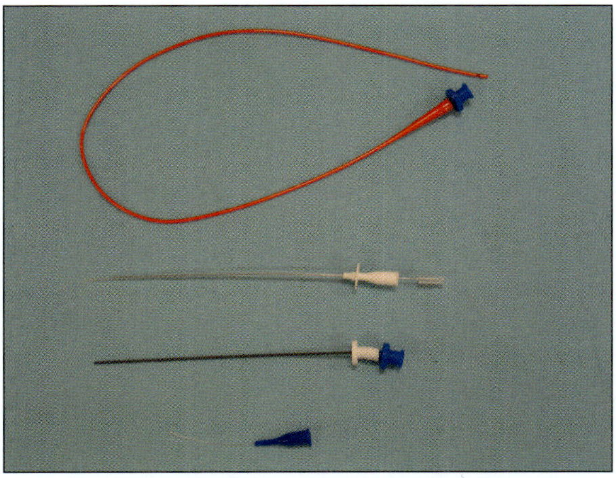

Figure App2.3 Three types of feline urethral catheter (from top to bottom): red rubber catheter; Portex® Jackson Cat Catheter; Slippery Sam®. A blue Little Herbert® adaptor is connected to the red rubber catheter and the Slippery Sam®. A lacrimal irrigating cannula is shown at the bottom.

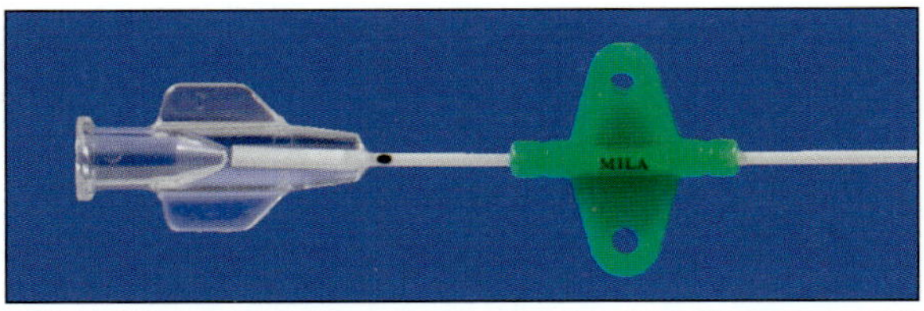

Figure App2.4 MILA International, Inc. Tomcat Catheter with suture wing.

usually necessary to use a rigid catheter to unblock the urethra initially. Although softer catheters can be made stiffer by placing them in the freezer, a rigid catheter such as the Portex® Jackson Cat Catheter (Smiths Medical International Ltd, UK) which is widely available in the United Kingdom is typically used for unblocking. It also has the advantage of a stylet that assists with catheterisation further. However it is preferable not to leave a rigid catheter in situ as there is a greater likelihood of exacerbating urethral and bladder mucosal damage and discomfort. The Jackson catheter is also not very long and can be too short to drain the bladder reliably in bigger tomcats. The rigid catheter should ideally be removed (flushing through the catheter repeatedly as it is pulled out) and replaced with a less traumatic one. MILA® Tomcat Urethral Catheters (MILA International, Inc., Erlanger, KY USA) are provided with optional stylets; they can therefore be used for unblocking and then left in situ. They have wings which can be separated from the catheter tube then repositioned at the appropriate length on the catheter once it has been measured against the cat. The two pieces are then attached together with a suture at each end of the wings, and the wings are sutured to the prepuce using dedicated suture holes (Figure App2.4). As such the catheter is essentially flexible in length. It is also soft and open-ended. Red rubber urethral catheters (3.5- or 5-French; e.g. Kendall Sovereign™, Tyco Healthcare Group LP, Massachusetts, USA) may also be used and are both soft and long. They are fixed to the preputial area using butterfly tapes. The Slippery Sam® (SurgiVet, Smiths Medical Inc., Wisconsin, USA) urethral catheter can be readily sutured in place and connected to a collection system via a suitable luer lock adaptor (e.g. Little Herbert®, SurgiVet, Smiths Medical Inc., Wisconsin, USA). However this catheter is not intended to be left in situ – the warning from the manufacturer at the time of writing is that the catheter and silicone hub are not permanently affixed to each other and it is advised not to leave the catheter in place for more than 6 hours.

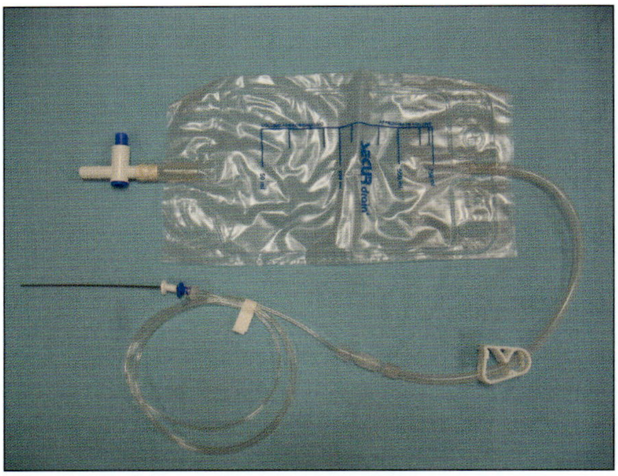

Figure App2.5 A Slippery Sam® connected to a closed system drainage set (Closed System Drainage Set (Drainset)®, Infusion Concepts, Halifax, UK) via a blue Little Herbert® adaptor.

Advantages of a closed urinary collection system include reduced risk of ascending infection, avoiding urine scalding of the perineal region, and overall improved patient welfare (see Figure App2.5). If a proprietary urine collection system is not available, one can be improvised using an intravenous fluid administration set attached to an empty fluid bag. The chances of success with such an improvised system can be maximized by prefilling the administration set (as when setting up an intravenous drip) before it is connected to the urinary catheter and by minimizing the amount of air that gets into the line subsequently. If a closed collection system really cannot be made to work reliably, the urethral catheter can be bunged and the bladder can be manually drained intermittently using aseptic technique. It is clearly essential that this is done regularly. If for some exceptional reason the urethral catheter must be left open, it is recommended to leave a short length of tubing connected to the catheter such that the voided urine will collect at a site away from the cat's perineum.

RETROGRADE UROHYDROPULSION IN MALE DOGS WITH URETHRAL OBSTRUCTION

Equipment required

- Four individuals usually required
- Clippers
- Surgical scrub equipment
- Sterile gloves (one pair) and nonsterile gloves (at least one pair for rectal palpation)

- Sterile lubricant
- Rigid canine urethral catheter of largest appropriate size (usually 6- to 12-French)
- Multiple syringes prefilled with sterile 0.9% sodium chloride (normal, physiological saline) – for dogs weighing less than 12 kg, each syringe should contain 5 ml/kg of saline; full 60 ml syringes should be used for dogs weighing more than 12 kg.

Procedure

- Place the dog in lateral recumbency.
- Clip fur from around the preputial opening as required.
- One individual should then extrude the penis and clean the tip thoroughly.
- A second individual should lubricate the urethral catheter generously and insert it gently to the level of the most distal obstructing calculus; this is often at the level of the os penis.
- The third individual should insert a lubricated finger into the rectum and compress the urethra (lies ventral to the rectum) against the pubis via pressure through the rectal wall. This therefore provides compression proximal to the obstructing calculus.
- A fourth individual should then rapidly flush sterile saline into the urethra via the catheter – it can be helpful to occlude the urethral orifice around the catheter during flushing to minimize saline leakage
- Once enough flushing under pressure has been performed to cause significant dilation of the urethra, proximal compression via rectal pressure is released by lifting off the finger and an attempt should then be made to advance the urethral catheter further. This will be possible if the build up and sudden release of pressure have dislodged the calculus, flushing it into the bladder or at least more proximally.
- The above procedure may need to be performed several times before successful catheterization is achieved. The bladder should be monitored for over-distension as a result of saline that may enter the bladder with each attempt.
- Once the obstruction is relieved, it may be appropriate to leave a soft urethral catheter connected to a closed collection system in situ.

Additional notes

Successful retrograde hydropulsion usually requires general anaesthesia or heavy sedation and must therefore only be attempted once the patient has received adequate stabilization of cardiovascular, electrolyte and acid–base status.

Retrograde hydropulsion is intended to flush urethroliths into the bladder and not to push them physically with the catheter. Great care must be taken throughout catheterization to minimize urethral trauma and avoid rupture.

Further reading

Books

Adams, L.G., Syme, H.M., 2005. Canine lower urinary tract diseases. In: Ettinger, S.J., Feldman, E.C. (Eds.), Textbook of veterinary internal medicine. Saunders, St Louis, pp. 1850–1874.

Bay, J.D., Johnson, L.R., 2004. Feline bronchial disease/asthma. In: King, L.G. (Ed.), Textbook of respiratory disease in dogs and cats. Saunders, St Louis, pp. 388–396.

Campbell, A., Chapman, M., 2000. Handbook of poisoning in dogs and cats. Blackwell Science, Oxford.

DiBartola, S.P., 2005. Routine urinalysis. In: Ettinger, S.J., Feldman, E.C. (Eds.), Textbook of veterinary internal medicine. Saunders, St Louis, pp. 1722–1727.

DiBartola, S.P., 2006. Disorders of sodium and water: hypernatremia and hyponatremia. In: DiBartola, S.P. (Ed.), Fluid, electrolyte, and acid–base disorders in small animal practice. Saunders, St Louis, pp. 47–79.

DiBartola, S.P., Autran de Morais, H., 2006. Disorders of potassium: hypokalemia and hyperkalemia. In: DiBartola, S.P. (Ed.), Fluid, electrolyte, and acid–base disorders in small animal practice. Saunders, St Louis, pp. 91–121.

Hendricks, J.C., 2004. Brachycephalic airway syndrome. In: King, L.G. (Ed.), Textbook of respiratory disease in dogs and cats. Saunders, St Louis, pp. 310–318.

Kittleson, M.D., 2005. Systemic arterial thromboembolism. In: Ettinger, S.J., Feldman, E.C. (Eds.), Textbook of veterinary internal medicine. Saunders, St Louis, pp. 1098–1104.

Martin, M., 2007. Small animal ECGs: an introductory guide, second ed. Wiley-Blackwell, Oxford.

Peterson, M.E., Talcott, P.A., 2006. Small animal toxicology, second ed. Saunders, St Louis.

Schaer, M., 2005. Diabetic ketoacidosis and hyperglycemic hyperosmolar syndrome. In: Ettinger, S.J., Feldman, E.C. (Eds.), Textbook of veterinary internal medicine. Saunders, St Louis, pp. 424–428.

Tilley, L.P., 1992. Essentials of canine and feline electrocardiography. Lea & Febiger, Philadelphia.

Tobias, A.H., 2005. Acquired pericardial disorders. In: Ettinger, S.J,, Feldman, E.C. (Eds.), Textbook of veterinary internal medicine. Saunders, St Louis, pp. 1107–1118.

Westropp, J.L., Buffington, C.A.T., Chew, D., 2005. Feline lower urinary tract diseases. In: Ettinger, S.J., Feldman, E.C. (Eds.), Textbook of veterinary internal medicine. Saunders, St Louis, pp. 1828–1850.

Williams, D.A., Steiner, J.M., 2005. Canine exocrine pancreatic disease. In: Ettinger, S.J., Feldman, E.C. (Eds.), Textbook of veterinary internal medicine. Saunders, St Louis, pp. 1482–1488.

Williams, D.A., Steiner, J.M., 2005. Feline exocrine pancreatic disease. In: Ettinger, S.J., Feldman, E.C. (Eds.), Textbook of veterinary internal medicine. Saunders, St Louis, pp. 1489–1492.

Articles

Adamantos, S., Boag, A., Hughes, D., 2008. Clinical use of a haemoglobin-based oxygen-carrying solution in dogs and cats. In Practice 27, 399–405.

Atkins, C.E., 1984. Disorders of glucose homeostasis in neonatal and juvenile dogs: Hypoglycemia – Part I. Compendium on Continuing Education for the Practicing Veterinarian 6, 197–208.

Atkins, C.E., 1984. Disorders of glucose homeostasis in neonatal and juvenile dogs: Hypoglycemia – Part II. Compendium on Continuing Education for the Practicing Veterinarian 6, 353–364.

Beal, M.W., 2005. Approach to the acute abdomen. Veterinary Clinics: Small Animal Practice 35, 375–396.

Boag, A.K., Hughes, D., 2005. Assessment and treatment of perfusion abnormalities in the emergency patient. Veterinary Clinics, Small Animal Practice 35, 319–342.

Boag, A., Hughes, D., 2004. Emergency management of the acute abdomen in dogs and cats. 1. Investigation and initial stabilisation. In Practice 26 (9), 476–483.

Boothe, D.M., 1992. Special considerations for drug and fluid therapy in the pediatric patient. Compendium on Continuing Education for the Practicing Veterinarian 14 (3), 313–317.

Boswood, A., 2001. Rationale for the use of drugs in the treatment of cardiovascular disease 4. Antiarrhythmic drugs. In Practice 23 (2), 63–73.

Boysen, S.R., Rozanski, E.A., Tidwell, A.S., et al., 2004. Evaluation of a focused assessment with sinography for trauma protocol to detect free abdominal fluid in dogs involved in motor vehicle accidents. Journal of the American Veterinary Medical Association 225 (8), 1198–1204.

Connally, H.E., 2003. Cytology and fluid analysis of the acute abdomen. Clinical Techniques in Small Animal Practice 18 (1), 39–44.

Davidson, B.J., Paling, A.C., Lahmers, S.L., et al., 2008. Disease association and clinical assessment of feline pericardial effusion. Journal of the American Animal Hospital Association 44, 5–9.

Gendler, A., Brourman, J.D., Graf, K.E., 2007. Canine dystocia: medical and surgical management. Compendium on Continuing Education for the Practicing Veterinarian 29 (9), 551–563.

Goggs, R., Humm, K., Hughes, D., 2008. Fluid therapy in small animals 3. Colloid solutions. In Practice 30, 136–142.

Herold, L.V., Devey, J.J., Kirby, R., et al., 2008. Clinical evaluation and management of hemoperitoneum in dogs. Journal of Veterinary Emergency and Critical Care 18 (1), 40–53.

Humm, K., Goggs, R., Hughes, D., 2008. Fluid therapy in small animals 2. Crystalloid solutions. In Practice 30, 85–91.

Jutkowitz, L.A., 2005. Reproductive emergencies. Veterinary Clinics: Small Animal Practice 35, 397–420.

Koenig, A., Drobatz, K.J., Brady, Beale, A., et al., 2004. Hyperglycemic hyperosmolar syndrome in feline diabetics: 17 cases (1995–2001). Journal of Veterinary Emergency and Critical Care 14 (1), 30–40.

Mathews, K.A. (Ed.), 2000. Management of pain. Veterinary Clinics: Small Animal Practice 30 (4), 703–970.

Mathews, K.A., 2005. Analgesia for the pregnant, lactating and neonatal to pediatric cat and dog. Journal of Veterinary Emergency and Critical Care 15 (4), 273–284.

Mathews, K.A., 2005. Analgesia for the pregnant, lactating and neonatal to pediatric cat and dog. Journal of Veterinary Emergency and Critical Care 15, 273–284.

McMichael, M.A., Dhupa, N., 2000. Pediatric critical care medicine: physiologic considerations. Compendium on Continuing Education for the Practicing Veterinarian 22 (3), 353–359.

McMichael, M.A., Dhupa, N., 2000. Pediatric critical care medicine: specific syndromes. Compendium on Continuing Education for the Practicing Veterinarian 22 (4), 353–360.

Prittie, J., 2004. Canine parvoviral enteritis: a review of diagnosis, management, and prevention. Journal of Veterinary Emergency and Critical Care 14 (3), 167–176.

Rush, J.E., Keene, B.W., Fox, P.R., 1990. Pericardial disease in the cat: a retrospective evaluation of 66 cases. Journal of the American Animal Hospital Association 26, 39–46.

Ryan, S.D., Wagner, A.E., 2006. Cesarean section in dogs: physiology and perioperative considerations. Compendium on Continuing Education for the Practicing Veterinarian 28 (1), 34–42.

Ryan, S.D., Wagner, A.E., 2006. Cesarean section in dogs: anesthetic management. Compendium on Continuing Education for the Practicing Veterinarian 28 (1), 44–54.

Schacter, S., Norris, C.R., 2000. Laryngeal paralysis in cats: 16 cases (1990–1999). Journal of the American Veterinary Medical Association 216 (7), 1100–1103.

Schaer, M., 2001. The treatment of acute adrenocortical insufficiency in the dog. Journal of Veterinary Emergency and Critical Care 11 (1), 7–14.

Smith, S.A., Tobias, A.H., 2004. Feline arterial thromboembolism: an update. Veterinary Clinics: Small Animal Practice 34, 1245–1271.

Spattini, G., Rossi, F., Vignoli, M., Lamb, C.R., 2003. Use of ultrasound to diagnose diaphragmatic rupture in dogs and cats. Veterinary Radiology and Ultrasound 44 (2), 226–230.

Verstegen, J., Dhaliwal, G., Verstegen-Onclin, K., 2008. Mucometra, cystic endometrial hyperplasia, and pyometra in the bitch: advances in treatment and assessment of future reproductive success. Theriogenology 70, 364–374.

Weisse, C., Soares, N., Beal, M.W., et al., 2005. Survival times in dogs with right atrial hemangiosarcoma treated by means of surgical resection with or without adjuvant chemotherapy: 23 cases (1986–2000). Journal of the American Veterinary Medical Association 226 (4), 575–579.

Worth, A.J., Machon, R.G., 2005. Traumatic diaphragmatic herniation: pathophysiology and management. Compendium on Continuing Education for the Practicing Veterinarian 27 (3), 178–191.

Zoran, D.L., 2006. Pancreatitis in cats: diagnosis and management of a challenging disease. Journal of the American Animal Hospital Association 42, 1–9.

Pyrethrins and pyrethroids

Hansen, S.R., 1994. Pyrethrins and pyrethroids in dogs and cats. Compendium on Continuing Education for the Practicing Veterinarian 16, 707–712.

Meyer, K.E., 1999. Toxicosis in cats erroneously treated with 45–65% permethrin products. Journal of the American Veterinary Medical Association 215, 198–202.

Richardson, J.A., 2000. Permethrin spot-on toxicoses in cats. Journal of Veterinary Emergency and Critical Care 10 (2), 103–106.

Whittem, T., 1995. Pyrethrin and pyrethroid insecticide intoxication in cats. Compendium on Continuing Education for the Practicing Veterinarian 17 (4), 489–492.

Metaldehyde

Firth, A.M., 1992. Part 1: Treatment of snail bait toxicity in dogs: literature review. Journal of Veterinary Emergency and Critical Care 2 (1), 25–30.

Firth, A.M., 1992. Part 2: Treatment of snail bait toxicity in dogs: retrospective study of 56 cases. Journal of Veterinary Emergency and Critical Care 2 (1), 31–36.

Richardson, J.A., Welch, S.L., Gwaltney-Brant, S.M., et al., 2003. Metaldehyde toxicoses in dogs. Compendium on Continuing Education for the Practicing Veterinarian 25 (5), 376–380.

Yas-Natan, E., Segev, G., Aroch, I., 2007. Clinical, neurological and clinicopathological signs, treatment and outcome of metaldehyde intoxication in 18 dogs. Journal of Small Animal Practice 48, 438–443.

Ethylene glycol

Connally, H.E., Thrall, M.A., Forney, S.D., et al., 1996. Safety and efficacy of 4-methylpyrazole as treatment for suspected or confirmed ethylene glycol intoxication in dogs: 107 cases (1983–1995). Journal of the American Veterinary Medical Association 209, 1880–1883.

Gaynor, A.R., Dhupa, N., 1999. Acute ethylene glycol intoxication. Part I. Pathophysiology and clinical stages. Compendium on Continuing Education for the Practicing Veterinarian 21 (11), 1014–1021.

Gaynor, A.R., Dhupa, N., 1999. Acute ethylene glycol intoxication. Part II. Diagnosis, treatment, prognosis and prevention. Compendium on Continuing Education for the Practicing Veterinarian 21 (12), 1124–1133.

Grauer, G.F., Thrall, M.A., Henre, B.A., et al., 1984. Early clinicopathologic findings in dogs ingesting ethylene glycol. American Journal of Veterinary Research 45, 2299–2303.

Thrall, M.A., Grauer, G.F., Mero, K.N., 1984. Clinicopathologic findings in dogs and cats with ethylene glycol intoxication. Journal of the American Veterinary Medical Association 184, 37–41.

Grapes/raisins

Eubig, P.A., Brady, M.S., Gwaltney-Brant, S.M., et al., 2005. Acute renal failure in dogs after the ingestion of grapes or raisins: a retrospective evaluation of 43 dogs (1992–2002). Journal of Veterinary Internal Medicine 19, 663–674.

Mazzaferro, E.M., Eubig, P.A., Hackett, T.B., et al., 2004. Acute renal failure associated with raisin or grape ingestion in 4 dogs. Journal of Veterinary Emergency and Critical Care 14 (3), 203–212.

Lilies

Langston, C.E., 2002. Acute renal failure caused by lily ingestion in six cats. Journal of the American Veterinary Medical Association 220 (1), 49–52.

Nonsteroidal antiinflammatory agents

Isaacs, J.P., 1996. Adverse effects of nonsteroidal anti-inflammatory drugs in the dog and cat. Australian Veterinary Practitioner 26, 180–186.

Kore, A.M., 1990. Toxicology of nonsteroidal antiinflammatory drugs. Veterinary Clinics: Small Animal Practice 20 (2), 419–430.

Lees, P., May, S.A., McKellar, Q.A., 1991. Pharmacology and therapeutics of nonsteroidal anti-inflammatory drugs in the dog and cat. Journal of Small Animal Practice 32, 183–193.

Paracetamol (acetaminophen)

Aronson, L.R., Drobatz, K., 1996. Acetaminophen toxicosis in 17 cats. Journal of Veterinary Emergency and Critical Care 6, 65–69.

Taylor, N.S., Dhupa, N., 2000. Acetaminophen toxicity in cats and dogs. Compendium on Continuing Education for the Practicing Veterinarian 22 (2), 160–170.

Wallace, K.P., Center, S.A., Hickford, F.H., et al., 2002. S-adenosyl-L-methionine (SAMe) for the treatment of acetaminophen toxicity in a dog. Journal of the American Animal Hospital Association 38, 246–254.

Webb, C.B., Twedt, D.C., Fettman, M.J., et al., 2003. S-adenosylmethionine (SAMe) in a feline acetaminophen model of oxidative injury. Journal of Feline Medicine and Surgery 5, 69–75.

Anticoagulant rodenticides

Murphy, M.J., 2002. Rodenticides. Veterinary Clinics: Small Animal Practice 32, 469–484.

Sheafor, S.E., Couto, C.G., 1999. Anticoagulant rodenticide toxicity in 21 dogs. Journal of the American Animal Hospital Association 35, 38–46.

Sheafor, S.E., Couto, C.G., 1999. Clinical approach to a dog with anticoagulant rodenticide poisoning. Veterinary Medicine 94 (5), 466–471.

Xylitol

Dunayer, E.K., 2004. Hypoglycemia following canine ingestion of xylitol-containing gum. Veterinary and Human Toxicology 46 (2), 87–88.

Dunayer, E.K., 2006. New findings on the effects of xylitol ingestion in dogs. Veterinary Medicine 101, 791–798.

Dunayer, E.K., Gwaltney-Brant, S.M., 2006. Acute hepatic failure and coagulopathy associated with xylitol ingestion in eight dogs. Journal of the American Veterinary Medical Association 229 (7), 1113–1117.

Todd, J.M., Powell, L., 2007. Xylitol intoxication associated with fulminant hepatic failure in a dog. Journal of Veterinary Emergency and Critical Care 17 (3), 286–289.

Index

Notes: Page numbers in **bold** refer to boxes, figures and tables.